Conscious and Unconscious Programs in the Brain

PSYCHOBIOLOGY OF HUMAN BEHAVIOR
Benjamin Kissin, M.D.

Conscious and Unconscious Programs in the Brain

Benjamin Kissin, M.D.

State University of New York
Health Science Center
Brooklyn, New York

Plenum Medical Book Company • New York and London

Library of Congress Cataloging in Publication Data

Kissin, Benjamin.
  Conscious and unconscious programs in the brain.

  (Psychobiology of human behavior; v. 1)
  Bibliography: p.
  Includes indexes.
  1. Consciousness. 2. Psychobiology. 3. Neuropsychology. I. Title. II. Series.
[DNLM: 1. Consciousness. 2. Neuropsychology. 3. Psychoanalytical Theory. 4. Psy-
chophysiology. 5. Unconscious (Psychology) WL 103 K61c]
QP411.K57   1986   153   86-12310
ISBN-13: 978-1-4612-9287-6   e-ISBN-13: 978-1-4613-2187-3
DOI: 10.1007/978-1-4613-2187-3

© 1986 Plenum Publishing Corporation
Softcover reprint of the hardcover 1st edition 1986
233 Spring Street, New York, NY 10013

Plenum Medical Book Company is an imprint of Plenum Publishing Corporation

To my wife
Eve
whose unfaltering support made possible the writing
of this book and all the other interesting enterprises
of my life

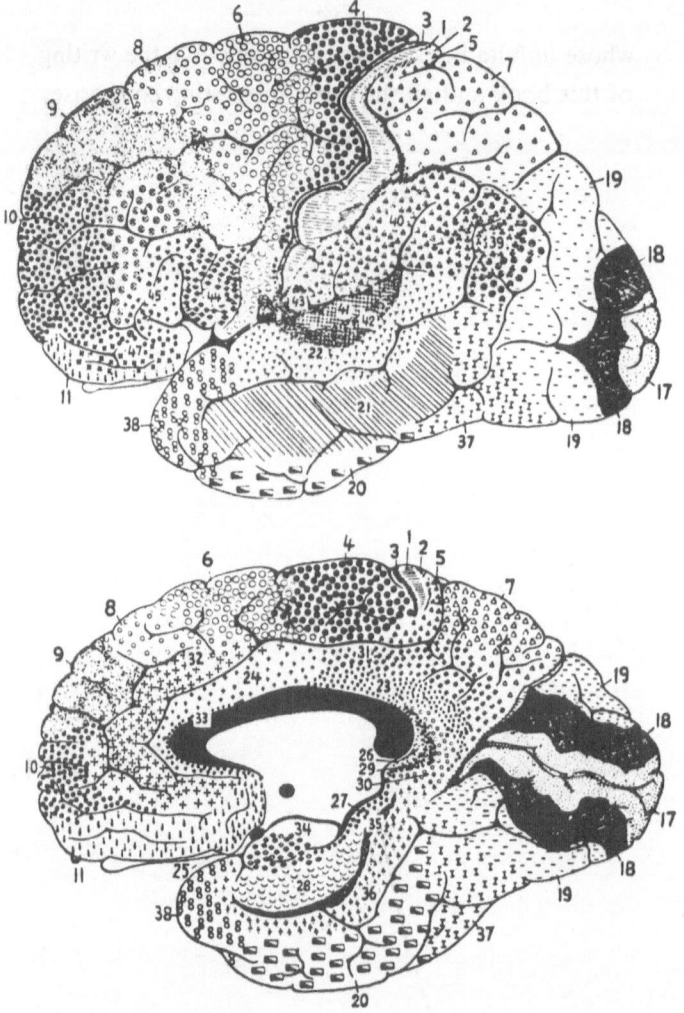

Cytoarchitectonic maps. From Brodmann, 1909.

Preface

For almost a century now, since Freud described the basic motivations and Pavlov the basic mechanisms of human behavior, we have had a reasonable concept of the forces that drive us. Only recently have we gained any real insight into how the brain really works to produce such behavior. The new developments in cognitive psychology and neuroscience have taught us things about the function of the brain that would have been inconceivable even ten years ago. Yet, there still remains a tremendous gap between the two studies—human behavior and brain function—a gap which often seems irreconcilable in view of the basic differences in the methodologies and approaches of the two fields. Students of behavior are frequently disinterested in the underlying neurophysiology while neurophysiologists tend to consider the concepts of psychiatrists and clinical psychologists too vague and theoretical to be applicable to their own more limited schemata. Several valiant attempts have been made by experimentalists to develop a theoretical context in which behavior is described, not separately from brain function but rather as its direct outgrowth. This present work is still another attempt to develop a theoretical system which, given the limitations of our present knowledge, will describe as completely as possible, the underlying brain mechanisms that influence and determine human behavior.

The main emphasis of this work, however, will be not on normal behavior but rather on more neurotic manifestations. The reasons for this are not only professional—neurotic behavior is presumably of greater interest to potential readers of these volumes—but even more, philosophic. It is my belief that the human mind, like all biological entities, is governed by opposing forces that, through continuous interaction, reach some intermediate level of function at which the organism can survive. This, of course, is the biological principle of "homeostasis." Observation of the normal, even in biological terms, is less revealing than observation of the extremes. For example, less would be learned about glucose metabolism by inspecting 100 normal serum glucose levels of 100mg/ml each than by observing a spectrum of 100 samples ranging from 20mg/ml to 400 mg/ml. It is the extreme variations in glucose levels that tell us about the opposing forces at work. Similarly, it is at the extremes of neurotic behavior that we can identify, in their purest form, the various opposing influences that govern human behavior.

Accordingly, the first three sections of this book will be directed toward developing a comprehensive psychobiological system which describes some of the mechanisms of human behavior, while the fourth section will apply those mechanisms to an analysis of the dynamics of various neurotic syndromes. However, these latter descriptions will necessarily be superficial, intended only to suggest how the psychobiological mechanisms considered in the earlier sections could be applied to real clinical conditions. In order to make the clinical applicability of this system more coherent, the present volume has been expanded into a series of four under the general title *Psychobiology of Human Behavior* with the last three volumes dealing directly with mechanisms underlying clinical psychopathology.

Volume 2 will concern itself with those neurotic syndromes in which psychoanalytic theory best describes the underlying dynamics. It will provide the vehicle for the further application of the psychodynamic mechanisms described in this first volume. Volume 3 will address the mechanisms of motivation and conditioning in addiction, perversion, and psychopathy where they are most pertinent. The principles of learning-theory psychology that are most applicable and consequently best illustrated in a clinical setting will be discussed. The central issue of interest of Volume 4 will be psychosomatic disorders in which the psychophysiology of emotions translates into physical disease. The theoretical descriptions in this present volume will hopefully achieve greater clinical significance in the following volumes. The presentation of a broad spectrum of neurophysiological dynamics in diverse clinical conditions should lead to a broader understanding of the interactions between neural and behavioral mechanisms. Within the context of these clinical descriptions, the basic neural mechanisms underlying normal as well as neurotic behaviors should also become more evident.

Because of the variety of readers for whom this work is intended—psychiatrists, clinical psychologists, and experimentalists—the presentation is directed more to a general view than to a scientific study in-depth. Minimum familiarity with neuroanatomy and psychophysiology is assumed. However, for those without such information, a brief review of the pertinent elements is included in Chapters 1–5 in sufficient detail to carry the argument of the book. New ideas are described in somewhat greater depth but with a minimum of references. Overall, I have attempted to make the material technical enough to support the general argument but not so technical as to obscure the central theme of the volume.

Despite recent advances, psychobiology is still in its early stage of development so that many of the mechanisms postulated in this volume remain unproven. Nevertheless, by tying together clinical material, psychological studies, and laboratory data into a single psychobiological synthesis, mechanisms described in one discipline often prove to be generally compatible with those in another. Such cross-disciplinary correlations do not necessarily prove a given hypothesis but they do tend to support it. Most important, the interdisciplinary approach opens up the possibility of applying psychobiological concepts and techniques to clinical case material; the ultimate test of the value of a particular theoretical system.

I wish here to thank those who helped me write this work. My long time friend and colleague, Henri Begleiter, directed me to many references pertinent to my argument which I might otherwise have overlooked. Any misinterpretations of those articles which may exist in this volume are, of course, entirely my own. I also want to thank my editor at Plenum, Janice Stern, for facilitating the production of this book and for arranging for the publication of the remainder of the series. Finally, my gratitude goes to the secretaries who struggled over the many versions of the manuscript—Sharon Blumenfeld, Phyllis Miller, and Susan Lefelstein.

Benjamin Kissin

Contents

III. Hierarchial and Hemispheric Origins of Repression and Other Defense Mechanisms

Introduction

Psychobiology is a relatively new science that deals with the neurophysiology of total behavior rather than with that of its individual components. Consequently it is more concerned with organismic phenomena such as conscious and unconscious thought processing and with functional entities such as the "self" than with the more orthodox considerations of perception, motivation, and emotional expression. Nevertheless, because complex behaviors derive from basic mechanisms, an understanding of those mechanisms is essential for the formulation of holistic concepts.

Another characteristic that differentiates psychobiology from physiological psychology (the study of basic mechanisms) is its relatedness to more clinical psychologies. Although the approach of psychobiology is predominantly that of neurophysiology, its interest in holistic behavior requires that it be philosophically based on some psychological system that views behavior organismically rather than fragmentarily. Both psychoanalysis and learning theory psychology fulfill that requirement. On the surface, learning theory would appear to make a more suitable marriage with psychobiology since the methodologies of both are quite similar. However, in what is becoming a major area of interest in psychology, the study of unconscious mental activity, learning theory is deficient while psychoanalysis is, if anything, overabundant.

Consequently it is not surprising to find psychobiologists involved in what in the past would have been considered esoteric research such as studies of dream content, hypnagogic productions, transcendental meditation, and so on. In a different direction, psychobiologists perform experiments exploring the physiology of defense mechanisms, an area vastly removed from that of physiological psychology and learning theory but integral to psychoanalysis. Freudian psychology also provides a better theoretical paradigm for personality formation and for the development of neurotic behaviors than does learning theory, making psychobiological research in these areas more feasible.

In a work like this, directed toward developing a comprehensive model of mental activity, a major problem is to take into full account the impact of experience. Despite my major interest in biological mechanisms I am not so prejudiced as to believe that they are the only influences molding human behavior. In the Freudian tradition, I am convinced that the dominant forces shaping human development and behavior are environmental; consequently I believe that personal experience must constitute an essential element in every psychological model.

Toward that goal it is necessary to describe the mechanisms through which experiences are transmitted into their neurological equivalents—so-called engrams. Several chapters in this book will be devoted to such descriptions. However, providing a physiological mechanism for such transitions is entirely different from considering how specific life events affect behavior. Such purely psychological explanations are not the subject matter of this book; nevertheless some provision must be made for incorporating such interactions into our physiological model. This is accomplished through a somewhat simplistic device in which experiences are categorized emotionally as either positive or negative where positive affective charge exercises one behavioral effect (approach behavior) and negative affective charge another (avoidance). Other stratagems such as the analysis of the reactions of different individuals to different types of stress provide another paradigm for studying the influence of experience on the development of personality and behavior. All of these devices are borrowed from learning theory which, together with psychobiology and psychoanalysis, form the understructure of this formulation.

This effort to incorporate the effects of maturation and experience into what is basically a physiological system of behavior enlarges the scope of psychobiology beyond the level of a laboratory science. It allows us to address questions of normal human development and behavior in physiological as well as in psychological terms. It provides mechanisms other than introspection for examining the complex operations of consciousness and the unconscious. Finally, because neurotic behavior is thought to be merely a distortion of normal behavior, we are able to examine it within the context of normal physiological and psychological mechanisms somehow gone askew.

The intent of this book is to define the field of psychobiology more specifically and to sharpen its parameters more clearly. The term psychobiology is not a new one. It has been used with the same connotations suggested here for a fairly long time but in a general sense, more or less as a synonym for physiological psychology and psychophysiology. The distinctions made here between psychobiology and physiological psychology are a useful start in these delineations. Later in this volume psychophysiology will be defined as the study of the visceral manifestations of emotional reactivities with particular reference to their significance in the pathogenesis of psychosomatic disease. On the other hand, the psychoses appear to constitute an entirely different category of biological psychopathology, the study of which is generally known as biological psychiatry. What biological psychiatry is to the psychoses and what psychophysiology is to psychosomatic illness, psychobiology should be to normal behavior and the neuroses.

Organization of the Book

This book is divided into four sections. The first, "Fundamentals of Psychobiology," is essentially a review of the subject matter of physiological psychology with special emphasis on those areas most pertinent to the larger issues of psychobiology. The first chapter presents a short review of the anatomy of the brain together with a description of those functional principles upon which the brain is organized. The following chapters on motivations and emotions emphasize the biological role these modalities play as well as the specifics of their neural connections. Two chapters on cognitive function deal largely with the questions of the neural representation of perceptions and memories in the brain—so-called engrams—since these are the stuff from which all higher psychobiological concepts ultimately derive.*

The second section, "Conscious and Unconscious Thought Processing," is the longest in the book because it deals with one of the most fundamental problems in psychology. Consciousness, with its implications of awareness and even more of self-awareness, has always been one of the major philosophical and psychological mysteries. With the new discoveries in psychobiology it is now possible to describe this unique phenomenon in terms of the interaction of discrete physiological systems in the brain. Similarly the concept of the unconscious has had a somewhat mystical quality that appeared to separate it from the realm of legitimate scientific fields of study. This too no longer applies. Recent advances in cognitive psychology and in the study of artificial intelligence have made it clear that unconscious mental activity is not only real but that it plays an immense role in governing all human and animal behavior.

In the course of these historical developments, two concepts of unconscious mental activity, the *cognitive* and the *affective,* have evolved. The earliest references to unconscious mental activity dealt mainly with its affective interactions, yet that aspect of the unconscious is still regarded as somewhat questionable. Conversely, as a result of recent work in cognitive psychology and artificial intelligence, the existence of a *cognitive unconscious* has become so well established as to be considered more or less axiomatic. For example, in a recent article on integrated circuits, Preston (1983), a computer scientist, writes:

> The uses of artificial intelligence have only recently begun to receive public attention, although this class of applications was foreseen by the pioneers of computer science. Some of the differences between the function (if not the structure) of the brain and the computer were also noted at that time, and indeed it is when we approach the task of designing computers to perform some of the functions of the brain with the tools of the analyst and the computer architect in hand that the awesome dimensions of the animal intellect become evident. Take, for example, the implied powers of trajectory extrapolation exhibited by athletes engaged in tennis, baseball, or football, in which such extrapolations are performed subconsciously in perfect ignorance of the laws of motion, or the human ability to recognize melodies—even with sections omitted—that have been transformed in key, tempo, and timbre. This latter power seems to defy explanation unless one postulates sophisticated data-abstraction algorithms in the brain that operate at the subconscious level on incoming sensory data. Comparable powers of subconscious abstraction and associative recall must operate on visual data, since one readily identifies a variety of objects in spite of changes in their orientations or partial obscuration. (p. 469)

It is interesting that a computer scientist should use the equivocal word "subconscious" rather than the more accurate term "unconscious" to describe a realm of

---

*Readers who are thoroughly familiar with the field of physiological psychology may prefer to skim this first review section (Chapters 1–5) since the real argument of the book begins with Chapter 6. However, many of the ideas presented in this section are essential to the understanding of the rest of the book.

cognitive activity that is completely distant from the domain of consciousness. Without being overly sensitive, one can detect an unwillingness (conscious or unconscious) to identify the apparent existence of a huge cognitive unconscious with the possible existence of a similarly large *affective unconscious*. Yet this position is clearly inconsistent. It is obvious that motivational and emotional forces are at least as significant as are cognitive mechanisms in determining unconscious behavior, animal or human. Hence the question should be not whether there is an affective unconscious but rather whether it works the way Freud said it does.

The third section of the book, "Hierarchical and Hemispheric Origins of Repression and Other Defense Mechanisms," confronts one of the most controversial issues, that of the putative psychoanalytic process of *repression*. It appears that with markedly negative affect there may be inhibitory effects that result in clinical and experimental suppression of the cognitive component of perceptions and memories. These activities, although deriving from mechanisms entirely different from the hypothetical Freudian repressive barrier, provide effects that are phenomenologically quite similar. The effects of these activities on unconscious cognitive processing provide important elements on which a model of a psychological unconscious may be constructed.

In the fourth section, "Psychobiology and the Pathogenesis of the Neuroses," a preliminary attempt will be made to apply some of the previously described psychobiological mechanisms to real clinical problems. A theoretical system that exists in a void may be of interest but is not readily subject to experimental verification. Since the purpose of this entire work is to introduce concepts that will ultimately be testable, some indication of the areas of applicability of such mechanisms to clinical material is essential. The few chapters devoted to this critical task can serve only as an introduction to the larger task. Psychobiological mechanisms applicable to the study of neuroses, addictions and psychosomatic disorders are merely touched upon. The greater elaboration of these concepts will be undertaken, as described in the Preface, in future volumes of this series. Another purpose of this study is to compare known physiological mechanisms of mental function with the psychodynamic principles enunciated by Freud and elaborated by his co-workers. It seems evident that a psychological theory that has exercised so important an influence on the thinking of our times would benefit if its methodology could be brought more in line with that of modern biological science. This is not meant in any way to impugn the psychodynamic method; rather it is an attempt to reconcile that method with approaches that are in many places considered more "scientific." One step toward accomplishing that goal could be through demonstrating that many of the formulations of psychoanalysis made by way of psychodynamic methodology are generally compatible with findings in experimental psychology and psychobiology. The approach of this volume will be to present the accepted psychobiological mechanisms that are pertinent to psychoanalytic thought and then in the final chapter to attempt to relate those mechanisms, positively or negatively, to those postulated in psychoanalytic theory.

Definitions

A word on terminology. The phrase *motivational–emotional,* used repeatedly throughout this book to connote those behaviors stemming from basic biological drives, is rhetorically somewhat clumsy and has generally been replaced in the literature by the term *affective*. The latter is both euphonious and fortuitous in that it fits so well in dichotomizing behavior into its affective and cognitive aspects. However, motivational–emotional and affective are not entirely synonymous since the first term is more comprehensive and represents the objective manifestations of the phenomenon whereas the second reflects rather than the subjective feelings associated with emotional behavior. Nevertheless throughout the text the two terms will be used more or less interchangeably. A similar situation applies in other behavioral parameters. For example, *need* represents biological requirements for survival while *drive* describes the mechanisms through which needs are fulfilled. In the same way *consciousness* constitutes the objective description of the phenomenon and *awareness* the subjective analogue. In each of these instances, the word pairs will be used more or less interchangeably with exceptions explained in their proper place.

One of the most difficult concepts to be dealt with in this book is that of consciousness. First there is the dichotomy between objective *alertness* and subjective *awareness* which raises the philosophical question as to whether they represent only different aspects of the same underlying mechanism or basically different mechanisms. This question is addressed at the beginning of Chapter 1. Second, there are the different varieties of consciousness along a spectrum ranging from normal alertness, through altered states of consciousness, to the dream states of REM sleep. Finally, as described in Chapters 10 and 11, alert consciousness is merely the overlay of total brain activity in which unconscious mechanisms contribute well over 99% of the total. Consequently, it is clear that consciousness is not, as we are accustomed to think, a single integrated phenomenon but rather a complex interaction among various mechanisms which results in a wide variety of phenomena.

Perhaps most confusing of all is the word *unconscious*, a term that has been largely pre-empted by psychoanalysis to signify the Freudian unconscious with all of its implications. In this volume the term unconscious carries only its most literal meaning, specifying *all* activities in the brain that at any moment are not in awareness. Thus the psychobiological unconscious describes a broad spectrum of nonconscious activities including such disparate entities as the *cognitive unconscious*, the *preconscious*, the *psychobiological dynamic unconscious*, the *visceral unconscious*, and still others, all of which will be described later (see Chapter 17). Of these, only the *decathected unconscious* will be designated as comparable to the Freudian unconscious. However, even though this segment is relatively small (probably less than 10% of the total), it is our thesis that it is of particular interest because like the Freudian unconscious it may account for much psychopathology of the neurotic type.

At the highest level of integration lies the psychobiological *self* which is the analogue of the psychoanalytic *ego*. This is the entity that includes in it more or less all of the other functional elements of individual psychology. Because conscious and unconscious activities each encompass the four basic modalities of behavior—motivation, emotion, cognition, and motor activity—one speaks of conscious or unconscious behavior with the full knowledge that all of the several behavioral components are involved. The concept of self goes one step further. It signifies the entire organism operating as a single entity rather than as a composite of various separate activities. Even though one may speak of the conscious self as opposed to the unconscious self, such a distinction is artificial and is used only as a device for explaining differences in function and operation. In normal individuals, the self is a single unifying functional entity, possibly showing different manifestations at different levels, the conscious and unconscious, but providing the all-encompassing rubric that establishes the organism as a separate and unique individual.

The ability to describe holistic functions such as the self in terms of the complex interactions of multiple physiological systems distinguishes psychobiology from physiological psychology. Nevertheless, in an analytic science, even so holistic a concept as the self must be broken down into its various components. Thus I will describe in Chapter 7 the elements of the self-system that provide the physical sense of self; in Chapter 9, its decision making functions; in Chapter 10, its conscious psychological elements; in Chapter 11, its role in the procedural unconscious; and in Chapter 12, its role in the cognitive unconscious. Only in the final chapters, when the psychobiological self is equated with the psychoanalytic ego, will the concept be treated wholly as a single unified entity.

I

Fundamentals of Psychobiology

I

Fundamentals of Psychobiology

1

Anatomical and Functional Organization of the Central Nervous System

The Brain–Mind Dichotomy

A major philosophic issue in the field of psychobiology is the question of the relationship of the brain to the *mind*. Some neurobiologists such as Eccles (1963) lean toward the view that the world of the mind and that of the physical are separate and distinct and relate only through a so-called psychophysical parallelism. In this theory, events in the two worlds are parallel but not equivalent. Other neurobiologists such as Kornhuber (1978) believe, with Spinoza, that "the mental and the physical are different aspects of the same thing" (p. 323). For myself, only the latter position makes philosophic sense and it is that position which rules this volume.

The mind, then, is the subjective analogue of the total objective activity of the central nervous system with particular reference to that activity centered in the brain. However, it is not merely the sum total of all random neural activity. The term *mind* implies a high level of organized neural activity that occurs paradoxically, both in full and impaired consciousness (e.g., the sense of awareness of self in alert consciousness and also in dreams). The mind is a highly structured entity where primitive functions are incorporated progressively into more complex ones and these sequentially, into the still more complex. The entire pyramid culminates in the concept of self, which provides both the subjective sense of a separate and distinct entity and the executive control for the entire organism. But these subjective and objective integrations do not occur in a physiological vacuum. They are merely the behavioral equivalents of the neural organization of the brain. At the lowest levels of neural structure are the primitive visceral, motor, and perceptive reactivities. These are progressively integrated in the higher tiers of neurological organization until, at the highest levels, the complex consciousness and self-awareness systems exercise the final subjective and objective integrating functions. The principles of organization in the brain are both hierarchical (i.e., simple systems become more complex as they ascend vertically) and hemispheric (differentiated horizontally by the different functions of the two cortical

3

hemispheres). It is with these two kinds of neural organization in the brain that this volume is mainly concerned.

A Brief Description of the Anatomy of the Central Nervous System

The central nervous system, of which the brain is the control organ, coordinates all cognitive and behavioral activities of the organism. The functional unit in the nervous system is the nerve cell or neuron. There are about 50 billion neurons in the brain proper and almost as many again in the cerebellum and the spinal cord. Neurons are organized in operational units called *neural centers* that are connected in longitudinally structured entities known as *neural systems*. No system works independently of the others so that the activity of each depends upon the activity of all. Interactions among systems, defined as *programs*, result in more complex functions.

The biological organization of the brain may be considered as a complex of individual neural systems. Each of these is responsible for controlling and sustaining a different function necessary for the survival and evolutionary development of the individual and the species. Most important is the motivational system which provides the drives to satisfy the biological needs of the individual. Emotional reactivities supply the adaptive and affective elements necessary to guarantee the effectiveness of motivational influences. Cognition allows the comprehending of the environment while motor activity permits behavioral control of that environment. Consciousness is a special cognitive and emotional state which has evolved in mammals; it provides for the greatest mobilization of biological resources to cope effectively with the moment-to-moment exigencies of living. The interaction of these systems with perhaps the highest neurological level of all, the self-concept system, results in the complex mental activities of all mammals, particularly those of man.

The central nervous system may be viewed as having two major components, the *afferent* and the *efferent*. Afferent systems collect data from the internal and external environments and bring them to the brain for analysis and integration. Efferent systems lead from the brain to peripheral organs such as endocrine glands and the musculature to implement decisions made centrally. The brain, which lies functionally between the two systems, translates afferent stimuli into a cognitive–emotional structure on the basis of which meaningful behavior can be exercised.

Thus the brain is the master control center for the nervous system and is responsible for coordinating all of the biological and behavioral activities of the organism. In terms of its anatomical and evolutionary development, the brain is divided into four major areas: the brain stem, the cerebellum, the paleocortex, and the neocortex. The cerebellum, a primitive structure, is involved mainly in muscular coordination and mechanisms of equilibrium that are only indirectly related to the present discussion (see Chapter 11). The other three areas and their interrelationships provide the major theses for our presentation.

The *brain stem* is biologically the oldest part of the brain in humans and as a consequence, in both structure and function, is not vastly different from that of the earliest vertebrate fishes. Although the brain stem represents only a small and primitive

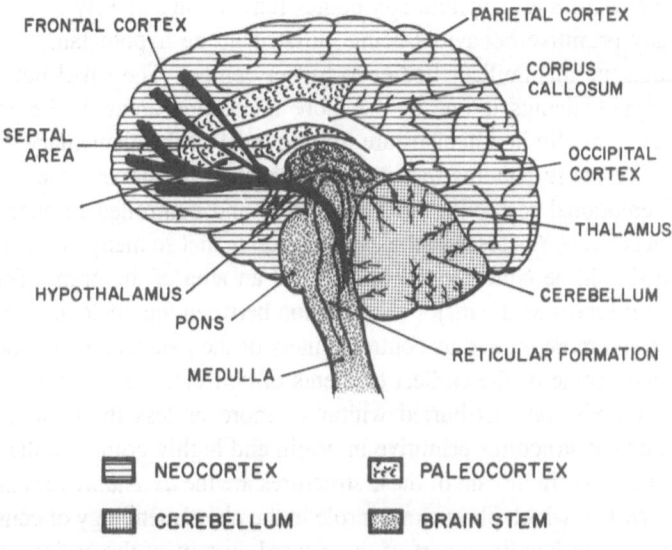

FRONTAL CORTEX

PARIETAL CORTEX

CORPUS
CALLOSUM

SEPTAL
AREA

OCCIPITAL
CORTEX

THALAMUS

HYPOTHALAMUS

CEREBELLUM

PONS

RETICULAR FORMATION

MEDULLA

NEOCORTEX   PALEOCORTEX

CEREBELLUM   BRAIN STEM

Figure 1-1 Functional anatomy of the brain. (Adapted from Routtenberg, 1978. Reprinted with permission.)

portion of the brain, many of the most important biological functions even in man have their control centers lodged there.

The brain stem is itself divided into two segments: lower and upper. The lower brain stem in turn is divided into two subsections, the *medulla* (an upward continuation of the spinal cord) and directly above it the *pons* (Fig. 1-1). Each of these centers plays a similar functional role in man to that in lower animals. The medulla contains the vital control centers for respiration and cardiovascular function; damage to this area carries the highest risk of death. The pons appears to regulate the wake–sleep cycle, is the source of many of the chemical systems that activate the brain, and also serves as a bridge between the rest of the brain and the cerebellum.

The upper brain stem, known also as the mesencephalon or midbrain, contains the *superior* and *inferior colliculi* which are important way stations in the processing of sensory stimuli. The superior colliculi are the lowest integrating centers for incoming visual stimuli while the inferior colliculi serve a similar function for auditory and somatosensory (bodily) stimuli. These centers make evaluations of a primitive type on incoming sensory impulses to determine their relative significance and then to initiate early decisions on the ultimate pathways for processing.

Riding on top of the brain stem is the *diencephalon*,* an area that from the behavioral viewpoint is one of the most important in the brain. While the brain stem serves in all vertebrates as the primitive control center for physiological reactions, the diencephalon initiates most of the primitive elements of behavior. The diencephalon has three major components, the *hypothalamus*, the *mammillary bodies*, and the *thalamus*.

---

*The diencephalon, technically speaking, is not a part of the brain stem. However, from an evolutionary point of view its functions are more closely allied to those of the brain stem than to those of the areas above it. Therefore, in the text, we shall consider it as part of the primitive "brain stem" complex.

The hypothalamus and mammillary bodies function in a closely coordinated fashion, with many primitive behaviors being initiated in the hypothalamus and directed upward through the mammillary bodies to higher centers. The small but structurally complicated hypothalamus is one of the more interesting areas of the entire brain. Within this relatively limited nucleus are located most of the elementary motivational and emotional response patterns that drive vertebrates. In humans, these basic motivational and emotional reactivities are modulated and controlled through influences from higher nerve centers; it is nonetheless remarkable that so many of the fundamental drives of life should be concentrated in so small an area of the brain. The thalamus directly above it serves as the major relay station between the nuclei of the brain stem and the larger and more numerous control centers of the paleocortex and neocortex; it may also contain some of the earliest elements of consciousness and awareness.

The brain stem contains buried within it, more or less throughout its length, several longitudinal structures primitive in origin and highly critical to the survival of the animal. The most significant of these structures are the *ascending reticular activating substance (RAS)*, which plays a major role in the phenomenology of consciousness; the *median forebrain bundle,* a part of the reward system of the brain; and the *periaqueductal gray,* which is responsible for the transmission of pain. Although these three brain stem tracts will not be described in detail until later in this volume, their functions, i.e., awareness and pain–pleasure motivation, are directly involved in all forms of behavior. A diagrammatic illustration of the course of the ascending reticular activating substance and the reward system is shown in Figure 1-1; the periaqueductal gray has a similar although not identical distribution to that of the reticular formation.

The *paleocortex* (old covering) is the oldest part of the superstructure of the brain (i.e., the part developing on top of the brain stem) and derives originally from the olfactory lobe in amphibia. In humans, it is a structure that fits like a thick cap over the upper thalamic end of the brain stem with its inner aspect comprising mainly the *basal ganglia* and its outer aspect the *rhinencephalon.* Each of these structures consists in turn of several nuclei involved in the elaboration of emotional reactivities. For the sake of simplification we will assume for the time being that the various nuclei of the basal ganglia act essentially as one. For the rhinencephalon, we will distinguish arbitrarily only between its four major nuclei: the *hippocampus,* the *septal area,* the *amygdala,* and the *cingulate gyrus.* The basal ganglia act synchronously with associated nuclei in the brain stem in a functionally integrated pathway known as the *nigrostriatal system.* The four elements of the rhinencephalon are involved with the hypothalamus, thalamus, and the frontal lobe of the cortex in a functionally integrated pathway known as the *limbic system,* the neural system largely responsible for emotional and attentional reactivities and perhaps the most important neural structure with which we will be dealing.

The *neocortex* (new covering) is readily seen in the illustration of the human brain in Figure 1-1 as the large mass (the cerebrum) covering the entire brain with the exception of part of the cerebellum. Although the paleocortex represents a significant element in the evolutionary growth of the brain, it is the neocortex that contributes the giant proportion. If one recognizes that the human brain as depicted in Figure 1-1 has a three-dimensional projection where the depth of the cerebrum is about equal to its height, then it becomes apparent that the neocortex constitutes about 95% of the total brain volume, excluding the cerebellum. Since the cerebellum is almost entirely a structure of motor coordination involved mainly with maintenance of body equilibrium and with the mechanics of body motion, it is not generally considered as part of the thinking or feeling brain and will be largely excluded from consideration until later in this volume (see Chapter 11).

The neocortex, more commonly referred to as the cortex, is divided in its lateral projection into four major lobes: reading from in front backwards, they are the *frontal,* the *temporal,* the *parietal,* and the *occipital* (see Fig. 1-1). The frontal lobe is, in turn, divided into two general segments, the most forward or *prefrontal* area and the posterior or *precentral* area. From an evolutionary perspective, the prefrontal lobe is the newest part of the brain and achieves its largest dimensions in man. It appears to be involved in the higher intellectual functions such as planning, judgment, and so on. The precentral area of the frontal lobe is old; in it lie the control centers for all voluntary motor activity. The temporal lobe is similarly divided into two anatomically adjacent but functionally discrete segments, the upper outer area which is the receiving area for sound and hearing and the lower inner area (the *inferotemporal lobe*) which is a higher control center for motivational and emotional expression. The parietal lobe is the receiving area for all of the tactile sensory stimuli in the body: touch, pain, and proprioception (body position). Finally, the occipital lobe receives and organizes all visual stimuli from the environment as they are reflected on the retinae.

The neocortex, like all of the other cerebral structures thus far described, is a bilateral symmetrical structure. However, it is unique in that the two sides are sharply separated from one another by a deep longitudinal fissure. This formation results in the creation of two apparently separate cerebral hemispheres, the left and the right. The two hemispheres are anatomically independent but functionally interrelated through heavy connecting communicating pathways that travel below the dividing fissure, close to the brain stem, from one hemisphere to the other. These connecting pathways are known as the *corpus callosum* and are shown in Figure 1-1 as a large structure covering the thalamus and the septum.

As opposed to the rest of the brain where both sides are more or less equipotential, the two cerebral hemispheres differ significantly, not so much in structure as in demonstrable function. The left temporal lobe does tend to be somewhat larger than the right; most children are born with this difference which appears as early as the 29th week of gestation. This difference in size is thought to be associated with the genetic presence of the speech center in the left cerebral hemisphere in over 90% of humans, a finding that often correlates with right-handedness as the dominant behavioral mode (since most sensory and motor functions on each side of the body are represented in the opposite side of the cortex).

The left hemisphere apparently tends to control the ability to read, write, speak, and do arithmetic. It also appears to be the more conscious hemisphere, in the operational sense at least that it is able to report to the experimenter its awareness. It is more analytic and verbal in its functions and contributes largely to sequential types of reasoning. The right hemisphere is more effective at three-dimensional visual pattern recognition, musical ability, and holistic reasoning. It almost certainly has its own type of consciousness and awareness such as that expressed by the emotional reactions to music, but it lacks the necessary verbal equipment to express that awareness. Nevertheless, despite convincing evidence of these disparate functions, it is clear that in the intact human, the two hemispheres do not operate independently of each other. The corpus callosum contains some 200 million nerve fibers, each of which carries some 20 impulses/second for a total of about 4 billion impulses/second traveling between the two hemispheres at any given time. As will be repeatedly emphasized, the brain does not function as distinct and independent anatomical and physiological units but rather as an integrated whole. The anatomy and physiology of the corpus callosum bears adequate witness to this.

Biological Homeostasis and the Nervous System

The dominant principle organizing all living behavior is biological homeostasis, the need to maintain the metabolic and physiological equilibria that characterize all living organisms. The principle of biological homeostasis is well-described in the following excerpt from Dubos (1959):

> The process of living involves the interplay and integration of two ecological systems. On the one hand, the individual organism constitutes a community of interdependent parts—cells, body fluids, and tissue structures—each of which is related to the others through a complex network of balance mechanisms. This intra-individual community operates best when its own *internal environment* remains stable within a barely narrow range characteristic of each species. On the other hand, each organism constantly reacts and competes with all the living and inanimate things with which it comes into contact. Under normal conditions the *external environment* changes constantly, in an unpredictable manner. Many of the modifications that occur in the outer world can have damaging effects. In order to survive and to continue to function effectively the organism must make adaptive responses to these modifications.

The nervous system is the major control system for maintaining biological homeostasis of both the internal and external environments. Because of the electrical nature of nervous system activity its effects are almost immediate so that all rapid reactions are carried out through its mechanisms. Long-term adaptations are most often accomplished through the slower biochemical means of the endocrine system. However, such effects may also be implemented by chronic changes in nervous system reactivities.

The nervous system may be divided anatomically and functionally into two major subdivisions that deal with biological homeostasis: the central nervous system and the autonomic system. These systems have different control centers in the brain and different peripheral nerve distributions. The central nervous system is predominantly responsible for all interactions with the environment. Particularly in mammals it is the much larger of the two. It comprises all of the brain as previously described plus the spinal cord and the vast network of peripheral nerves that spread to all parts of the body.

The autonomic nervous system has major responsibility for maintaining metabolic and physiological equilibrium of the internal environment; it is also known as the *visceral* nervous system. It has two components; the sympathetic nervous system which has its control center in the posterior hypothalamus and the parasympathetic nervous system which has its control center in the anterior hypothalamus. Each system has its own separate network of peripheral nerves that are independent of the peripheral nerves of the central nervous system.

In general the parasympathetic nervous system is responsible for the *anabolic* (tissue building) activities of the living organism while the sympathetic nervous system is responsible for *catabolic* (tissue breaking down) activities necessary in emergencies. The continual interaction of these two nervous systems determines the state of the internal environment. Long-term effects are also accomplished through a balance of discharge of anabolic and catabolic hormones from the endocrine system.

The Biological Organization of Behavioral Modalities

The nervous system is functionally organized to insure the maintenance of biological homeostasis in the internal and external environments. The complex demands of this intricate process may essentially be reduced to four basic reactivities. First there is the necessity to identify the basic needs of the living organism, so-called motivation. Secondly there is the necessity for internal mechanisms that will insure the gratification of these basic needs, so-called emotional reactivities. In coping with the external environment, it is essential that the organism be informed of significant events (food, sex, or danger); these effects are accomplished through perception and cognition. Finally the survival of the organism depends upon its ability to respond appropriately to the perceived event (to attack or flee); this activity is accomplished through the motor system. Hence the four major categories of behavior are motivation, emotions, cognition (including perception), and motor activity.

Although it is convenient (and from a physiological point of view perhaps necessary) to categorize behavior into four separate components, such compartmentalization is really artificial and invalid. Actually, all behavior must have within it all four modalities. For example, although overt behavior is defined by some coordinated motor response, there is no such thing as behavior without motivation, without emotional reactivity, or without perception and cognition. Consequently the compartmentalization of behavior into its four separate components is done purely for the sake of description.

There is, however, one practical justification for considering the four behavioral modalities as more or less distinct entities (as we shall do in subsequent chapters). It appears that each behavioral modality is represented in a separate and distinct neuronal system which can be differentiated positively through stimulatory experiments and negatively through lesioning studies. The fact that stimulation of a particular neural system produces objective and subjective evidence of a particular behavioral modality while lesioning removes all evidence of such experience does lend credibility to the principle of *neurological specificity.** This principle states that specific neuronal systems in the brain are responsible for the specific subjective and objective experiences of a given behavioral modality. In this paradigm, hunger is perceived when there is

*See caveat at end of this chapter.

activity in the hunger system; pleasure when there is activity in the pleasure system; and pain when there is activity in the pain system.

How is it possible for each behavioral system to exist separately and yet for all behavioral modalities to be so intimately interrelated as to constitute almost a single entity? The answer lies in the nature of brain activity. Especially during consciousness when subjective reactions are most manifest, neural activity involves the entire brain so that the various systems, although anatomically separate and distinct, are physiologically elements in a single functional process. Although we may describe the various behavioral modalities independently, it must be emphasized that during both conscious and unconscious brain activity, the activity of each can be understood only within the context of the activity of all. Hence behavior must be considered as a single functional entity: an amalgam of the four modalities into a single motivational–emotional–cognitive–motor event in which each modality is individually recognizable but only as a function of the interaction between itself and the others.

In mammals (and perhaps in some lower vertebrates) still another division of activities can be noted—that between conscious and unconscious behavior. This is particularly evident in humans who subjectively recognize both mental activities of which they are aware and mental activities of which they are not aware. As will be described in later chapters consciousness is a special biological state, the purpose of which is to cope most effectively with the immediate demands of the internal and external environments. But consciousness and unconsciousness are not separate behavioral modalities such as motivation, emotions, cognition, and motor activity. They are rather different biological states of functional organization of the brain provided to fulfill the behavioral needs of the organism under different unique circumstances. Behavior is defined by the motivational, emotional, cognitive, and motor activity of the brain and remains so defined regardless of the conscious or unconscious state of the brain. Hence one can speak of conscious or unconscious behavior, but the interaction of the four modalities under each of these conditions remains unchanged.

Nevertheless, like the other behavioral modalities, the conscious–unconscious dichotomy is also represented anatomically and physiologically by a single neurological system in the brain: the so-called consciousness system. This system is responsible both for activating experience to a state of consciousness and for inactivating it to a state of unconsciousness. Depending on the state of activation in the consciousness system, representation of one or another behavioral experience will either exist or not exist in the subject's awareness. Thus there can be conscious or unconscious perception of pleasure, pain, hunger, sensory experience or motor movements, where each behavioral activity either may or may not reach the awareness of the individual.

The phenomenology of consciousness itself illustrates another important characteristic of neurological specificity, namely the fact that behavior is accomplished physiologically in small modules, most often at an unconscious level, and then integrated into what appears to be a single conscious event. In this way all of the elements deriving from different behavioral modalities are independently derived within their specific physiological systems and are then integrated within the consciousness system. Consciousness itself consists of many disparate elements that are integrated into the sense of a single event at some higher level of the brain.

The modular arrangement of brain function suggests that the brain, although operating as a single entity, allocates specific functions to specific low-level neural units, the activities of which are integrated at some higher neural center. An excellent example of such modular arrangement occurs in vision which is broken down into two phases: the first a "structural" one, in which the raw data of vision are organized so that they can be cognitively processed, and the second the "episodic," in which actual cognitive processing for meaning occurs.* Structurally, the outline of a visualized object is determined by neural programs in the retina, its estimated distance from the observer by stereoscopic mechanisms in the superior colliculi, and its differential color discrimination in cortical area 17. Concomitantly episodic processing occurs and ultimately all information is integrated at higher levels in the brain.

Generalized versus Localized Organization of Brain Function

The principle of neurological specificity is by no means universally accepted. In 1950, Karl Lashley reported that learning in the rat could not be allocated to any specific areas in the brain but was related to the total mass of intact neural tissue. This remarkable finding gave rise to a new theory that considered neural activity is an electrical field phenomenon occurring in masses of brain tissue rather than as discrete electrical circuits operating through specific neurons and their interconnecting synapses. This idea was further extended by John and co-workers (1973) who interpreted the electrical patterns of evoked potentials (see Chapter 4 this volume) as field phenomena only indirectly related to the underlying nerve cells. Recently this approach has been extended even further to include the concept of holography, or three-dimensional electrical fields in the brain representing the neural equivalents of perceived stimuli.

At the opposite theoretical extreme are those anatomists and neurophysiologists who assign control of different mental functions to specific localized areas in the brain. These investigators relate specific behavioral losses of function to localized brain lesions and conclude that the lost function was normally under the control of the now-damaged center. It was in this way, for example, that the localization of the speech centers in the left hemisphere was first uncovered. This line of reasoning is unfortunately marred by the fact that lesions in the pathways connecting interacting centers will often produce the same behavioral deficiencies as those in the centers themselves, thus confusing the picture.

Recent evidence suggests that most brain functions are neither as generalized as proposed by Lashley and John nor as localized as suggested by those assigning specific functions to specific neural centers. Instead, most brain functions are now thought of as being organized in systems, generally running longitudinally upward and downward and organized according to biological principles of homeostatic control. Hence there

---

*See Chapter 11 for further discussion of "structural," "procedural," and "episodic" processing.

are afferent sensory systems reaching from the periphery to the cortex and efferent systems from the cortex to the periphery, each controlling a separate function but each intimately intertwined with all the others. The overall effect is that of a large network of interacting nerve fibers which sometimes appears to function as a single pulsating entity. But that view would be erroneous. Even this diffuse structural arrangement postulates specific nerve centers and nervous systems for specific functions.

Within this context the ancient argument for localization versus generalization of function in the brain has little meaning. The following statement by Gregory (1975) best expresses both the nature of the separation of function between the microscopic and macroscopic levels and simultaneously the nature of the interaction:

> The brain is not a homogeneous mass. The anatomy, physiology and psychobiology of the brain all attest to some degree of differentiation of function that has evolved for the many macroscopic nuclei. On the other hand, no nucleus acts as the unique locus of any mental function. Obviously, neither radical localization nor radical homogeneity theory is adequate. The emerging new perspective supports a theory in which networks of interacting nuclei must collectively operate to control any facet of behavior. Within the networks of nuclei, the psychological states are represented by networks of neurons. (pp. 688–689)

The Biological Origins of Motivated Behavior

Motivation is the driving force that energizes all animal behavior. The main biological drives in all organisms are to survive, to grow, and to procreate, but the specific formula adopted to accomplish these universal goals vary markedly from species to species. In man the evolutionary devices to achieve these ends have become so complex as to have become goals in themselves. Chief among these are the demands of a social environment in which man, a social animal, must endure. In this milieu even basic biological drives such as the will to survive and to procreate may be sacrificed to the greater good.

The complexities in man resulting from the conflict of basic biological drives with social demands are even more complicated by the fact that the individual's psyche becomes the battleground between these frequently opposed forces. Thus man is not a biological animal alone, but is rather simultaneously a biological, psychological, and social organism. The psychoanalytic view of the conflict of the id (the biological) and the superego (society) in the realm of the ego (the psyche) reflects this basic formulation.

Motivational drives are activated by complex sensory impulses that come into the brain from the external environment (the smell and taste of food, the fear invoked by lightening and thunder), from internal bodily end-organs (hunger from contracting stomach musculature, thirst from hypothalamic osmoreceptors), or from more complex activities within the brain itself (memories). The number and variety of motivational drives is immense, ranging from the most physiological (the need for oxygen, the need for a stable body temperature), through the combined physiological and psychological (hunger, thirst, sex), to the most psychological (the need for power, for recognition, for nurturance). Each of the physiological drives is represented by a specific physiological system, elegantly designed to maintain biological equilibrium. Psychophysiological drives such as food foraging and sex are based on the functions of innate biological systems that are translated through complex interactions with cognitive experience into more psychologically controlled activities. Purely psychological motivations consist of cognitive equivalents of physiological and psychophysiological needs. Although these are largely independent of their biological sources, they are never completely so and always retain some dependence on underlying primitive physiological mechanisms. Social drives derive entirely from experience and as such are largely independent of primitive biological motivations. Most often they are actually in conflict with them.

Classification of Drives

Drives may be classified generally into seven major categories ranging from the most biologically determined to those that have their origins mainly in psychosocial interactions. The most primitive biological drives may be called *homeostatic drives* such as hunger, thirst, the need for sleep, and the need for temperature control. These are represented in specific neurological systems in the brain which provide the mechanisms through which physiological and metabolic homeostasis of the internal environment is gauranteed. Equally primitive are the *pleasure–pain reactivities* that define experience as either pleasurable or unpleasurable; these determine the direction of behavior (approach behavior to seek pleasure or avoidance behavior to avoid pain or tension). Closely related to the pleasure–seeking drives (and to a large extent controlled by them) are the *sexual and sensual drives*. These not only provide specifically for the propagation of the species but also contribute to the satisfaction of the homeostatic drives (e.g., the taste and smell of food; the sight, sound, and feel of the opposite sex). A more recently recognized category of drives are the *developmental* which insure the satisfactory growth and maturation of the individual. These drives include a variety of stimulatory experiences that lead to increased development and maturation through the effective exercise of the sensory and motor apparatus. *Survival drives,* the so-called instinct of self-preservation, are among the most complex biological drives since they involve the entire spectrum of emotional (affective) reactivities. *Psychological and behavioral drives* such as need for nurturance, power drives, and the need for self-realization derive from biological reactions to social experiences and are necessary to guarantee the integrity of the self. Finally, so-called *social drives* are determined by the continual interaction of the individual with his immediate social environment; they are differentially determined at different levels of social interaction (the child–mother dyad, the family, the community, and the nation).

Drives are represented subjectively as in feelings of hunger, thirst, sexuality, curiosity, or patriotism and objectively as in behavior directed toward gratifying those subjective feelings. The subjective and objective representation of primitive biological drives are defined by specific neuronal programs in the brain (see section on homeostatic drives). Those of the more complex developmental, behavioral, and social drives constitute more diffuse mental operations which are not readily described in terms of neurophysiological mechanisms.

The Homeostatic Drives (Metabolic)

Since biological homeostasis is perhaps the single most important mechanism characterizing all living organisms, the drives that insure internal homeostasis are the most primitive and the most elemental. The physiological representations of these primitive biological drives exist in genetically hard-wired anatomical formations in the brain. In a rigorous sense, *drives* are not the same as *biological needs* even though one tends to use the terms interchangeably. Needs exist as theoretical constructs; drives are the built-in physiological mechanisms through which biological needs are realized. Thus hunger and thirst are drive mechanisms that ultimately assure the fulfillment of the organism's need for metabolic homeostasis.

Functionally, drives may be conceptualized as the sensory components in a more complex constellation called *motivated behavior*. For example, an animal will feel hunger when there is increased activity in a variety of end-organs (increased stomach contractions, low blood sugar, etc.) which results in increased activity in the hunger center of the hypothalamus. Depending on the intensity of the latter activity, hunger signals either do or do not reach awareness in a system originating in the brain stem and radiating upward (the consciousness system). In either case (aware or unaware), increased activity in the hunger center of the hypothalamus causes organized reactions in the nearby basal ganglia which prepare the animal for food foraging or hunting activities. These ultimately involve all higher centers in the cortex. However, the basic patterns of behavior still stem fundamentally from the primitive control centers in the hypothalamus, thalamus, and basal ganglia. Homeostatic motivated behaviors are usually initiated by some metabolic instability within the organism and continue until a metabolic balance is restored.

Because homeostatic drives are so vital to organismic survival, they are usually represented redundantly in a variety of mechanisms. Thus at the peripheral sensory control level, the sensation of hunger may be produced either by stomach contractions or by a lowered level of blood sugar. Similarly, thirst sensations can be caused either by local dryness of the mouth, by an increase in blood concentration, or by a decrease in blood volume. In each case a kind of physiological or chemical rheostat in the hypothalamus responds to physiological (stomach contractions or dry mouth) or chemical changes (low blood sugar or high blood concentration) to produce sensations of hunger or thirst, respectively. The mechanisms for temperature control are similar, with exposures to either excessive heat or cold triggering corresponding feelings associated with appropriate behavioral responses.

The sensations of hunger, thirst, heat, and cold are basically cognitive experiences that are transmitted through mechanisms similar to those involved in perception and cognition (see Chapter 4). It is an interesting anatomical observation that although homeostatic drives derive largely from visceral events, these stimuli are carried to the brain not through the autonomic nervous system (which has no afferent sensory component) but rather through the same tracts in the central nervous system that receive messages from the external environment. There is sometimes the tendency to speak of motivation as separate and distinct from cognitive activity. As will be stressed repeatedly throughout this volume, there can be no motivational experience without a cognitive component, just as there can be no cognitive experience without a motivational component.

The subjective experience of awareness of a motivational drive (hunger, thirst, etc.) is activated in the same way as that for affect (the emotions) and for cognitive experience (seeing, hearing, etc.). It involves stimulation of the awareness system which arises in the reticular activating system and has major sensory representation in the thalamus. Activation of the awareness system takes place in the brain stem and limbic system through the interaction of motivational and consciousness neural elements (see Chapters 3 and 6).

An efferent discharge of visceral reactivities is simultaneously triggered with the stimulation of motivational centers. These homeostatic functions are implemented through the autonomic nervous system. Visceral reactivities include such reactions as increased salivation associated with hunger, shunting of the blood from the periphery inward in conditions of extreme cold, and sweating associated with excessive heat.

Involuntary muscle responses associated with motivational activities are controlled by the nigrostriatal motor system which has its neural centers in the substantia nigra of the brain stem and the striatum of the basal ganglia. Involuntary muscle responses associated with motivational behavior include shivering (cold), restlessness (hunger), and listlessness(heat). A variety of other primitive visceral and muscle responses associated with the adaptive components of motivational behavior are described in the next chapter.

Pleasure–Pain Systems (Affective)—The Reward System

All of the homeostatic drives, hunger, thirst, temperature control, sex, and so forth, differ from one another in their anatomical and physiological representations and in their associated behavioral patterns. All have in common the necessity for some built-in criteria on the basis of which a drive can be evaluated as fulfilled or unfulfilled. Whereas the physiologies of different drives vary markedly, the mechanisms for assessing drive satisfaction are relatively few. Since these higher-order mechanisms, expressed in terms of pleasure or displeasure, ultimately define the satisfaction of all bodily and psychological needs, they can be regarded in a sense as the most basic of all drives: to seek pleasure and to avoid displeasure.

A pleasure–displeasure continuum introduces a new dimension into the consideration of motivational mechanisms since pleasure–displeasure are affective reactivities that are generally considered emotional rather than motivational. Indeed, this interaction points up the inherent fallacy in separating motivational from emotional reactivities.

Search for pleasure and avoidance of pain or tension are the affective parameters against which all other drives are measured. Each of these three parameters is represented by a specific physiological system in the brain. The experimental basis for the concept that there are specific areas in the brain responsible for the experience of pleasure stems from the work of Olds and his co-workers (1958). These investigators demonstrated that rats with electrodes implanted in certain parts of the brain stem would bar-press for self-stimulation to the exclusion of all other activities, eating, drinking, or sex, until they died of exhaustion. Stimulation of similar areas of the brain in conscious humans (during surgical procedures) results in highly pleasant sensations; for the purpose of this volume, it seems reasonable to extrapolate the same feeling of pleasure to lower animals as well.

The specific pathways that define the brain reward system have been worked out predominantly by Olds (1958), Routtenberg (1978), and Stein (1977), using the Olds' paradigm of intracranial self-stimulation (ICSS) in animals. Electrodes are implanted at various sites in the brain and experimental procedures are established in which bar-pressing by a given animal results in stimulation of that site in the brain. Where the animal continues to bar-press to the exclusion of all other activities (food, water, sex), the reward system is said to be powerfully represented; where the bar-pressing response is moderate or slight or absent, the representation of the reward system is designated accordingly; where the animal responds with active aversion to bar-pressing, the pathway is considered to represent part of the discomfort or pain system. In humans, the brain reward system has been mapped through stimulation of various sites during brain surgery in conscious patients where the criterion is the level of pleasure (or displeasure) experienced by the individual. In this way, physiological anatomical systems have been delineated for humans. These were illustrated in Figure 1-1. The validity of these conclusions has been supported in experiments in which similar pathways are destroyed either electrolytically or chemically in rats, after which the self-stimulation responses disappear.

The brain reward system consists of several centers in the brain. Its innervation is predominantly through the median forebrain bundle. This nerve tract rises in the locus coeruleus (Fig. 2-1), radiates upward through the midbrain stem through the hypothalamus and thalamus to the basal ganglia and limbic system, and from there upward to the frontal cortex. In each area, it activates a specific center of the brain reward system. Recent work using a variety of neurochemical and pharmacologic techniques has demonstrated that the brain reward system, rather than being a single discrete anatomical entity, actually consists of all of these different centers, each activated by a different neurotransmitter system and each serving a different function in the transmission of the pleasure–displeasure impulses (Table 2-1).

Particulary important in this system is the septal area of the limbic system (see Fig. 2-3). This was the first area identified by Olds and Milner (1954) as being critical in the brain reward system; subsequent work has reinforced this impression. Heath (1963) observed that stimulation of the septal area in alert humans blocked uncontrollable rage and substituted for it a sense of markedly pleasurable euphoria. There is some evidence that stimulation of the septal area produces a more euphoric type of sensation than the ordinary sense of pleasure associated with stimulation of lower portions of the brain reward system. The significance of this finding in transcendent experience and in drug addiction is reviewed in Chapter 21.

The relationship of the various neurotransmitter systems to the different behavioral functions in which the brain reward system is involved is suggested in Table 2-1, modeled after Stein et al. (1977) and Pradhan (1974). The chemical innervation of the brain reward system is thought to be highly related to the activity of the monoaminergic neurotransmitters, dopamine, norepinephrine, and serotonin. This viewpoint is supported by the evidence of the distribution of these chemical systems in the brain which closely follow the neural distribution of the reward system, the reticular activating system, and the pain system (Fig. 1-1 and 2-1). In drug addicts, the search for ecstatic and euphoric experience is achieved chemically through stimulation of the brain reward system by the use of different drugs (cocaine, morphine, etc.). These latter effects are described in Chapter 21.

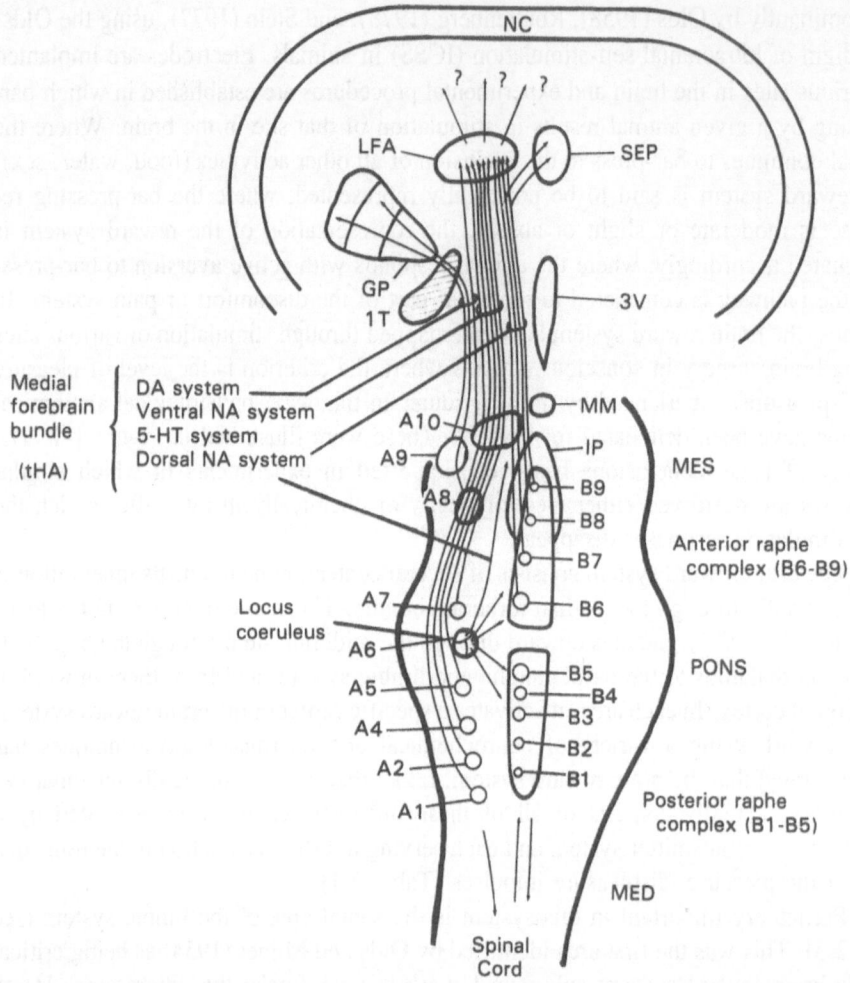

Figure 2-1 Chemical systems in the brain stem and paleocortex. (From Morgane, 1975. Reprinted with permission.)

Pleasure–Pain Systems (Affective)—The Pain System

From an evolutionary viewpoint, an equally or perhaps even more important element in external sensory reception is the perception of pain, the response to nociceptive stimuli. The animal organism is so constructed that painful stimuli are almost always dangerous or actively destructive to the organism's integrity so that the learning of aversive or avoidance behavior is critical to the animal's survival. The pain pathways arise in the nerve endings of end-organs and after reaching the spinal cord through afferent peripheral nerves, ascend in the spinothalamic tract. In transmission of pain (Fig. 2-2), two routes innervate the cortex, the *direct* through the medial lemniscus via the specific nuclei in the thalamus, and the *indirect* from the medial

Table 2-1 Relationship of Neurotransmitter Systems to Behavioral Functions of the Brain Reward System

Neurotransmitter System	Behavioral Function
Dopaminergic (dominant in median forebrain bundle)	Motivational incentive
Enkephalin (central gray)	Motivational fulfillment
Noradrenergic (septal area and hippocampus)	Passive avoidance conditioning
Serotonergic (amygdala)	Active avoidance conditioning
Benzodiazepine (cingulate nucleus)	Reduction of displeasure reactions

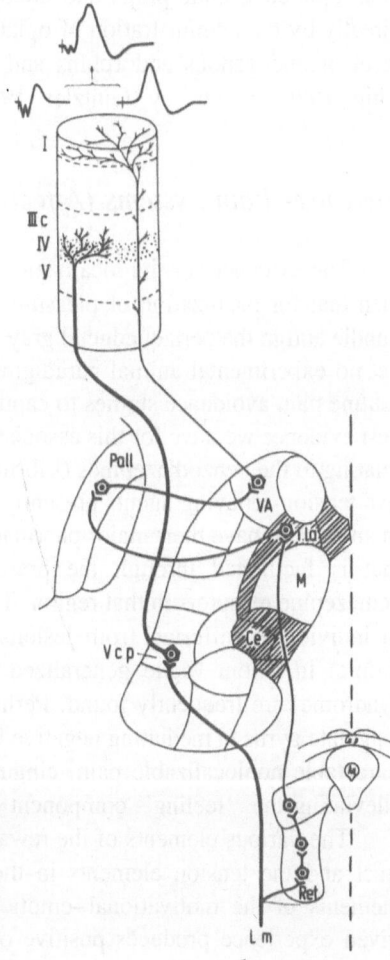

Figure 2-2 The thalamic–basal gangliar complex. Abbreviations: Lm, medial lemniscus; Vcp, specific nuclei in the thalamus; Ret, reticular activating system; M, median thalamic nucleus; ila, truncothalamic nucleus; Pall., globus pallidus: VA, anterior thalamic nucleus; areas 1, 2, 3, parietal cortex. (From Hassler, 1978. Reprinted with permission.)

lemniscus to the reticular activating system to the median thalamic nucleus to the truncothalamic nucleus to the globus pallidus to the anterior thalamic nucleus and thence to the parietal cortex. The cortical evoked potentials generated by the *direct* route (top of diagram, left) and by the *indirect* route (top of diagram, right) coalesce to form a single evoked potential (top of diagram) indicating an integration and merging of the two sensory inputs. The direct route accounts for sensory components of the experience while the indirect route contributes the element of subjective feeling. Like the evoked potential, both separate effects are integrated into one.

The indirect spinothalamic tract branches off from the main neural trunk in the brain stem and forms a separate pathway in the periaqueductal gray (Liebeskind et al., 1973). This tract provides the feeling component for pain similar to that of the reward system for pleasure. The periaqueductal gray ascends from the medulla through the core of the brain stem to the thalamus where it connects with radiations to the rhinencephalon (cingulate nucleus) and thence to the prefrontal cortex (see Fig. 2-2). The neurons of the periaqueductal gray have been demonstrated to be particularly rich in opiate receptors which are activated both by exogeneous opiates and by the endogenous opiatelike endorphins and enkephalins. Pain reactivities can thus be lessened directly by the administration of opiate narcotics or indirectly by increasing the brain level of endogenous endorphins and enkephalins as in acupuncture (Pomeranz and Chin, 1976), pregnancy (Gintzler, 1980), and stress (Willer et al., 1981).

Pleasure–Pain Systems (Affective)—The Tension System

The evidence for the localization of tension in the limbic system is less concrete than that for localization of pleasure and pain, respectively, in the median forebrain bundle and in the periaqueductal gray. This is probably due to the fact that there are as yet no experimental animal paradigms such as Olds' self-stimulation for pleasure or routine pain avoidance studies to capture the phenomenology of tension. Probably the best evidence we have for this association comes indirectly from pharmacological data relating to the benzodiazepines (Librium, Valium, etc.), drugs that are the most effective tension-relieving agents presently available. These drugs have been demonstrated in animals to have their major pharmacologic activity in the cingulate gyrus, an action that is facilitated through the presence of large numbers of drug-specific benzodiazepine receptors in that region. These conclusions are further supported clinically in individuals suffering from lesions in the limbic systems (Dejerine-Roussy syndrome) in whom vague generalized bodily sensations of discomfort (the thalamic syndrome) are frequently found. Perhaps the best evidence for the special role of the cingulate gyrus in mediating negative feelings of tension is the fact that in patients with intractable nonlocalizable pain, cingulotomy is the single most effective method for alleviating the "feeling" component of such pain.

The various elements of the reward system, together with the pain system neural tract and the tension elements in the limbic system, represent the most primitive elements of the motivational–emotional system, those which determine whether a given experience produces positive or negative affective valence. Experiences with positive affective valence are responded to behaviorally with "approach"; those with negative valences elicit "avoidance" responses. In learning (to be discussed in Chapter 5), positive valence is associated with positive reinforcement with a rapid improvement in performance. With highly charged negative affective valence, the opposite is true and harmful activities are carefully avoided. Hence the affective element in motivational–emotional behavior provides the index of the pleasure/displeasure ratio for every experience, the index that ultimately determines all behavior.

The Limbic System as the Seat of ''Feeling''

The cingulate nucleus, which together with the hypothalamus and thalamus is responsible for much of the feeling component of basic motivational drives of pleasure, pain, and tension (and as will be seen in the next chapter, of the emotional reactivities), is part of the limbic system, first described by Papez (1937) as the seat of the emotions. Papez wrote (as reported in Winson, 1985):

> It is thus evident that the afferent pathways from the receptor organs split at the thalamic level into three routes, each conducting a stream of impulses of special importance. One route conducts impulses through the . . . thalamus . . . to the corpus striatum (the basal ganglia, a group of subcortical nuclei associated with action of movement). This route represents ''the stream of movement.'' The second conducts impulses from the thalamus . . . to the lateral cerebral cortex. This route represents ''the stream of thought.'' The third conducts a set of concomitant impulses through the . . . thalamus by way of the mammillary body and the anterior thalamic nuclei to the gyrus cinguli, in the medial wall of the cerebral hemisphere. This route represents ''the stream of feeling.'' In this way, the sensory excitations which reach the lateral cortex . . . receive their emotional coloring from the concurrent processes of hypothalamic origin which irradiate them from the gyrus cinguli. (p. 725)

The general outlines of the limbic system as delineated in this excerpt from Papez are illustrated in Figure 2-3. However, the core of this program lies in the thalamic–basal gangliar complex (Fig. 2-2), an integrated structure connecting various elements

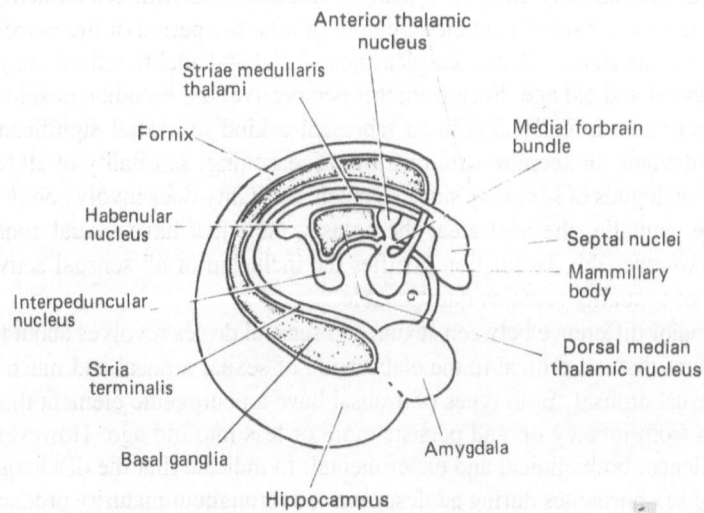

Figure 2-3 Anatomy of the limbic system. (Adapted from Kupferman, 1981.)

of the thalamus, the anterior thalamic nucleus and the median thalamic nucleus, with the globus pallidus of the basal ganglia. This complex, together with the hypothalamus, provides the most basic elements of "feeling" and as a consequence, of "consciousness" (see Chapter 6). Such "feelings" are activated through stimulation of the reticular activating system (*Ret* in Fig. 2-2) and are elaborated in parts of the limbic system (the system and cingulate nucleus) before ascending to the cortex.

The limbic system is shown in general outline in Figure 2-3. Included but not shown in this illustration are the hypothalamus, the cingulate gyrus (peripheral to the fornix), and the elements of the basal ganglia (shown in Fig. 2-2). Input from the hypothalamus to this system is through the mammillary body; the connections between the thalamus and basal ganglia are illustrated in Figure 2-2. The amygdala and hippocampus which form the major portion of the rhinencephalon are thought to be activated at a later state of information processing and are less involved in the "feeling" aspect of experience. On the other hand, they are critical in more cognitive functions such as attention, memory, and awareness. These latter processes are discussed in detail in Chapters 7 through 10.

Sensual and Sexual Drives

Of all ordinary events in normal behavior, sexual excitement and gratification certainly provide the most highly charged positive affective experience. It appears that a similar sensation can be evoked by the effects of intravenous injection of drugs (cocaine or heroin) or by direct electrical stimulation on the reward system in the brain, but these procedures are neither biological nor ordinary. The extraordinary level of pleasure felt in sexual orgasm is hardly ever otherwise experienced in ordinary living. As a consequence, sex and its related activities have achieved a special significance disproportionate even to its essential biological function. As an index of pleasure, it remains the ultimate standard against which all other experiences must be measured.

At the biological level, only a few activities offer amounts of pleasure which can begin to be meaningfully compared with those associated with sexual activity. Even these tend to be most significant either before or after the period of life associated with active sexual experience. Hence the pleasures of oral and anal functions are greatest in early childhood and old age. Seen from this perspective, the Freudian position that oral and anal activities in early childhood represent a kind of sexual significance seems much less deviant. In keeping with this line of reasoning, sensuality of all forms may be seen as analogues of sexuality since so much sensuality does involve body areas (the mouth, the genitalia, the anal area, the breasts, etc.) that have sexual connotations. However, whether this association justifies the inclusion of all sensual activity under the rubric of sexuality remains questionable.

The major difference between sexual and sensual drives revolves about the role of sex hormones that are critical to the elaboration of sexual arousal and much less so to that of sensual arousal. Both types of arousal have a neurogenic element that presumably exists from infancy on and persists more or less into old age. However, there is ample evidence, both clinical and experimental, to indicate that the discharge of large amounts of sex hormones during adolescence and throughout maturity produces a level of sexual desire far and above that sustained by neurogenic sensuality alone. On the other hand, the occurrence of infantile masturbation at one end of the age spectrum and of active sexuality in the 70s and 80s at the other end are evidence enough for the importance of the neurogenic sensual element of sexuality.

Developmental Drives (Stimulatory)

Motivational drives such as hunger, thirst, temperature regulation, and sex drives are the prototypical mechanisms through which organisms fulfill their biological needs to survive and to procreate. All of these activities are characterized by the need to reduce drive tensions. Drives of a more active nature are involved in the processes of growth and development; these express themselves mainly as various requirements for physiological stimulation: sensory and/or motor. These reactivities have been well-documented experimentally in a series of studies on the need for stimulation for effective growth and development in the visual system (Blakemore and Cooper, 1970), in sensory motor coordination (Held and Hein, 1963), and in general brain development (Rosenzweig, 1970). Lack of stimulation results in physiological underdevelopment and in psychological depression. The need to be hugged and caressed has been shown to be one of the most important, so that such experience is essential for the normal development of infant monkeys and infant humans (Spitz, 1945; Harlow and Zimmerman, 1959). It now appears that the various needs for stimulation may be just as important for the psychological growth of the individual as is satisfaction of the basic physiological needs for his physical growth. How these developmental drives are implemented physiologically is not known. Presumably activity of the motor and sensory apparatus is associated with stimulation of the pleasure system while inactivity is associated with a notable lack of such pleasure (Boddy, 1978; Chapter 7).

Developmental drives are manifest in such universal drives as playfulness in children, curiosity, and the general need for activity to escape boredom. At some other levels, these developmental drives are translated into a need for challenging experiences which is further transformed into a need to control the environment (Piaget, 1978). How much such needs are involved in the development of power drives are questions of both theoretical and practical significance.

The Instinct of Self-Preservation—The Need for Survival

Of all needs, that for survival must certainly seem the most primitive as well as the most biological; consequently, it must be surprising to find it at the bottom of the list for biological drives. Certainly among primitive animals the mechanisms serving the so-called instinct for self-preservation are elemental, existing at the most basic physiological levels. But this is not entirely true in mammals and most particularly not true in man. Here, innate but extremely complex mechanisms exist to guarantee survival not only at the biological level but also at the social level since the environment in which the individual exists and upon which he is dependent is frequently more social than it is biological.

The instinct of self-preservation differs in a variety of ways from the biological drives previously described. Those, by and large, were directed toward satisfaction of needs stemming from the internal milieu: metabolic homeostasis, pleasurable gratification, and stimulation. The instinct of self-preservation is directed mainly toward the external environment both in terms of implementing positive goals (approach behaviors) and in terms of escaping negative dangers (avoidance behaviors). Toward the accomplishment of these goals, higher animals are equipped with a large repertory of special responsivities, each appropriate to a corresponding positive or negative situation. These special responsivities are known as emotional reactions and are designed to permit the organism to cope with the various exigencies—positive or negative—that the environment offers.

Emotional reactions are of course a subject in themselves and will constitute the subject matter of the next chapter. Here it is enough to say that they provide both in their variety and in the magnitude of their intensity some of the most important forces determining mammalian and particularly human behavior. Emotions derive their impetus from the biological mechanisms underlying the other primitive drives. However, the intensity of their reaction is enormously multiplied by the fact that the neural, endocrine, and muscular systems (and all other visceral systems) are mobilized in emotional expression. Thus the various emotional reactivities act as magnifiers of lesser stimuli, immensely increasing their significance. Although emotions are of greatest importance in facilitating avoidance survival activities (fear for flight, rage for attack, disgust for discomfort, and so on), they are also of importance for approach reactivities (passion for sexual involvement, appetite for food, and so forth).

Another factor distinguishing the instinct of self-preservation from the more primitive biological drives is implied in the very term, "self-preservation." Here for the first time is introduced among biological configurations the concept of "self"—i.e., of the entire organism. Metabolic homeostasis, the pleasure principle, stimulatory, sensual, and sexual drives, are all governed mainly by the pervasive presence of an inner sense of glow or darkness. With survival drives, the possibility of external danger must be translated into a sense of danger to oneself. But the concept of "safety of the self" implies sophisticated reaction systems to support it, more complex than those provided to insure implementation of biological drives. Thus the instinct of self-preservation, insofar as it involves an awareness of self and is not merely a collection of instinctive reactivities, is only a mammalian characteristic.

In lower mammals, the instinct of self-preservation subsumes all of the other biological drives since, in the self-aware animal, the violation of any primitive need signals a danger to the entire organism. In humans, where both the self-image and higher psychosocial motivations are well-developed, the instinct of self-preservation may be bent away from the biological and toward the psychosocial. Only through such complex interactions can the self-destructive behavior of soldiers in war begin to be understood.

Psychological Drives

Psychological drives are best considered as deriving from one or another of the biological drives described in the preceding five categories but elaborated through experience to a more complex structure. Many psychological drives have been so changed through the process of their evolution that they seem remote and almost unrelated to the primitive drives from which they originated. For example, the need for affection probably stems originally from the basic physiological need to be touched. However, during development it becomes overladen with psychological needs, to be attended to, to be cared for, and to be loved for oneself. These additional considerations obviously involve a whole series of constructs that are not biological in nature but which have been derived through complex cognitive experience. Although the origins of psychological drives are inherently biological, their development is largely cognitive and experiential.

How primitive drives evolve into psychological drives is extremely pertinent to our considerations and will be discussed in the following sections. Here it is only necessary to enumerate the various types of psychological drives and to describe some of the mechanisms involved in their manifestations.

A partial, certainly not all-inclusive, list of psychological drives includes the need for nurturance, power drives, the need for experience, and the need for self-realization and ego-ideal gratification.

Need for Nurturance

This stems from childhood experience where some basic physiological drives are early recognized as dependent on outside forces for their fulfillment. The primitive drives include need for feeding, need to be cleaned and made comfortable, need for human touch and warmth, and need for stimulation. As previously described, these basic drives are translated through development and experience into dependency needs, the need for physical affection, and finally the need for unequivocal love and acceptance.

Power Drives

These drives stem in part from biological aggressive tendencies and in part from the developmental drives (Piaget's need to control the environment). They are elaborated through development and experience into various power manifestations that may be interpersonal, professional, political, or economic.

The Need for Experience

This stems largely from the developmental drives and is translated into an interest in athletics, travel, entertainment, and so on. The psychological need for sexual experience derives of course from the biological sex drives.

The Needs for Self-Realization and Ego-Ideal Gratification

These stem not so much from the primitive biological drives thus far discussed but from those processes associated with the development of the sense of self. As will be described in Chapter 7, the physical sense of self derives from physiological reactivities based on the reception in the self-awareness system of the multiple impressions associated with internal and external sensory experience. Consequently, the sense of self is originally an essentially physiological entity. With experience, it becomes elaborated into a complex cognitive entity one might label the "self-image," stemming from the physiological sense of self but incorporating all pertinent life experience.

The fact that "sense of self" is involved both in the biological survival drives (instinct of self-preservation) and in the psychological needs for self-realization forms an important bridge between these two generally disparate groups of motivations. It implies that the need for self-realization is more than psychological and that it is really firmly based in the biological instinct of self-preservation. It also implies that the implementation systems for both of these sets of drives are the same, namely the array of emotional reactivities (see Chapter 3).

Although the concept of self has been invoked only for the instincts of self-preservation and the need for self-realization, it is obvious that it applies equally to all psychological drives. In each instance, nurturance, power, or experience (sexual or otherwise), it is the total individual rather than some organic system within him that is involved. Similarly, the response system for all of these reactivities is again that of the generalized emotions rather than that of any reactivity at a more local level.

Social Drives

Social drives resemble psychological drives in their dependence on the emotions but are radically different from them in mode of derivation. Like psychological drives, social drives are complex cognitive–motivational constructs evolved through experience and lodged predominantly in the highest cognitive centers of the cortex. Whereas psychological drives stem from and are closely related to biological drives in the brain stem and paleocortex, social drives derive solely from cognitive–emotional experience. Thus social drives represent that major category of behavioral experience where the driving motivation comes not from within the individual but from the society without.

It is apparent that even the most socially advanced human will not knowingly behave in a way calculated to deprive himself of the satisfaction of an important need, or even worse to harm himself, unless there is fear of some greater punishment that society may impose. The starving man who will not steal a loaf of bread and the soldier who fights knowing that he may be killed repress their biological drive (to take the bread, to flee) in the face of a greater fear. Here cognitive–emotional complexes, existing at the highest cognitive level (the neocortex) and only distantly related to primitive impulses coming from the primitive brain (the brain stem and paleocortex), inhibit strong motivational impulses stemming from the old brain. The mechanism through which the higher levels of the brain control stimuli coming from lower levels is generally described as hierarchical control and constitutes one of the most important principles of motivational and emotional control in mammalian (but especially human) behavior (see Chapter 3).

The derivation of social drives, divorced as they are from biological forces innately centered in the brain, constitutes one of the more difficult physiological reconstructions with which we will deal in this volume. The formulations underlying social motivational constructs are completely cognitive in origin. Not only are they not based on biological drives but most often, because of the nature of societal regulations, they are directed toward inhibiting or otherwise thwarting basic biological motivations. Nevertheless, they ultimately assume a level of influence sufficient to overcome even the most powerful biological drives.

Social drives like psychological drives are associated with two fundamental reactivities: the essential presence of the self-concept and the use of the emotional system as the instrument of evaluation and implementation. In addition, both share a heavy reliance on developmental and experiential influences, as will be described in the following section.

The Elaboration of Biological and Psychosocial Drives

These descriptions of the biological and psychosocial drives speak largely to their derivation and little to their developed state in the mature adult. The elaboration of even the most biologically derived drives such as hunger and thirst into their final adult shape is the product of the ongoing effects of development and experience. These effects are so enormous as to almost confound those of biological origin. Thus the civilized man will frequently not eat when he is hungry, not drink when he is thirsty, not sleep when he is sleepy, and most remarkable, not flee when he is terrified.

These effects result from the elaboration of even the most biological drives into complex constellations in the brain. In this way, hunger becomes elaborated into gourmet tastes and the need for warmth into "haute couture." The complexities surrounding sexual drives are vastly complicated by psychological and social mores. The instinct of self-preservation, often considered the most biological of drives, is elaborated into such a maze of personal, economic, social, and nationalistic complexities as to permit its frequent abrogation. In the same way, every biological drive is shaped and elaborated into a form that frequently bears little resemblance to the original.

The physiological processes through which these changes take place can only be hinted at. As previously described, the afferent components of visceral stimuli progress to the brain through the same afferent elements of the central nervous system as do cognitive stimuli. They are presumably organized in the same way and with the same degree of complexity. In this way, even nonemotional experiences are changed during development into vastly different patterns.

But even stronger than these essentially cognitive effects are those related to emotional charge. As previously described, no motivational activity takes place in an emotional vacuum; the very nature of motivation proscribes such a possibility. Motivational behavior by definition is the most emotionally charged behavior there is since every motivational experience shapes that particular drive positively or negatively. Development and experience not only affect the cognitive elaboration of given drives but even more importantly determine the specific patterns of responsivity associated with those drives. Where in the brain this occurs is not entirely clear but presumably these changes occur in the specific cortical areas (the inferotemporal lobe) where cognitive and emotional stimuli are integrated.* As a result of such interactions, behavioral responses to even biological drives may be significantly changed.

The mechanisms through which these inhibitions (because they are primarily inhibitions) of biological urges are accomplished are thought to be activated through neural pathways leading from the highest levels of the cortex (i.e., the prefrontal lobe) down upon the limbic system, the hypothalamus, and other portions of the brain stem. These influences are supported by the anatomical demonstration of such tracts and by strong physiological evidence of such inhibiting influences, especially from the prefrontal cortex onto the hypothalamus and other portions of the limbic system (see Chapter 13).

The Interaction of Biological and Psychosocial Drives

The two sets of drives, the biological and the psychosocial are, by nature of their derivation, often strongly facilitatory and often strongly antagonistic. It is a mistake to think of biological drives and psychosocial drives as always in conflict. Indeed, it must be apparent that most adult behavior, activated as it is by psychological and social drives, is designed to satisfy biological drives. Nevertheless, it is equally true that by the very nature of their origin and elaboration, biological and psychosocial drives not infrequently strive toward antithetical goals, giving rise to considerable motivational conflict.

Such conflict is engendered by the opposition of energy flow in the two types of drives. The neurological representations of biological and psychosocial drives in the brain are not vastly different. Biological drives are anchored in the brain stem and elaborated in the neocortex; psychosocial drives are mainly anchored in the neocortex but have attached to them strong emotional influences radiating up from the brain stem. The major differences between biological and psychosocial drives is in the direction of apparent flow of the relative dominant energies. Drives in which the flow of energy appears to be mainly upward from the brain stem and paleocortex (basal ganglia and rhinencephalon) may be designated as more biological. Those in which the energies appear to flow mainly from the neocortex downward may be designated as more psychosocial. Ultimately it is the level of brain stem arousal associated with either that determines the relative strength of drives.

The Freudian formulation of id and superego drives and of the conflict between them is readily translated into these anatomical and physiological analogues. Id drives could be conceptualized as arising from the first five categories of motivational drives described in this chapter, i.e., the metabolic, the affective, the sensual, the developmental, and the survival. These derive and are activated almost entirely from biologically innate mechanisms in the brain stem and limbic system, even though they are susceptible to modification by experience. The last two categories of motivational drives, the psychological and social, derive almost entirely from experience; their

---

*For a detailed description of the processes involved in the organization of perceptual and cognitive stimuli, see Chapters 4 and 5.

physiological representation is mainly in the neocortex. The putative interaction between primitive id drives, striving upward from the brain stem and limbic system, and the experientially derived superego drives, exerting their inhibitory influence downward from the neocortex, is fully compatible both with the Freudian concept of id–superego conflict and the psychobiological concept of hierarchical feedback control in the motivational system. However, the Freudian id as conceptualized is different from the general reservoir for biological drives in the sense that only the most socially controversial biological drives (usually sexual) are repressed and relegated to the unconscious. These distinctions are elaborated upon in Chapter 18.

3

Adaptive and Affective Roles of the Emotions

All motivational and emotional reactivities are part of a single behavioral system established to insure the satisfaction of the basic motivational needs. Motivation and emotions may be seen as two sides of a single coin where all motivational experiences have an emotional component and all emotional experiences a motivational component. For example, hunger, usually identified as a purely motivational state, is almost always associated with a generalized state of bodily tension (restlessness, discomfort, and so on) the relief of which is the major driving force in food-seeking behavior. Similarly fear, most often considered an emotional reactivity, is usually associated with some motivational drive (fear of pain, of danger, of falling) or even, as in anxiety, fear of fear. In each case the emotional component plays a strong organizing physiological role in facilitating behavior that will satisfy basic motivational drives—to obtain pleasure, to relieve an internally produced tension, or to avoid pain.

If motivation existed only as needs without provision for fulfilling those needs, the species would soon die out. Consequently, the emotional apparatus which has developed to fulfill those needs must be considered as an integral segment of the motivational system. Responses of this type fall into two main categories: (1) the physiological reorganization of the internal environment appropriate for the fulfillment of particular motivational drives (the adaptive function), and (2) affective reactivities that define underlying pleasure–displeasure parameters on the basis of which drive fulfillment may be evaluated (the affective function). Both of these types of responses are built into the structure of the brain stem and paleocortex in so-called emotional reaction patterns. These reaction patterns are what the individual feels as emotional states; the latter are the subjective equivalents of the total physiological expression of particular patterns of adaptive and affective reactivities.

Emotional reactions are most clearly delineated as specific states of physiological reactivity associated with powerful subjective feelings. These states run the entire gamut from most pleasurable (ecstasy) to least pleasurable (terror) and as such are the most powerful determinants of behavior. Experience that results in strongly negative affect is assiduously avoided while that resulting in strongly positive affect is constantly pursued. Most emotional reactivities to environmental experience are thought to be innate but the conditions that evoke complex emotional reactivities are learned. The emotional charge on experience, in the sense of eliciting a traditional emotional response such as fear, anger, rage, and so on, is the most important element in determining positive or negative psychological and social motivation and behavior.

Adaptive Aspects of the Emotions*

The adaptive function of emotions provides the necessary organismic reorganization that will enable the animal to deal most effectively with its own needs in a manner that is compatible with the demands of the environment. Under the rubric of adjustment to environmental influences, emotions are considered (1) as a means of maintaining physiological homeostasis; (2) as a source of psychological energy; (3) as a mechanism for preparing motor intervention; and (4) as a positive influence on performance.

Emotions and Physiological Homeostasis

The physiological mechanisms through which emotions change the metabolic internal milieu to adapt to environmental demands involve the autonomic nervous system for rapid changes and the neuroendocrine system over more prolonged periods of time. The autonomic nervous system responds rapidly to varying conditions. For example, the cholinergic parasympathetic nervous system (the vegetative nervous system), the control center for which is in the anterior hypothalamus, shows greatest activity during periods of anabolic activity. Such are the internal adjustments that accompany eating (shunting of the blood from the skeletal musculature to the gastrointestinal tract), sexual activity (shunting of the blood from the skeletal musculature to the erogenous zones), or changes in temperature (shunting of the blood from the skin to the internal organs and vice versa). In these conditions there is a concomitant shift in the activity of the endocrine system toward the anabolic side (e.g., sex hormones).

On the other hand, in the course of most animals' lives critical situations constantly occur that demand the mustering of all of the organism's resources for some life-saving effort. The most common of these emergency situations involve the need for an animal to defend itself from imminent destruction by some other animal. Consequently, aggressive (fight) and defensive (flight) behavior are essential elements in the survival kits of all animals. These are accomplished by a sudden, explosive discharge of the catecholaminergic sympathetic nervous system (the emergency nervous system), the control center for which lies in the posterior hypothalamus. Metabolic processes are quickly shifted from tissue building and energy storage (anabolic) to tissue tearing

---

*The term "adaptive" as used in this volume carries the meaning of acute physiological adjustments to sudden changes in the environment rather than the more customary connotation of long-term adjustments to slow changes in the environment.

down and energy expending (catabolic). Heart rate and respirations are increased, blood is shunted from the intestinal tract to the skeletal musculature, motor activity necessary for running is initiated, and the animal flees or stands and fights. During such stressful periods, particularly when they are prolonged, there is an endocrine shift in activity away from the anabolic hormones (testosterone, estrogen) and toward the catabolic (cortisone).

Emotions as the Source of Psychological Energy

The second adaptive function of the emotions is best illustrated in the process through which adaptive influences provide the physiological and psychic energies that drive the organism to action (the dynamic principle). The physiological energy level of the organism which is translated objectively into behavioral energy and subjectively into psychic energy is determined by the levels of metabolic activity in the body and electrical activity in the brain. This parameter is known as the arousal level of the organism and can be measured on a variety of peripheral physiological indices. Posner (1975) has described the relationship of arousal to motivational–emotional influences as follows:

> The term arousal has its origin in the idea of a general drive state which potentiates all behavior. The idea is that all activity must be driven by some internal energy and the availability of this energy corresponds to the arousal level of the organism. (p. 444)

The arousal level of an organism is one of its most important behavioral parameters, setting the quantitative limits of response as opposed to the qualitative aspects which are motivationally determined. Behaviorally, the level of arousal in the brain is reflected in the level of consciousness in the animal as well as in its emotional state. The kinds of brain activity associated with these two behavioral correlates, i.e., emotional arousal and level of consciousness, are intimately related one to the other but are sufficiently different to warrent consideration as similar but not quite identical phenomena. Thus in this volume, the electrical activity of the brain associated with consciousness will be referred to as *activation* while the energy level of the organism associated with the intensity of the emotional state will be referred to as *arousal*. These two parameters, arousal and activation, are quite similar and indeed are considered by some authors to be identical (Duffy, 1962), but the differences between them appear to be sufficient to warrent their separate nomenclature (see Chapter 6).

The level of arousal generated by motivational–emotional (ME) states is closely related to the ratio of sympathetic to parasympathetic activities. The general principle is that high sympathetic nervous system (SNS) activity produces high levels of arousal (as in anger, fear, etc.) while high levels of parasympathetic nervous system (PNS) activity produce low levels of arousal (as in the postprandial state, relaxation, sleep, etc.). Since SNS and PNS activity levels tend to vary inversely, the arousal level is more or less directly related to the level of SNS activity. This is probably also true for the association during stress over prolonges periods of time between activity levels of catabolic hormones (cortisone) and levels of arousal.

The control of activation (i.e., the level of electrical activity in the brain) by the

ME system is accomplished through the influence of the brain stem centers of that system in the hypothalamus, thalamus, limbic, and nigrostriatal systems upon the reticular activating system (RAS), the specific control mechanism for activation. Activity of the PNS is associated with inhibitory stimuli from the anterior hypothalamic nuclei to the RAS with consequent reduction in the level of consciousness (drowsiness, sleep, etc.). Conversely, activity in the SNS centered in the posterior hypothalamic nuclei is associated with increased excitation of the RAS, increased levels of activation in the brain and consequently increased levels of behavioral excitation (hyperalert states).*

Musclar Patterns of Adaptation

The third adaptative function of emotions involves preparation of the motor system for the behavioral responses appropriate to the situation. In general such preparatory organization of the musculature occurs along two parameters: (1) increased or decreased general muscle tone, and (2) increased flexor or extensor muscle activity. Increased or decreased general muscle tone are associated, respectively, with high or low emergency situations. Increased flexor activity is usually associated with fear or withdrawl reactions while increased extensor activity characterizes rage and aggressive reactivities. The control center in the brain for these muscular reaction patterns is in the basal ganglia (the nigrostriatal or involuntary muscle control system). These reaction patterns are elicited in conjunction with adaptive responses previously described for metabolic reorganization and for elicitation of the appropriate level of arousal. Parasympathetic activity is most often associated with inhibitory stimuli from the limbic system to the basal ganglia of the paleocortex producing a general reduction in the tension level of the organism (muscular relaxation, etc.). Conversely, sympathetic activation is usually associated with excitatory stimuli from the same limbic system to the basal ganglia with a consequent increase in general bodily tension (increased muscle tone). Different emotional states are characterized by different patterns of emotional expression.

The Relationship of Emotions to Performance

The interaction between motivation and emotions in a tight motivational–emotional complex has not always been well understood. In this connection, Izard (1980) has written:

> There is still a prevailing tendency to view emotions in terms of disrupting and disorganizing phenomena or as the negative consequences of ongoing sequences of behavior. As a result, relatively little attention has been given to the organizing and guiding functions of emotions. (p. 194)

Much of the confusion on the role of emotions arises from the apparent paradox

*See Chapter 6 for further elucidation of these mechanisms (Figure 6-2).

that adaptive responses constitute a positive organizing effect in animal behavior while emotion, particularly excessive emotionality in humans, is often disruptive to well-organized, purposive behavior. The dynamics of this interrelationship are illustrated in Figure 3-1. As may be seen, very low levels of emotional arousal are associated with poor performance as are also very high levels of emotional arousal. On the other hand, moderate levels of emotional arousal are associated with optimal performance. The principle that too little or too much activity in a given system may have serious detrimental effects upon the organism is characteristic of most biological systems and constitutes the principle of homeostasis. It is well illustrated by the activity of the immunological system in humans. Underactivity of that system, as in agammaglobulinemia, is associated with death due to infections while marked overactivity of the immunological system can be associated with death due to allergy, as in asthma or anaphylactic shock. Among other examples of the danger of extremes, are low blood pressure and high blood pressure, anemia and polycythemia, hypoglycemia and hyperglycemia, hypothyroidism and hyperthyroidism, and so forth. Homeostasis, or physiological stabilization at a middle level, is the biological law of life so that it is not surprising that it applies to behavioral events as well.

Figure 3-1 indicates that there is an optimal range for level of arousal and that behavioral activities outside of this range may be characterized by impaired performance. This principle of behavioral homeostasis is pertinent to the conceptualization of the neuroses which frequently are characterized by either too high or too low levels of excitatory or inhibitory activities. The diagram in Figure 3-1 is known as the inverted U-shaped curve; in describing the relationship of levels of arousal and of performance it is a standard reference in psychological studies. It will be referred to frequently in this volume.

Affective Aspects of Emotions

Like motivations, emotions carry a strong affective valence so that each emotional reaction pattern may be categorized as weakly or strongly pleasant or weakly or

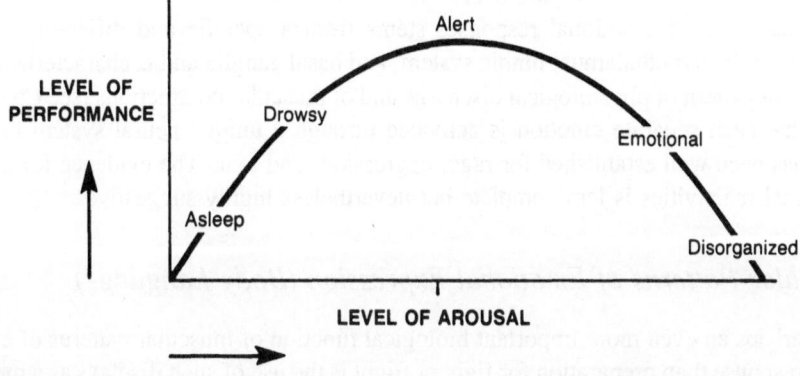

Figure 3-1 Inverted U-curve of relationship between arousal level and performance. (Modified from Hebb, 1966.)

strongly unpleasant. Affect, as defined by the pleasure, pain, or tension parameters described in Chapter 2, equally characterizes both motivational and emotional reactivities so that to assign its meaning to one or the other of these modalities alone would be erroneous. It is for this reason that in this book discussions of these types of behavior will describe them as motivational–emotional since this term offers a more precise definition of the phenomenon than the more commonly used affective.

The broad implications of the affective aspects of emotions will be considered here under three headings: (1) general patterns of emotional expression, (2) muscular patterns of emotional expression, and (3) subjective analogues of emotional reactions.

General Patterns of Emotional Expression

Emotions may be categorized by physiological and muscular patterns, by the level of arousal, and, as previously described, by positive and negative polarity where positive emotions tend to produce approach behaviors and negative emotions withdrawal behaviors. Of these three variables, emotional polarity is the most important since it defines the direction of subsequent behavior, i.e., approach or avoidance. Positive polarity is presumably initiated through stimulation of the brain reward system while negative emotional polarity is aroused through activation of the pain or tension systems in the brain. The intensity of both the subjective feeling and of the subsequent response are determined by the intensity of the emotional reaction and more specifically by the level of arousal elicited. In general, negative emotions are associated with higher levels of emotional arousal than are positive emotions, a condition sometimes associated with paradoxical consequences.*

Positive affective responses run a gamut from mild to extreme in a rather regular spectrum ranging from quiet contentment to a sense of pleasure to a sense of happiness to joy to sexual excitement. In this spectrum feelings are qualitatively similar but vary quantitatively with the level of emotional arousal. Negative affective responses run in the opposite direction from shame/shyness, to contempt to guilt to anger to fear. Here it appears that responses vary independently across a qualitatively broader spectrum. In any event, affective responses are defined both qualitatively and quantitatively (intensity of associated arousal). Different emotions are associated with different patterns of responses as illustrated in Figure 3-2.

Each of these emotional responses stems from a specific and different neural complex in the hypothalamus, limbic system, and basal ganglia and is characterized by a different pattern of physiological discharge and of muscular contractions (see Chapter 20). That each separate emotion is activated through a unique neural system in the brain has been well established for rage, aggression, and fear. The evidence for other emotional reactivities is less complete but nevertheless highly suggestive.

Muscular Patterns of Emotional Expression (Body Language)

Perhaps an even more important biological function of muscular patterns of emotional response than preparation for fight or flight is the use of such displays as a means

*See discussion on repression in Chapter 13.

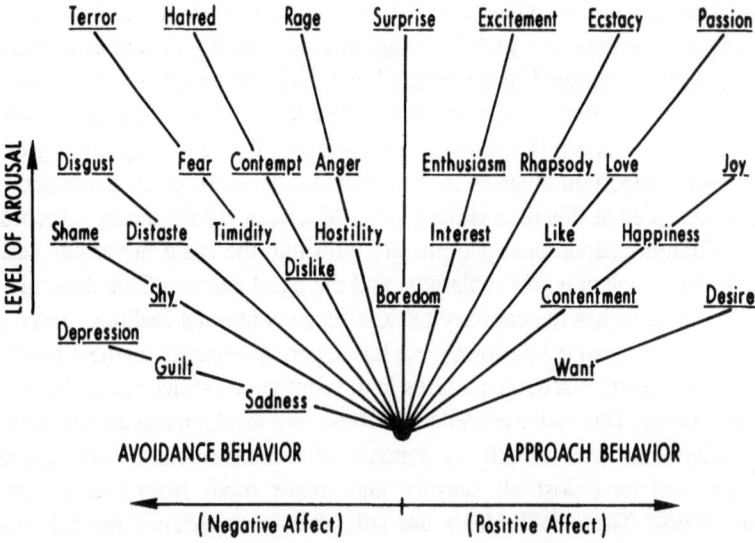

Figure 3-2 Positive and negative spectra of affective reactivities.

of social communication. For example, the aggressive stance of generalized extensor dominance is completely opposite to the stance of generalized flexor responsivity (curling itself up into a bundle) adopted in fear. These signals are abundantly clear and whatever their offensive or defensive value may be, they do prevent nature from becoming excessively ambiguous.

In man, the multifaceted behavioral patterns of affective reactions are most readily apparent in the various facial patterns of emotional expression. These were postulated by Darwin to be biologically derived and thus universal for all races of men. Recent work by Izard (1980) has effectively demonstrated that such facial patterns can already by recognized in early infancy, corroborating their essentially biological origin. Such reactivities are certainly modified by social influences but the basic response patterns do appear to be both consistent and universal. Patterns of bodily reactivities in a variety of emotion-provoking situations have given rise to studies in body language with similar implications to those for facial expressions. The essentially unconscious control of these motor reactivities by the involuntary nigrostriatal motor system rather than by the voluntary pyramidal motor system is evidenced in strokes where muscles of the face, paralyzed to voluntary motor control, will respond unconsciously in emotional situations (as in smiling or frowning).

The Subjective Analogues of Emotional Reactions

Through the interaction of various neural systems in the brain (the hypothalamic control centers, the hypophyseal–pituitary endocrine control system, the basal gangliar muscle control system, the limbic system, the RAS consciousness control system, and the neocortex), adaptive physiological reorganizations are translated into awareness as different emotional reactions. The readiness-for-flight syndrome is accompanied in humans (and we assume, in other mammals) by an awareness of palpitations, breath-lessness, and muscle tension which is designated as a feeling of fear or anxiety. The readiness-for-fight syndrome is accompanied by a different pattern of awareness where the palpitations and breathlessness are somewhat less and the muscle tensions of a different nature; this pattern is designated as a feeling of anger or rage or aggressivity. There are several important theories as to how emotional feelings are generated but the most widely accepted at this time is the Papez–MacLean (1937) theory. According to this model, efferent adaptational patterns are built into the brain in various structures involving the hypothalamus, the thalamus, and the basal ganglia. This thalamic–basal gangliar complex also has the capacity to experience emotional feelings, based in part on sensory feedback from the periphery but based perhaps equally on the direct transla-tion of the local efferent discharge patterns in the contiguous structures of the brain into sensory equivalents. The major evidence for these two mechanisms comes from quad-riplegics, individuals who usually as a result of a neck fracture have severed the cervical cord and have lost all sensory and motor input from and to the body (Hohmann, 1966). These individuals are still able to experience the full range of emotional expression, although there is evidence that sexual feelings and those of fear and rage are somewhat decreased. The Papez–MacLean theory fits most of the avail-able experimental evidence on emotional experience and constitutes the general frame of reference of this presentation.

Papez (1937) proposed the limbic system as the site of the brain in which the subjective sensations of emotional feelings were experienced and also as the control center for the efferent discharge of emotional expression. He wrote:

> It is proposed that the hypothalamus (mammillary body), the anterior thalamic nuclei,
> the gyrus cinguli (cingulate gyrus), and the hippocampus and their connections con-
> stitute a harmonious mechanism which may elaborate the functions of the central
> emotion, as well as participate in emotional expression.

The elaborations of this basic statement into a more complex formulation have already been presented in Chapter 2 and summarized in Figures 2-2 and 2-3. There the descriptions were predominantly for the "feeling" component of motivational drives; here it is for the emotions.

Thus the physiological nucleus for the manifestation of emotional feelings is centered largely in posterior hypothalamus, in the dorsal median thalamus, in the anterior thalamus, in the limbic system (particularly the cingulate gyrus), and in the neighboring basal gangliar nuclei. Lesions of this part of the thalamus in humans lead to aberrations of emotional sensation (Dejerine–Roussy syndrome) or in more extreme cases to a complete lack of emotional reactivity (akinetic mutism). The thalamic–basal gangliar complex plays a central role both in subjective emotional feelings and in the sensation of consciousness (see Chapter 6).

Hierarchical Control of Objective Emotional Behavior

As described in Chapter 2, the hierarchical organization of motivational brain functions is one of the central facts of behavioral control. This is equally true for the emotions. Every emotional impulse derives from influences at some biologically prim- itive level in the brain stem, most often the hypothalamus, and is then both elaborated cognitively as it passes upward into the centers of the neocortex and controlled by downward impulses from those same centers. These constant interactions account for the enormous complexities of mammalian behavior and apply to all aspects of behav- ior: cognitive, motor, and motivational–emotional. However, nowhere are these ac- tivities better demonstrated than in the motivational–emotional system; within that system they are best illustrated by the neural relationships in the elaboration of emo- tional reactions, particularly those of anger and rage.

The brain neurophysiology for the expression of aggressive behavior in animals has been tentatively defined. The basic attack response appears to be formulated in the more lateral hypothalamic nuclei; there is some evidence that this attack behavior is inhibited by stimuli from the most medial nuclei of the hypothalamus. Attack behavior in cats has been analyzed by Flynn et al. (1970) as falling into two categories: the first carefully structured toward killing prey and the second more in the nature of a blind undirected rage reaction. The first reaction appears to originate from the extreme lateral hypothalamus while the second involves an intermediate area of the hypoth- alamus, possibly the dorsomedial nuclei (see Fig. 3-3).

The activity of these two attack systems appears likewise to be under the direction of two higher level control systems in the limbic system, one stimulatory and the other inhibitory. For example, stimulation of the lateral aspects of the dorsomedial nuclei of the thalamus will facilitate attack behavior while stimulation of the more medial aspects of the same nuclei will inhibit such behavior. A similar duality of effects can be elicited by stimulation of the amygdala, with the anterior medial portions inhibitory and the posterolateral area facilitory (Pradhan, 1975). The septal area, on the other hand, exercises predominantly inhibitory influences on the hypothalamic rage reaction and lesions to this area result in the so-called septal rage syndrome. Both the hippo- campus and the frontal cortex exercise predominantly inhibitory influences upon the attack reaction. It has been demonstrated that the frontal cortical inhibitory influences upon hypothalamic attack behavior are mediated through pathways traveling through the lateral segment of the dorsomedial thalamic nuclei, the same area that, when stimulated, inhibits hypothalamic rage reactions.

The critical role of the amygdala in determining the balance within this hier- archical control system and thus setting the level of aggressivity is best demonstrated through the work of Rosvold, Mirsky, and Pribram (1954) in monkeys. These authors assessed aggressivity in the monkeys on two behavioral variables: aggressivity toward the human experimenters and that toward each other. The latter parameter of aggres- sion was evaluated by observing the order of social dominance in an experimental group of eight male monkeys living together in a single large enclosure. After the initial order of dominance was established, the most dominant monkey, Dave, was subjected to a bilateral amygdalectomy. Subsequent to surgery, Dave became the least dominant member of the group, each of the others moving up one notch. After bilateral amygdalectomy of the new leader, Zeke, he became subservient to all the others including Dave, the others also moving up a notch. The same surgery on the now dominant leader, Reva, unfortunately for the theory, had no significant effects. This aberration is explained by the authors as the consequence of either inadequate surgery

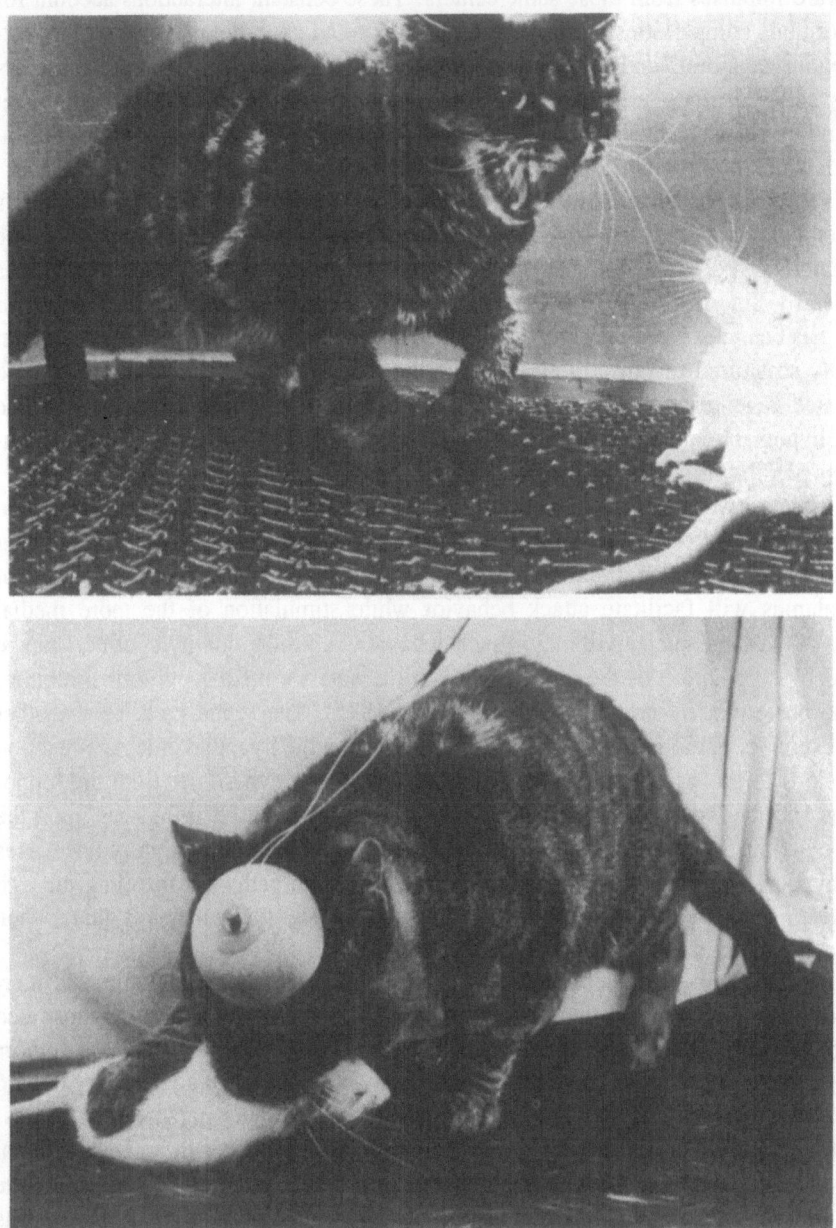

Figure 3-3 Patterns of emotional reactivities. (From Flynn, 1967. Reprinted with permission.)

or possibly as being due to the mild unthreatening manner of the new number-two monkey, Herby.

The role of the neocortex in controlling the behavioral manifestations of aggression was first elaborated in 1937 when Klüver and Bucy published their unique findings on the behavioral effects of bilateral removal of the temporal lobes in rhesus monkeys. The results were so remarkable and so revealing as to the function of the temporal lobes in the control of emotion and motivation that the resultant behavioral pattern has become known as the Klüver–Bucy syndrome. The behavioral effects may be divided into two types of responses: those involving reactions to environmental stimuli and changes in sexual and emotional behavior.

After bilateral removal of the temporal lobes, the animals developed a strong approach interest in all objects in their environment, examining closely even objects that in the past they would have avoided such as a lighted match or a hissing snake. They would test everything with their mouth and attempt to eat inedible objects. In general, it was as though they had lost all recollection of the learned emotional or motivational significance of objects. Klüver and Bucy labeled this reaction "psychic blindness." In addition to these changes, the animals became hypersexual, not only in actual performance but also in the character of the objects approached sexually. Finally, the previously fierce, aggressive animals became tame and placid.

The removal of both temporal lobes involves the removal of much of the limbic system, particularly the amygdala and the hippocampus, as well as the surrounding neocortex. As became evident after further experimentation, different elements in the Klüver–Bucy syndrome were probably the result of lesions in different anatomical areas. For example, psychic blindness is presumably due to removal of inferotemporal neocortex where cognitive stimuli are organized (see Chapter 4). The demonstrated oral behavior is probably related to the removal of the inhibitory control areas for rhythmic chewing, licking, and so forth located in the inferotemporal lobe. The docility and hypersexuality, on the other hand, are probably the result of the extirpation of the posterolateral amygdala and of the anterior cingulate gyrus, both areas that when stimulated electrically cause facilitation of the hypothalamic rage reactions.

The symptomatology displayed by monkeys in the experimentally induced Klüver–Bucy syndrome has been replicated in human patients with temporal lobe epilepsy who have undergone surgery for this condition. Temporal lobe epilepsy is associated with evidence of electrophysiological hyperexcitability stemming from foci of hyperirritability in that part of the cortex; surgical excision of the temporal lobe frequently produces amelioration of the epileptic episodes. Prior to surgery these patients show a clinical picture characteristic of overactivity of the temporal lobe while after surgery they show clinical patterns characteristic of underactivity of that lobe.

Blumer (1970) has described the clinical symptomatology associated with neural overactivity (prior to surgery) and of underactivity (postsurgical) in patients treated with temporal lobectomy for epilepsy. He found that prior to surgery, individuals with evidence of hyperirritability in one temporal lobe or the other were characterized by hyposexuality and irregular outbursts of temper and violence. After surgery and relief of epileptic symptoms, several previously hyposexual individuals became manifestly hypersexual while most subjects lost their preoperative hyperaggressive irritability. This pattern of behavioral aggressivity and hyposexuality prior to surgery in these patients and of behavioral passivity and hypersexuality after surgery has been confirmed by Walker (1973).

The frontal lobes probably represent the highest level in the hierarchical sequence of control centers in the motivational–emotional system. However, in addition to its influence in that system, the frontal lobes play a major role in cognitive, attentional, and decision-making processes, without an understanding of which the significance of their influence on motivational–emotional activity would be lost. Consequently, a fuller description of frontal lobe activity will be postponed until Chapter 9.

Behaviorally, Deets et al. (1970) found that prefrontal lobectomy in monkeys resulted in a generally lower level of aggressive behavior with occasional outbursts of socially inappropriate behavior. Kling (1976), also working with monkeys, found that bilateral ablation of the dorsolateral frontal cortex resulted in a general increase in aggressive behavior but with a general decrease in the usual concomitants of such behavior (hostility, anger, etc.). These behavioral effects are presumably produced by the removal of strong inhibitory tracts that run from the prefrontal cortex to the hypothalamus, thalamus, and other neural centers of the limbic system (see Chapter 13).

The Role of Cognition in Motivational–Emotional Behavior

There is no question that in motivational and emotional experience, one is acutely aware of emotional feelings. But emotional feelings do not exist in a vacuum, separate and distinct from all other feelings and sensations. In almost every instance an emotional reaction is a response to some cognitive event. Thus fear is usually fear of something or someone; anger is usually anger at someone; and disgust is disgust at some specific event. Even free-floating anxiety must be conceptualized as anxiety at some unrecognized threat, generated at the unconscious level. Thus there can be no emotional reaction except in a cognitive context.

There is an excellent anatomical explanation for this principle. The autonomic nervous system is the biological neural system specifically provided to implement motivational–emotional activities. Yet the autonomic systems, both sympathetic and parasympathetic, are essentially efferent in their anatomical and physiological distribution. These efferent fibers innervate all organs, endocrine glands, and various types of receptors (osmoreceptor, baroreceptors, and so on). At the opposite pole, the afferent sensory elements of motivation and emotions such as those notifying the individual of hunger, thirst, visceral pain, and so forth rise to the brain, not through afferent sensory tracts in the autonomic nervous system (there are none), but through the same afferent sensory tracts of the central nervous system utilized by the somatic body. Consequently, with few exceptions, almost all motivational–emotional and other visceral sensations are received into the regular afferent sensory tracts of the central nervous system, are encoded in the brain in similar fashion to somatic sensory experiences, and are ultimately utilized in much the same fashion.

Since it is the afferent sensory pattern of stimuli that provides information to the brain about any given behavioral modality and since that information is encoded and delivered through normal cognitive tracts, one can see why it is impossible to sepak comprehensively of motivational–emotional activity without involving the cognitive system. These implications are particularly noteworthy for the discussion in Chapter 2 on the elaboration of biological and psychosocial drives. It should be obvious that they apply equally to the elaboration of emotional reactivities. Therefore, (1) since motivational–emotional activities can be understood only in terms of their cognitive content, (2) since cognitive activities can be comprehended only as they are influenced by motivational–emotional influences, and (3) since cognitive material represents the major constituent of conscious experience, we shall apply the next two chapters to a broad exploration of cognitive function.

Perception, Learning, and Engram Formation

Perception and cognition subsume all the processes by which multiple simple, apparently unrelated sensory stimuli from the environment are categorized, analyzed, consolidated, and finally utilized in the brain in their new neural representations to permit effective behavioral responses. Perception and cognition are effectuated anatomically through a complex sensory apparatus and functionally through a genetic set of neurophysiological abilities: to abstract, to remember, to learn, and to use symbols. These anatomical and functional organizations create an innate grammar, syntax, and logic which are reflected in man as the universal abilities of language and mathematics (Chomsky, 1965).

Progressive Encoding of Sensory Stimuli

The major afferent pattern of physiological organization is that of progressive sensory encoding. It involves the sequential processing of afferent stimuli (sensory data from the internal and external milieus) as they travel successively from lower centers to progressively higher ones. The organism's ability to make appropriate responses depends on the adequate input and interpretation of information from the surrounding environment. The transduction of sensory information from raw physical stimuli into neural patterns of abstraction (engrams) is one of the most essential functions of the central nervous system.

All cognitive systems are organized structurally and functionally according to the principles of progressive encoding; these characterize all functions in which significant learning occurs. Among these organizational principles are the following (after Uttal, 1978):

1. Progressive processing or sensory encoding results behaviorally in the ability of organisms to abstract generalizations from sensed experience and to consolidate multiple perceptions of a given object or event into a single idea. The

neurological representation of that idea in the brain has been called the *en-gram*. Recent evidence suggests that progressive processing of perceptions produces the engram mainly through the microscopic structural device of convergence. This is a sequence in which multiple stimulated cells at the lowest level converge on a single cell or complex at the next higher level, which in turn, in combination with similarly stimulated cells at the same level, converge on a single cell or complex at the next higher level. In this way, the essence of an object or an event may be progressively abstracted and finally stored in either a single cell, or as is more likely, a complex of cells at the highest level of processing. Convergence results in a step-by-step sequence known as "serial processing."

2. Continuous progressive abstraction as the stimuli travel from one nuclear center to the next higher is associated with a process of consolidation. This is mediated by first functional and then organic changes at the synaptic connections that facilitate the transmission of the stimulus train. Because of the mechanism of convergence, neurons and neuronal complexes at the higher levels of progressive processing are more likely to develop the functional and organic synaptic changes characteristic of consolidation than are those at the lower levels. Thus, the engram, i.e., the neural representation of a given idea, is represented in specific constellations of stimulated neurons or neuron groups in the higher centers of progressive processing. With consolidation, engrams are transmuted into *memories*.

3. Concomitantly with convergence, there is, paradoxically, divergence in the process of engram formation. Because of the generalized nature of the neuronal syncytium in the neocortex, convergence of the engram occurs not upon a single cell at the highest levels of progressive processing but rather on multiple cells or groups of cells scattered diffusely throughout the brain. Thus, in keeping with Lashley's (1950) concept of the diffuse geography of learning, engrams of a given idea are represented redundantly throughout much of the neocortex rather than being concentrated in a specific localization. Divergence is associated with "parallel processing" of sensory stimuli as opposed to the "serial processing" characteristic of convergence.

The sequence represented by these mechanisms of sensory encoding, convergence, synaptic facilitation, and divergence, is a product of the generalized structural and physiological organization of the entire brain. Thus the brain functioning more or less as a whole is able to perform more difficult operations than would be possible if it were organized along lines of strict functional localization.

Functional Organization of Sensory Processing Systems: Serial and Parallel Processing

The mechanisms deriving from the physiological organization of the brain just described account for the initial encoding of sensory data from the external or internal environments as they impinge upon the central nervous system. The sequences of progressive encoding result in the production of a myriad of sensory memories, first as more or less unstable entities in the various receiving areas of each sensory modality and then, when the stimulus train continues, as more and more complex and stable configurations at higher functional levels of the brain. Because the level of refinement of this type of physiological organization is greatest in the visual system and because it is in that system that the greatest detail has been elucidated, it is most convenient to use visual activity as the prototypical system. Nevertheless, it must be understood that similar although not identical structural organizations exist for hearing, touch, proprioception, motivation, emotions, and for all other behavioral parameters that have cognitive dimensions.

There are two major types of pathways through which sensory stimuli are processed in the brain. The first may be called the primary classical pathways and are those described in most neuroanatomy texts. They are sequential in nature as the impulse travels upward from center to center and they produce predominantly convergent effects. The second, the parallel sensory tracts, consist of auxiliary sensory pathways that run parallel to the primary tract and to each other; they largely contribute the divergent functions of cognitive processing. Processing through the primary classical pathways is serial and hence better focused. It occurs characteristically in conscious perception and thought. Processing through the secondary parallel pathways may take several routes simultaneously. It is more diffuse and less focused than classical processing but may be more comprehensive in scope. Classical (controlled) processing is always accompanied by parallel (automatic) processing, but the latter can occur without the former. The functional relationships of these pathways will be expanded upon in Chapter 11; here it is enough to describe the differential anatomical structures of the two systems.

The two systems, the primary classical and the parallel processing, subserve different functions in visual activity. The first system provides the cognitive mechanisms for the encoding of visual information; the second provides most of the machinery for the complex mechanics of vision itself. Each of these processes comprises a separate and distinct spectrum of activities, operating on the same perceptual data in different manners and under different conditions. For example, the mechanical system that makes visual processing possible (e.g., discerning individual objects) operates almost entirely at the unconscious level; the encoding system that translates visual experience into neurological equivalents (e.g., recognizing individual objects) operates optimally at the conscious level but also, less efficiently, at the unconscious level. Mechanical visual processes are known as "procedural" or "structural" operations; encoding processes involve "episodic" events. These distinctions will be elaborated upon later.

Our major interest in this volume is with the encoding of episodic events since these are the elements that constitute life experience and hence are the more important elements of mental activity. However, recent developments in the understanding of the mechanics of vision which have evolved from studies in cognitive psychology, artificial intelligence, and computer science, are equally significant for they offer insights into the operations of at least one kind of unconscious activity. David Marr (1984) has presented an important analysis of the procedural features of the visual system that make "seeing" possible. He has described a variety of neurophysiological "modules," each of which provides a different function in the breakdown of the visual scene into object and background. For example, there are special neurophysiological mechanisms in the brain for outlining objects, special mechanisms for stereoscopic vision, and special mechanisms for discerning the textures of different surfaces. The integrated interaction of all of these mechanisms permits the identification of a given visual object and its separation from the background. Only after such procedural identification occurs can the processes of encoding significant visual information into episodic equivalents begin by the primary classical visual system.

These general principles are illustrated more specifically by a description of the functional anatomy of the visual system. In gross anatomical terms the first step in the coding of visual stimuli begins in the sensory receptor, i.e., the eye; further organization of the total mass of afferent stimuli in the visual modality continues in the brain stem and thalamus. In the brain stem, sensory stimuli also come into contact with the reward and tension systems and with the reticular activating system as a consequence of which, depending on quantitative and qualitative factors, those stimuli gain affective (positive or negative) and consciousness dimensions. From the brain stem, the stimuli advance to the thalamic nuclei where they achieve both feeling and further cognitive organization (see Fig. 2-3).

In primary classical processing, cognitive structuring continues with the arrival of the sensory stimuli in the primary cortical receiving area, e.g., area 17 for visual impulses. From the primary cortical receiving area, the impulses spread to the secondary and tertiary receiving areas where further convergent processing occurs (for vision, areas 18 and 19). From these areas, the impulses spread to the posterior associative areas in the inferotemporal and medial temporal lobes and also to the anterior associative areas in the prefrontal lobes. Finally, after further extensive processing, appropriate responsive behavior is taken through the influences of the various motor control systems in the brain. This sequence is illustrated in Figure 4-1.

In Figure 4-1, the main impulse is seen progressing sequentially from lower to successively higher centers (black lines), at first on the opposite side of the brain, later spreading to the ipsilateral side through the commissures (corpus callosum). There are also parallel ipsilateral pathways that travel directly from brain stem superior colliculus

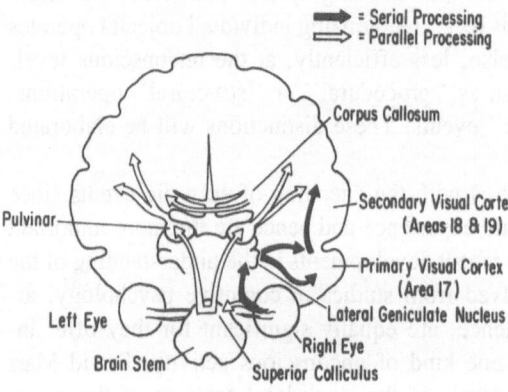

Figure 4-1 Serial and parallel processing in the visual system (left hemifield stimuli to right eye).

to secondary association cortices (Lennie, 1980). These permit parallel processing of stimuli in addition to the sequential processing of the primary system. The superior colliculus appears to be an important juncture where the two types of pathways, primary classical and secondary parallel, diverge.

Certain primitive but essential visual functions are already accomplished at these early levels. For example, the ability to visually separate an object from the surrounding environment is accomplished by two important mechanisms, one in the retina, the other in the superior colliculi. In the retina, a mechanism discovered by Kuffler (1953) provides that the stimuli from neurons at the periphery of an area illuminated by a circular light are transmitted onward at a higher intensity than are those deriving either from the darker surrounding environment or from the equally lighted inner area of illumination. This provides an outline of transmission for the illuminated circle regardless of where it falls on the retina. It also provides an outline for the object regardless of whether the image is white on black or black on white. This constitutes an unconscious procedural or structural operation which makes the object available for further abstractive episodic processing.

Another important mechanism for delineating an object from its background is stereoscopic vision, provided by integrating the images received from both eyes. The interactions through which binocular vision identifies the distance of a given object in the field as opposed to the receding background are not completely understood but are known to be initiated at the level of the superior colliculi. They are further elaborated in the columns of the visual cortex (Bishop, 1973). This is another unconscious procedural or structural operation necessary to prepare perceptual information for further episodic processing.

Abstraction in the Primary Classical Visual Pathway

The convergent functions of the primary classical pathways are carried out in a series of physiological processes at the microscopic level. Visual stimuli consist of reflected light from objects in the environment that is focused by the lens onto the retina where the spatial arrangement of the observed environmental scene is reconstituted. There are about 130 million cells in the retina that converge onto about one million ganglion cells, the axons of which form the fibers of the optic nerve. These carry the visual impulse from the eye to the brain stem (the superior colliculi) and then up to the lateral geniculate body of the thalamus whence it continues to area 17, the primary visual cortex receiving area. Convergence of retinal and thalamic fibers onto many specific cells in area 17 continues the process of encoding.

Some of the specific cellular mechanisms of progressive encoding became evident through the remarkable research studies of Hubel and Wiesel (1965) who were able to demonstrate elegantly the processes through which simple neuronal patterns of activity in the thalamus were transformed into the more complex physiological equivalents of visual experience in the cortex. Hubel and Wiesel differentiated four types of receiving neurons in the visual cortex: simple, complex, hypercomplex, and higher-order hypercomplex cells. Area 17, the first part of the visual cortex to be stimulated, contains mainly simple and complex cells. Simple cells respond to line stimuli that are relatively immobile in the field of vision. Complex cells also respond to line stimuli, mainly to those moving across the field of vision. It is clear that complex cells must receive projections from many retinal neurons that connect to ganglion cells in the retina to converge on a single optic nerve fiber. Many optic fibers must in turn converge on lateral geniculate body neurons, the axons of which converge on a single complex cell in the cortex to permit continuous firing when a line stimulus moves across the visual field.

Even more complicated patterns of visual stimuli are required to activate the so-called hypercomplex neurons of the visual cortex. Hypercomplex cells are usually found in the secondary and tertiary receiving areas of the visual cortex, areas 18 and 19 of the occipital lobe that subtend, in series, the cells in area 17. In Figure 4-2A is shown the firing rates of a hypercomplex neuron in area 19 that responds to movement of a right angle stimulus across the central portion of the visual field. In Figure 4-2B, stimuli of various angles are moved across the central visual field and those stimuli closest to a right angle evoked the highest firing rates. Thus complex reaction patterns of responses to visual stimuli are located in specific cells that fire at a significant rate only when appropriate constellations of retinal cells are stimulated in the proper spatial and temporal configuration. Through such stimulus coding, retinal images are projected onto the visual cortex in a highly complex relationship.

Still more complicated response patterns can be concentrated in the higher-order

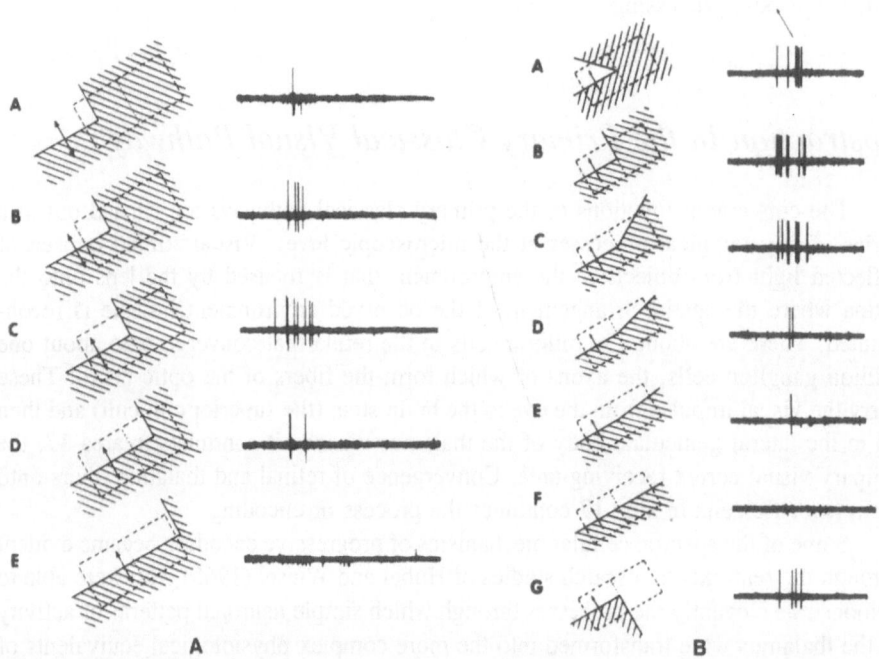

Figure 4-2 Reaction of a "right angle" hypercomplex neuron in area 19 of the visual cortex. (From Hubel and Wiesel, 1965. Reprinted with permission.)

hypercomplex neurons which are found mainly in the posterior association area and the inferotemporal lobe, the anatomical areas that subtend in series the neurons in areas 18 and 19. For example, Thompson et al. (1970) have reported neurons in the visual association cortex of the cat that appear to code number. These cells fire only on the sixth presentation of a given stimulus; the neurophysiology would appear to be the summation of six postsynaptic graded potentials before the action potential is discharged. Gross et al. (1972) reported an even more complicated neuron in the inferotemporal lobe of the monkey that fires most strongly when stimuli resembling a monkey's hand are presented (see Fig. 4-3). The presence of such presumably inherent neurological reaction patterns in monkeys lends some credibility to the reports of the ethologists of innate reactions in newborn birds to either threatening or reassuring visual patterns.

The Physiological Representation of Simple Engrams

Despite the attractive simplicity of the single neuron concept of engram formation, it appears extremely unlikely that sufficiently complicated higher-order hypercomplex cells can exist that will incorporate within their single-cell bodies the capacity to recognize and respond to the immensely complex patterns of stimuli that are constantly impinging upon the brain. On the other hand, neural circuits encompassing different types of higher-order hypercomplex cells in anatomically reinforced patterns, so-called microcircuits (Shepherd, 1978), could more readily contain the innumerable engrams capable of being stored in the brain. Recent work has established that such neural networks do exist in the brain and that they have developed both anatomical and physiological stability through the elaboration among them of dendro-dendritic connections (Rakic, 1975). Furthermore, these neural networks appear to have achieved greater physiological temporal stability through the propagation of reverberatory stimuli that circulate through these circuits for clinically significant time periods as opposed to the markedly transitory periods of single neuron activity (Hebb, 1949; Burns, 1958). Consequently, these so-called reverberatory neural circuits are now considered as a plausible physiological mechanism which offers a much greater possibility for abstracting complex engrams and for maintaining them electrophysiologically over clinically significant time periods (Uttal, 1978). Alternative descriptions of engram structure have been presented. Erickson (1984) has suggested that networks of brain neurons operating in different patterns of individual neuronal activities may provide physiologi-

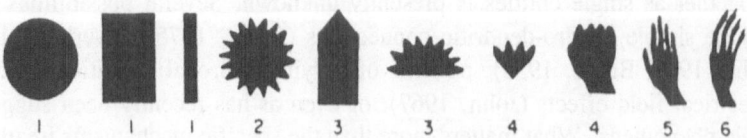

Figure 4-3 Higher-level-order hypercomplex neurons. (From Gross et al., 1972. Reprinted with permission.)

cal representation for engrams, while E. Roy John (1967) has advanced general fields of electrical activity as his candidate for engram structure. In any event, redundancy in engram storage capacity [multiple storage sites as demonstrated by Lashley (1950)] is more feasible with any one of these types of circuits among specific higher-order hypercomplex neurons than were one to postulate the simpler concept of engram storage in single neurons alone.

The convergence of simple neurons upon continually more complex ones in areas 17, 18, and 19 and so on is only one method of encoding. The cells in the visual cortex as in other sensory receiving areas are arranged in layers and in columns, permitting still other modes of encoding information. For example, impulses from the lateral geniculate body of the thalamus spread in a divergent manner onto area 17, so that a single cell in the lateral geniculate will connect to a column of cells in the various layers of the visual cortex. The cells in each layer of area 17 diverge onto a variety of more complex cells in areas 18 and 19 of differing functions, producing a three-dimensional spatial arrangement together with a multidimensional functional arrangement (Zeki, 1976; Mountcastle, 1978a). In this way, the engram is not only enriched by the multiplicity of representations, but it is also widely distributed, accounting for Lashley's inability to localize the engram in a limited area.

The other major significance of the columnar and layered structure of the visual and other sensory cortices lies in the enhanced possibilities of parallel processing. Such processing, as opposed to the more classical serial processing, already characterizes sensory pathways at the brain stem level (Fig. 4-1); however, it is even more evident at the cortical level. The divergence of a stimulus from a single geniculate cell onto a layered column of area 17 neurons and then onto a variety of functional treatments (i.e., onto different kinds of complex and hypercomplex neurons in areas 18, 19, the posterior association area, and the inferior temporal lobe) creates parallel processing of a multitude of partial engrams, constituting a remarkably enriched total engram. The existence of this type of parallel processing together with the more widespread diffusion of visual impulses activated through the superior colliculus (Fig. 4-1) underlies an entirely different form of simultaneous processing than the sequential type represented in the classical system. Parallel processing, because it is more diffuse and hence less replicable, lends itself less readily to the experiences of learning and memory to be described, but for those very same reasons permits a broader, more global type of engram processing than is possible through the primary classical sensory pathways.

The question of just how the engram is physiologically represented in the brain is one of the more important psychophysiological issues yet to be resolved. The anatomical and physiological evidence thus far presented seems to establish beyond question that engrams exist as constellations of electrical activity involving large numbers of different neurons in different parts of the brain. The nature of the forces holding the circuits together as single entities is presently unknown. Several possibilities exist. They may be simple dendro-dendritic connections (Rakic, 1975), reverberatory circuits (Hebb, 1949; Burns, 1958), patterns of varying neuronal activities (Erickson, 1984), electrical field effects (John, 1967), or even as has recently been suggested, holographic phenomena. What matters more than the specific mechanisms involved is the evidence that engrams are represented as some kind of circuits with widespread distribution in the brain. More specific evidence for this interpretation will be presented in the form of cortical evoked potentials to be described later in this chapter. Here it is enough to accept the general description.

Learning and Memory

As a consequence of the physiological sequence of progressive processing associated with consolidation of patterns of abstraction, especially in the primary classical pathways, experiences can be generalized, learned, and retained. The formation of engrams depends on repeated progressive abstraction from a series of identical or similar experiences. The retention of these engrams for future utilization in learned responses depends on their physiological and anatomical consolidation. Such consolidation, like most other nervous system functions, occurs on a continuum ranging from slight to marked. Consolidated engrams anywhere on that continuum are the physiological representation of events of which *memories* are the behavioral counterparts.

The translation of engrams into memories is a process simultaneous with the abstraction process itself. Memories are first laid down as memory traces that result from the electrophysiological facilitation among neurons through which reverberatory neuronal circuits are formed (Duncan, 1949; Kandel and Schwartz, 1982). These are then consolidated into long-term memories through the proliferation of dendritic interconnections to form anatomically stable neuronal circuits (Rosenzweig et al., 1972). Memory formation thus consists of two phases, the physiological and the anatomical, both of which should be viewed as sequential stages in a single process.

The stability of memory traces varies with the level of consolidation which in turn varies with the level of progression to the higher centers of cognition. Iconic visual memory traces occur to very brief stimuli as presented on a tachistoscope and persist for periods of significantly less than a second (200 msec). Evidence has been presented that in the brief period of duration of an iconic memory trace, the train of sensory stimuli into the cortex cannot have reached past the primary, secondary, or tertiary receiving areas where it is thought iconic memory traces are briefly retained (Averbach and Sperling, 1961). The auditory analogues of visual iconic memory traces are called echoic memory traces.

Short-term memory traces are those that last for a few seconds, like a briefly remembered telephone number. The rate of decay for short-term memory traces in humans is similar to the time course for electrophysiological recovery cycles over association areas of the cortex in humans recorded from the overlying scalp. The identity of the time course of primary memories and of recovery cycles for association cortex neurons suggests strongly that these two processes represent the behavioral and physiological equivalents of the same phenomenon. Lumsden and Wilson (1981) label these only slightly consolidated memory traces "intermediate image stores" and reserve the term short-term memory for engrams retrieved from long-term memory during cognition, a practice we shall adopt (see Fig. 5-4).

Intermediate image stores are translated into longer-lasting memories through repetition of the same stimulus. This occurs presumably through the strengthening of multiple reverberating circuits, either through mobilization of increased numbers, through facilitation of existing neural circuits, or most likely through some combination of both of these. The evidence for the electrophysiological nature of this short-lived effect comes from an experiment in rats by Duncan (1949), who using electroconvulsive shock treatment (ECS) at various intervals after learning, was able to demonstrate that such learning could be obliterated provided that ECS treatment was given early enough. Shock treatment given 20 sec after the learning experience obliterated about 80% of the memory experience. Electroconvulsive shock treatment given 40 sec after the learning experience obliterated 50% and at 15 min about 20%; after an interval of 1 hr or longer it had no effect.

The sequence of events through which the repeated stimulation of experience is translated into structural anatomical changes, although not completely understood, appears to involve a series of chemical reactions, early (Kandel and Schwartz, 1982) and late (Rosenzweig, 1972). The latter investigators first demonstrated the effects of learning on brain development, both chemically and structurally. Litter mate rats were exposed to either an enriched environment with lots of activities available or to an impoverished environment in which they were kept isolated in empty cages. After a period of such experience, both sets of rats were sacrificed and their brains examined. The rats that had the enriched experience had significantly larger and heavier brains, had higher concentrations of acetylcholinesterase per unit of brain tissue, and showed marked proliferation of glial cells. Their neurons, while no more numerous than in the "impoverished" rats, showed many more dendritic spines along the dendrites. Thus it appeared that increased exposure to learning experiences results in the development of increased memories which are the behavioral equivalents of the physiological changes going on in the brain as revealed by (1) increased number of synapses, (2) increased acetylcholinesterase levels, (3) increased glial proliferation, and (4) increased dendritic spine development (Globus et al., 1973).

The important work of Kandel and Schwartz (1982) suggests that the phenomena of learning may be accounted for more by chemical changes at the synapses involving cyclic AMP and biogenic amines than by those postulated by Rosenzweig and co-workers. In any event, such chemical changes almost certainly account for the early physiological stage of memory formation previously described. More recently, Lynch (1985) has implicated calcium ions as critical in the early stage of synaptic facilitation while Shashoua (1985) has described specific brain proteins called "ependymins" which are involved in the later organic stage of development of new synaptic connections.

The process of structural consolidation of intermediate and long-term memories apparently occurs as a sequel to electrophysiological stimulation, where such stimulation has been concentrated onto specific synapses. Consequently, it is not surprising that structural consolidation should tend to occur anatomically later in the cognitive sequence where a given sensory experience is funneled repeatedly through convergence onto a few specific synapses and not early in the sensory train where, as in the retina, almost all cells are involved in almost all perceptions. Long-term memories tend to be retained in the higher associative areas (e.g., for vision, the posterior associative area and the inferotemporal lobe) and less so in the brain stem and primary receiving areas of the cortex.

The distribution of visual memories of lesser or greater complexity in the cortex has been experimentally defined. Less specific visual memories tend to be stored in the primary receiving area (are 17), somewhat more specific memories in area 19, and most specific memories in area 21, the inferotemporal lobe. The evidence for such localization stemmed originally from the studies of Penfield and Rasmussen (1957) who electrically stimulated different parts of the brain in conscious patients undergoing brain surgery. Patients reported different types of memory depending on the site of stimulation.

Associative Learning

The development of unisensory engrams (memories) has been presented under the rubric of progressive encoding, but indeed this is merely a term for one type of "learning." Abstraction of multiple sensory experiences and their transduction into physiological engrams is the process through which external and internal events are translated into usable stimulus patterns to which the organism may meaningfully respond. Events are processed mainly in terms of the needs of the organism; experiences in all sensory modalities are brought together in patterns that are dynamically and cognitively meaningful.

The basic underlying cognitive principle that determines the formation of more complex multisensory engrams is associative learning. This apparently results from the development of neural interconnections among memories in different sensory modalities. Engrams are associated through a variety of influences which include contiguity in space or time; similarity in shape, color, or function; or conversely "oppositeness" in shape, color, or function.

Although the general mechanisms through which physiological interconnections among engrams are established can be conceptualized, the specific neural organization that determines the cognitive principles of associative learning are still speculative. Certainly, conditioning experiments show conclusively that temporal contiguity is an important factor in sucessful conditioning; such associative learning can be hypothesized to be dependent on the simultaneous interaction of activated circuits for associated engrams in short-term memory. Presumably similarity in formal characteristics (shape, color, distance, sound alikes, etc.) play the same role in establishing associative links (the developmental stage of memory) as they do in recognition (the retrieval stage, Chapter 9). Finally, the motivational and emotional charge on given percepts will determine in large part whether they will be learned or remain unlearned.

Even though the physiological mechanisms involved in associative phenomenology are unknown, they can be hypothesized. If one postulates that all hypercomplex engrams consist of an integrated aggregate of simpler constituent engrams, then two related hypercomplex engrams could be assumed to have at least one simple engram in common. Under those circumstances, excitation of either hypercomplex engram would result in at least partial stimulation of the associated hypercomplex engram through the offices of the shared simple engram. The strength of association would then vary with the number of shared simple engrams. Oden and Massaro (1978) have shown that in processing auditory information, the human brain uses "fuzzy logic" so that related phonemes are distinguished by an almost trial and error method. In a similar way, stimulation through mutually shared component simple engrams may form the basis of general associative phenomena.

The cellular mechanisms involved in associative learning are probably similar to those that characterize simple engram formation, and presumably involve two different types of processes: (1) the physiological interaction of engram circuits, first functionally and then structurally, and (2) the activation of certain specialized associative cells that serve a role in associative learning similar to that of hypercomplex neurons in engram formation. An example of specialized associative cells is shown in Figure 4-4 (Morrell, 1967). As described in the legend under the figure, this is a visual cortical cell in the associative area that responds not only to visual stimuli (L), but also to somatosensory stimuli (S), with a different spectrum of firing for each. When both stimuli are presented simultaneously (L & S), the cell shows a combined pattern of firing. After a sufficient number of paired trials, the cell will give the combined response when the visual stimulus alone (L) is presented. This is an excellent illustration of classical conditioning at the cellular level. However, such reactivities involve only about 10% of cortical cells (Morrell, 1967). Furthermore, one would have to

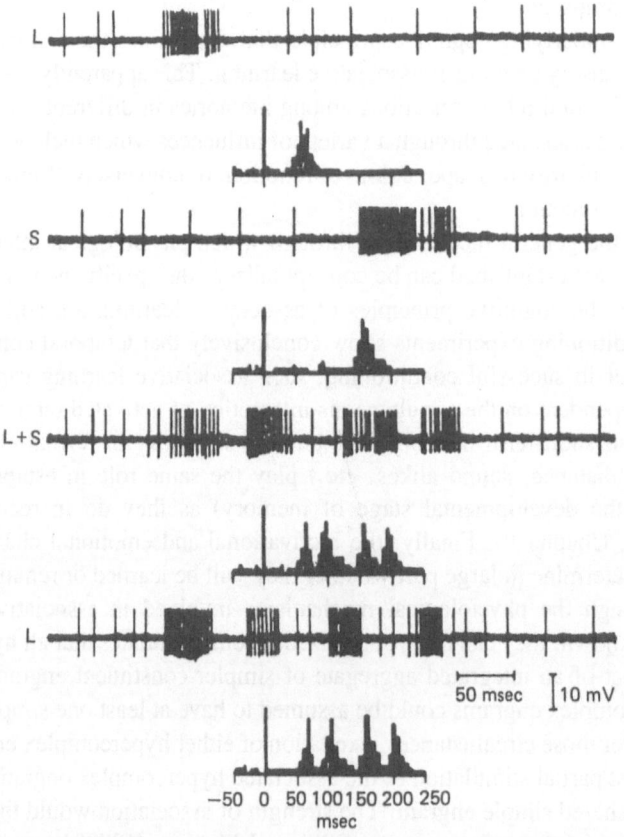

Figure 4-4 Associative neurons. L, visual stimuli; S, somatosensory stimuli. (From Morrell, 1967. Reproduced with permission.)

postulate that associative cells of this type must also include among them higher-level hypercomplex neurons to account for the association among more complex engrams. Although the evidence for associative and higher-level hypercomplex neurons is concrete and simple and thus provides the basis for a neat hypothesis for learning, that hypothesis would appear to be overly simplistic and incapable of accounting for the more complex behavioral patterns. These are more readily explained by the interacting engram circuits hypothesis.

The Posterior and Anterior Sensory Association Areas

The cortical areas that lie between the major sensory receiving and processing centers of the brain provide the largest virgin territory for multisensory association to be established and ultimately consolidated. Most important of these is the so-called posterior association area that subtends the contiguous visual cortex (areas 17, 18, and 19 in the occipital lobe), the auditory cortex (areas 22 and 23 in the temporal lobe), and the somatosensory cortex (areas 1, 2, and 3 in the parietal lobe). Two characteristics enable the posterior association area to hold within itself the major initial associational connections among these three sensory modalities. First, there is its geographic anatomical location, central and equidistant to the processing area for these sensory modalities. Second, there is the fact that at birth the association area is almost virginally clear of any innate synaptic connections. With experience and with the exposure to widespread engram formation encroaching simultaneously from the three contiguous sensory processing areas, there is essentially no limit to the number of complex multidimensional engrams that may be formed.

Accordingly, the posterior association area may be considered as the major reservoir of complex cognitive engrams in the brain. In no way is this meant to imply that all of those engrams are contained within that area. That is certainly not true. Rather, to be found here are the focal connections that tie together the unisensory engrams that exist predominantly in their own sensory processing areas. Nevertheless, because of the multiplicity and variety of engrams possible, the posterior association area must be considered the repository of the activation nodes for much of the cognitive information in the brain.

The anterior association area serves a function similar to that of the posterior but modified somewhat because of the nature of the processing areas it subtends. These are again the auditory and somatosensory but include also the cortical center for voluntary pyramidal motor function in the precentral frontal lobe. The nature of cognitive function in the anterior association area is less well understood both because of its connections to the motor cortex and also because of its connection to the prefrontal area. Some recent work has suggested that cognitive material from the posterior association area is funneled through the anterior association area where cognitive information is both tied into motor activity and more importantly fed into the prefrontal lobe for major integrative involvement.

More recently, another portion of the brain, the so-called entorhinal cortex, has been identified as still a higher level of cognitive consolidation (Van Hoesen, 1982).

Evidence has been cited that cognitive information from both the posterior and anterior association areas converge on the entorhinal cortex, together with motivational–emotional material from the inferior temporal lobe. Since the entorhinal cortex surrounds the hippocampus, its input into limbic system activities, particularly attention, is highly significant (see Chapters 8 and 9).

The Various Types of Engrams

The passage of stimuli through successively more sophisticated levels of abstraction and the development of multiple associations among related engrams results in the formation of new types of mental constructs. Through the processes of convergence, divergence, and learning, more complex cerebral engrams are developed which reconstitute in a neural transformation, the external and internal environments. Reality is then represented in the brain in at least three neural modes: the original, the abstraction, and the symbol. Premack (1975) has described three types of elements used in communication that essentially represent the types of engrams that constitute cognitive function; he has labeled them the veridical, the abstract,* and the symbolic. Veridical engrams consist of the primary sensory data involved in direct perception. Abstract engrams are formalized abstractions that come to represent the conceptualization of simplified versions of veridical engrams, as in line drawings of a face, a dog, or a house. Symbolic engrams are more complex entities that encompass an entire class of objects, actions, or ideas and are represented by such artificial symbols as words or flags.

Veridical engrams presumably constitute the memories residing in the consolidated higher-order hypercomplex cells and reverberatory circuits of the associative areas of a given sensory modality. They may encompass even more complex images involving several sensory modalities, possibly in the association areas connecting those sensory modalities (for example, area 39 between visual and auditory cortices, area 9 between visual and somatosensory cortices, and area 40 between auditory and somatosensory cortices). In general, imagery (i.e., the evocation of veridical engrams) is most often unimodal; multimodal images, although less common, are not impossible.

The physiological configurations and anatomical sites of the next higher level of abstraction resulting in concepts or so-called abstract engrams, are more difficult to even speculate on. The concept of a "dog" presumably ties together in a huge network all the veridical engrams relating to "dogness" (visual, auditory, somatosensory, emotional, etc.) that the individual has ever experienced (McGaugh, 1968). Furthermore, the entire constellation of consolidated memories, not only in their separate sensory configurations but in the total associative network, must be able to be reactivated by stimulus inputs through any one of the sensory channels—visual, auditory, somatosensory, smell, and so forth. From a physiological point of view, one must conceptualize multiple immense reverberatory circuits encompassing essentially all of

---

*Premack uses the word "iconic" here. I have substituted the term "abstract" to avoid confusion with the more common use of iconic as connoting extremely brief visual memory traces.

the brain to represent the abstract engrams of any concept. This phenomenon must exist in the absence of language because it is clear that both animals and prelanguage human infants are fully capable of developing and reacting to abstract engrams.

Evoked Potentials as Indices of Brain Activities

The evidence for some such widespread configuration of brain activity as the necessary underlying mechanism for the existence of concepts (abstract engrams) comes mainly from evoked potential data. The evoked potential is an electrophysiological technique illustrated in Figure 4-5 (after Hillyard and Woods, 1979) for exploring brain activity. It involves tracing the course of a sensory stimulus (visual, auditory, somatosensory) from the time it enters the brain stem until that time when it has been fully processed in the cortex. Through sophisticated techniques, the electrophysiological response to a series of sensory stimuli is recorded at electrodes on the scalp, resulting in a record of the wave train; each wave component represents the responsivity of a given nerve center in the course of transit of those stimuli. In Figure 4-5 (top portion) is outlined a typical wave response to a series of auditory clicks. The time dimension is represented logarithmically with the first panel constituting the first 10 msec, the second panel 10–100 msec, and the third panel 100–1000 msec. The waves in the first panel, numbered in Roman numerals, represent transit of the stimuli through various neural centers in the brain stem; those in the second panel, transit in the thalamic radiations to the cortex; those in the third panel, processing in the cortex. It is this last segment that is of immediate interest here. The N_1 wave (also known as N_{100} since it occurs at about 100 msec) signifies arrival of the stimulus in the primary receiving area of the auditory cortex. P_2 is thought to indicate processing in the posterior associative cortex while N_2 perhaps represents processing in the frontal associative cortices. P_3 (also known as P_{300} because it occurs at about 300 msec) has a special significance since it represents integration of the cognitive process with motivational–emotional influences, a phenomenon to be described in detail in Chapter 8. It is thought to derive from the amygdaloid–hippocampal complex. The bottom portion of Figure 4-5 correlates behavioral and physiological functions with corresponding anatomical centers reached in the course of stimulus processing as indicated in the evoked potential.

Studies with the evoked potential technique have contributed greatly to our understanding of the functional physiology of the brain and will be alluded to at some length in later chapters. Here it is sufficient to note that the overall shape of the evoked potential is a function of the relative activities of different centers in the brain, as a consequence of which different configurations of electrical activity in the brain produce differently shaped evoked potentials (John et al., 1967).

Returning to the question of the neurophysiological representation of concepts or abstract engrams in the brain, the previous analysis based on general physiological considerations would have predicted that such engrams should occupy more or less the entire brain in a network or multiple consolidated reverberatory circuits. Evoked potential data in both animals and humans tend to support the general thesis of abstract

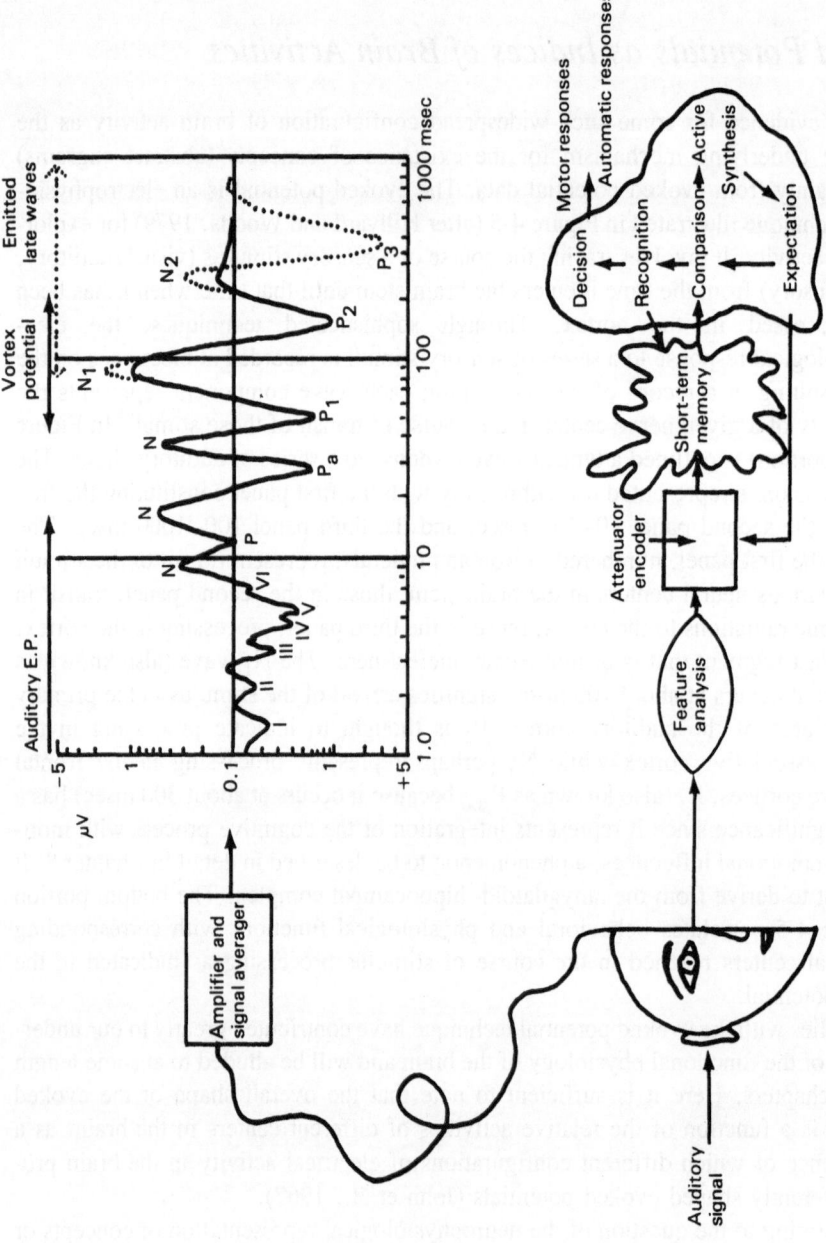

Figure 4-5 Auditory EPs and correlated neurophysiological events. (From Hillyard and Woods, 1979. Reprinted with permission.)

engrams as being associated with generalized electrophysiological configurations in the brain. John et al. (1973) have presented evidence that concepts are expressed neurophysiologically through the activity of electrical fields. John trained cats to respond to visual stimuli of two different frequencies (colors) with different behaviors. He studied the brain evoked potentials that were associated with the two frequencies and found them to differ in shape. He then compared the evoked potentials under conditions where the animal responded correctly and where the animal responded incorrectly, i.e., confused the two signals. If the evoked potentials to a stimulus of a given frequency always remained the same whether the animal responded correctly or incorrectly, it would indicate that evoked potentials reflected only extraneous input. However, John found that the shape of the evoked potentials during errors were those of the opposite wavelength so that the animal was responding not to the actual light flashes but to its conception of what the light flashes were. Hence, John concluded that the engrams existed in the animals' brain as specific electrical patterns independent of the actual visual stimulation.*

John concludes from data such as these that the essential element in the elaboration of concepts is the electrical field itself rather than any underlying neuronal configuration established through learning. To me, such an interpretation appears to introduce an unnecessary complication since the multiple engram circuit theory provides for similar electrical fields anchored in specific neuronal circuits rather than in nonspecific neuronal masses (see p. 52).

Another example of the eliciting of different abstract engrams with the same external stimulus is offered in the experiment of Teyler and co-workers (1973) as illustrated in Figure 4-6. The same verbal stimulus "rock" produced different auditory evoked potentials when presented as a noun ("a rock") or as a verb ("to rock"). Apparently, a single symbolic engram (a word) was associated with two different abstract engrams which in turn might be associated with entirely different motivational–adaptive and motor engrams. Depending upon the prevailing "set" or "meaning," different sequences of interconnecting engram circuits were activated, resulting in correspondingly different forms in the evoked cortical potential. Consequently, the Teyler et al. (1973) experiment strongly suggests that even with the presentation of the same word, different abstract and probably veridical engrams with which it is associated may be evoked.

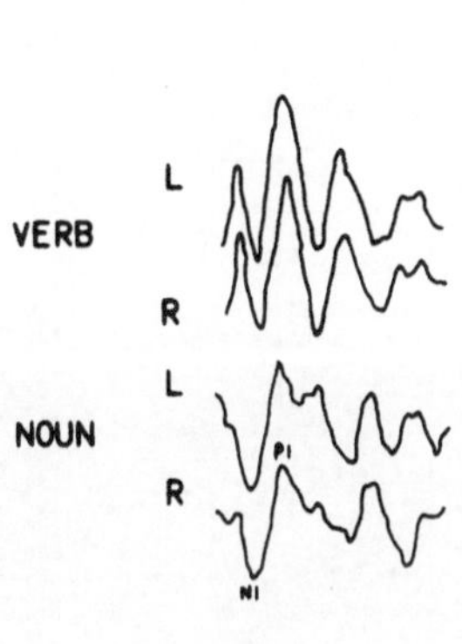

Figure 4-6 Evoked potential to same word with different meaning. (From Teyler et al., 1973. Reproduced with permission.)

---

*See discussion on mental set in Chapter 9.

The perceptual and cognitive mechanisms described in this chapter, complex as they may seem, represent only the simplest elements in the dynamics of cognition. In the next chapter will be described some of the mechanisms through which apparently disconnected engrams can be tied together in a meaningful flow of rational thinking.

Language and the Higher Cognitive Processes

The dual processes of abstraction and of association described in the last chapter result in an immense number of engrams represented anatomically throughout the brain. Whether these engrams exist as reverberatory circuits (Hebb, 1949), as specific patterns of neurons differentially activated (Erickson, 1984), as diffuse field effects (John et al., 1973), or indeed in still some other physiological structure, is not critical to our considerations at this point. What seems true almost beyond question is that engrams, regardless of their nature, must have a diffuse representation ultimately incorporating all of the neocortex.

The picture then is one of an immense number of engrams, either veridical or abstract in character, anatomically and physiologically diffused throughout the cortex. Connections between engrams are associational in nature based psychologically on such connecting links as similarity in meaning and spatial or temporal contiguity, and physiologically based on shared neuronal circuits among constituent components of the larger associated engrams. But such interactions, although sufficient for thought processing and even behavior, are insufficient for communication; consequently, for human speech some shorthand and symbolic representation of these diffusely represented engrams becomes essential. That symbolic representation is of course language.

Language represents the highest form of symbolization in which an engram for an arbitrarily selected word has come to represent the entire constellation of abstract engrams associated with the concept underlying that word. Word engrams are uniquely symbolic not only in their unrelatedness in form and content to the engrams with which they are associated, but also in the high level of abstraction which they represent. The written or spoken word "dog" describes in a way no original perceptual engram could replicate the total class of dogs. Since language is the ultimate instrument of communication, it is important to explore in what form the engrams represented by words exist and are utilized.

The Anatomy of Language

In about 95% of individuals, the anatomical locus of language lies in the left cortex in two major areas, one motor (Broca's area), the other auditory (Wernicke's area). These areas and the tract connecting them, the arcuate fasciculus, are illustrated in Figure 5-1. Destruction of Broca's area by strokes, tumors, and so forth produces a so-called motor aphasia in which the individual understands language but is unable to speak. Destruction of Wernicke's area, on the other hand, produces a complete loss of understanding of spoken language as well as difficulty in verbalization. The angular gyrus connects the visual association areas with Wernicke's area; lesions here have no effect on speech but produce impaired reading and writing abilities, so-called alexia. Finally, lesions of the arcuate fasciculus permit comprehension of language (since Wernicke's area is intact) and speech (since Broca's area is intact) but speech is incoherent and disconnected because of the isolated activity of the two important language areas.

Neurophysiologically, it would appear that the semantic connections between the spoken word and its related abstract engrams are made both in Broca's and in Wernicke's area while those between the written word and its related abstract engrams are made in the angular gyrus. It is interesting to explore the putative form and anatomical placement of the engrams representing words as well as the type of connections between word engrams and the abstract engrammatic complexes of the concepts represented by them. On the first issue, it would seem that word engrams themselves would be relatively simple in form since the symbols themselves are relatively simple. The spoken word would presumably involve simple neuronal activity in the auditory (sensory) and motor (speech) areas while the written word would involve similar neuronal

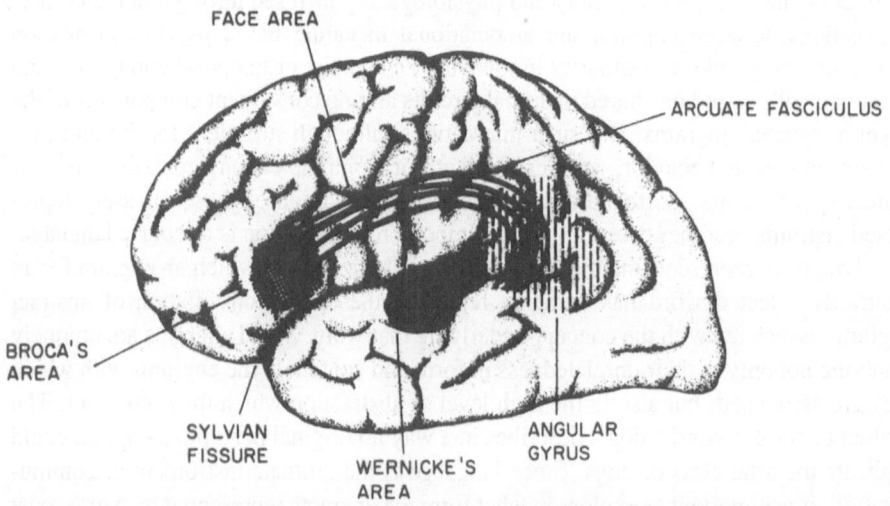

Figure 5-1 Important language areas in the brain. (From Thompson, 1975. Reprinted with permission.)

configurations in the visual (reading) and motor (writing) area. The total word engram then would consist mainly of these four elements.

However, there must be a certain amount of ambiguity as illustrated in the Teyler et al. (1973) study where the single word "rock" elicited different evoked potentials when presented in different contexts (Fig. 4-6). Such ambiguity could stem from two different types of developmental mechanisms: (1) ambiguity of a particular word engram as the result of its usage in different cognitive situations (e.g., rock) and (2) ambiguity due to a multiplicity of connections of a specific word engram to subcomponents of a multiplicity of associated word engrams. It is little wonder then that meaning in language can be so ambiguous. The number of engrams represented by a single word can be quite substantial as can also be the variety of meanings that a given word might have in different situations and to different people.

Thus there is both redundancy in representation and substantial variation in the anatomical placement of different elements of word engrams. There is, in addition, a wide distribution of associations of word engrams with different areas of the brain encompassing different underlying abstract engrams. The question is whether word engrams are as physiologically diffuse and widely represented in the brain as are the abstract engrams they represent. The evidence appears to suggest that they are not. This interpretation stems from two sets of clinical experience associated with vascular damage to the brain.

In the first place, strokes hitting specific localized areas of the language complex in the brain (Fig. 5-1), produce, as previously described, very specific language deficits. This does not necessarily mean that the word engrams of the particular type affected lie specifically in the damaged area; however, the probability is that some particular anatomical component of the word engram affected may lie there. As with other lesion experiments, it may also be that some connecting tract between the word engram and the abstract engram represented by it is affected rather than any word engram population itself. In either event, the specificity of language deficits associated

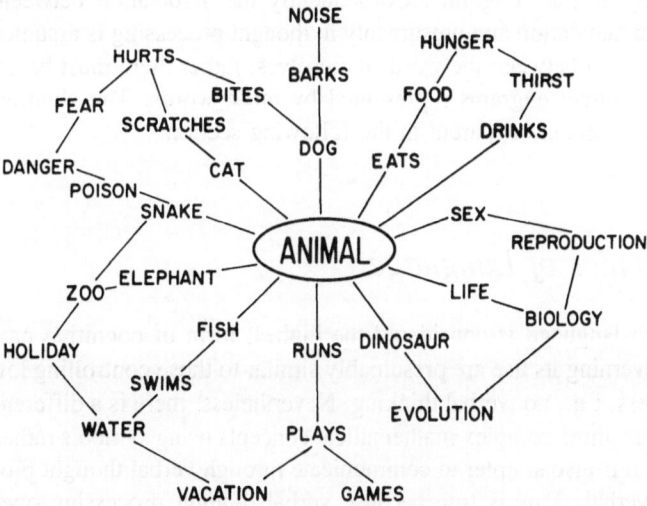

Figure 5-2 The association network.

with strokes of different parts of the language system does speak for a concentration of the connecting tracts leading from the various abstract engrams to word engrams located in the area of the language centers.

Equally pertinent to the question of the anatomical and physiological characteristics of word engrams is the consideration of another type of vascular lesion, the diffuse involvement of the brain produced by innumerable very small vascular infarcts. This process, often mislabeled as senile arteriosclerosis of the brain, is a not uncommon finding in older people and is associated with the general forgetfulness characteristic of certain senile dementias. It is interesting to note the order of things in which older people with this condition tend to have difficulty in remembering. The first class of thoughts that tend to cause difficulty are proper names; the second class are words; the last to go are memories of events. Since the anatomical defect here is a diffuse one, it seems reasonable to speculate that names are represented in the most concentrated and least redundant form (name engrams), words in a somewhat less concentrated and more redundant forms (word engrams), and events (essentially abstract engrams), in the least concentrated, most diffuse, and most redundant form.

This conclusion seems somewhat at odds with the interpretation of the Teyler et al. (1973) experiment (Fig. 4-6) where the word "rock" elicited a general widespread evoked response seemingly from the entire brain. But on further consideration there is no contradiction. There the word engram, wherever it might be located, was assumed to be connected to its corresponding abstract engrams which were presumed to occupy the entire brain. If there had been a lesion in Wernicke's area, the word "rock" would probably not have elicited either one of the corresponding evoked potentials, either because a significant component of the word engram was itself destroyed or because some critical connection to the language system had been destroyed.

The Teyler et al. (1973) experiment does, however, illuminate another characteristic of language; that is the relationship of word engrams to their corresponding abstract engrams both in communication and in thought. It appears from that experiment that the expression of word engrams is always associated with the stimulation of the underlying abstract engrams. Consequently the association between words that occurs in communication and presumably in thought processing is assumed to be more than a relationship between the words themselves; rather there must be an association between the abstract engrams represented by those words. The significance of this conclusion will become apparent in the following section.

The Dynamics of Language

Although language is considered the highest form of cognitive processing, the principles governing its use are presumably similar to those controlling lower forms of thought process, i.e., nonverbal thinking. Nevertheless, there is a difference. Just as it is simpler to examine complex mathematical concepts using symbols rather than verbal descriptions, it is also simpler to communicate through verbal thought processing than through nonverbal. This is true because verbal thought processing operates at two levels: at the word level, but additionally at the level associated with processing of the associated abstract engrams, the same engrams as those involved in nonverbal thinking. Consequently, verbal and nonverbal thought processing are identical except that the first is implemented at two levels, the symbolic and the abstract, while the second operates only at the abstract.

Most important is the conclusion that language, despite its symbolic structure, is processed not only through words but also through abstract engrams. That this is true is particularly evident in the phenomenology of association. The association network of a given word "animal," as illustrated in Figure 5-2, covers a vast range of direct and indirect connections. However, in the example shown, none of these connections are to the word engram itself, i.e., "animal," but all rather are to abstract engrams related to that word. Direct associations among word engrams themselves would depend on similarities in the structures of the words themselves as, for example, between the words "dog" and "bog" or between the words "cat" and "bat." But such associations seem remote and infrequent as opposed to the more semantic relationships expressed and illustrated in Figure 5-2.

In addition to translating abstract engrams into symbols that, like mathematical symbols, are both parsimonious and easily manipulated, language has another important characteristic, the inherent logical syntax and grammar that appear universally in all human speech. Chomsky (1965) has defined this inherent characteristic of language in his "generative and transformational linguistics" as a function that derives from the anatomical and physiological organization of the brain. Lennenberg (1967) and Uttal (1978) have further ascribed this quality as deriving from the microscopic neural organization of the brain. In their systems, the process of abstraction and engram formation contains within itself an internal logic that is as implicit as the process of abstraction itself. Whereas the neurophysiology of abstraction is readily traced to the structural organization conferred by convergence, that of linguistic grammar is somewhat more obscure.

The best evidence to support Uttal's and Lennenberg's position that linguistic grammar is, like abstraction, a function of the microscopic organization of the brain, comes from studies in different types of aphasia. In general, a more complete breakdown in grammatical logic occurs in diffuse functional or organic disruptions of the brain as in schizophrenia or senile dementia than it does in the more severe but highly localized destruction of the speech centers, as with strokes or tumors. This evidence suggests that the physiological function underlying grammatical logic is similar to that in learning (diffusely structured) rather than to speech (highly localized in the brain).

Perhaps the most profitable strategy toward understanding the biological basis of grammar is to assume that it springs from the same kinds of anatomical and physiological structures and functions that underlie abstraction. Indeed, since that type of microscopic anatomy and its physiological operations are characteristic of concept formation, it seems at least reasonable to speculate that the organization of grammar is itself a function of the abstraction process, but one step further along. To pursue this line of reasoning, it is necessary to examine the structure of language. Since symbolic language is the last step in the abstraction process, then somehow the logic of grammar should lie in that same process.

The Structure of Language

The science of language structure and production is known as linguistics and is subdivided into three major sections: phonetics, semantics, and syntactics. *Phonetics* deals with the mechanisms of speech production, specifically of the sounds used in auditory communication, the level at which speech presumably originated. *Semantics* deals with the meaning of words. It is the study of the mechanisms through which symbolic words, either spoken or written have come to represent the abstract engrammatic constructs in the brain. The neurophysiological foundations of semantics are presumably those involved in the formation of the three forms of engram, the veridical, the abstract, and the symbolic. *Syntactics* is the study of the interactions of various types of words—nouns, adjectives, and verbs—in sequences that meaningfully transmit information. Its linguistic expression is in syntax or grammar in which words connoting different categories of acting or being are woven together in meaningful sentences to communicate more complex pieces of information. For example, using an analogy from mathematics, in the equation $E = mc^2$, semantics would define the meaning of each symbol while syntactics would describe the specific relationships among them.

Hayakawa (1941), in a concept called the "abstraction ladder," has illustrated how, by means of the neurophysiological processes of abstraction described in these chapters, experiences are translated into words which in turn are abstracted into other words of more and more general meaning. In Figure 5-3, the "process" level of activity (equivalent to the process of veridical engram formation) leads to the "object" level (abstract engrams) which in turn leads to "word" level (symbolic engrams), in this example the words for each of several lower level concepts. The abstraction of the general category of "sex" is portrayed in this formulation as a linguistic one, i.e., carried out through the office of words. However, it is more likely that neurophysiologically, abstractions of this kind occur even in the absence of language so that the one-year-old probably accomplishes refinements of this type at the level of abstract engrams. On the other hand, higher levels of abstraction are more apt to be achieved through the direct manipulation of words, i.e., symbols as illustrated in the abstraction ladder (Fig. 5-3). More importantly, the future direction on the abstraction ladder (as conceptualized by Korzybski) to either "humanity" or "biology" is apparently accomplished largely through the direct usage of words and symbols and only indirectly through the utilization of abstract engrams. Perhaps that is why our conceptualizations of highly abstract ideas are so often vague and undefined because they derive from other word engrams and not directly from the simpler abstract engrams that underlie them.

It is at the highest levels of abstraction that words appear to escape from their close association with the abstract engrams underlying them and begin to assume a life of their own. At the middle level of abstraction even a vague word like "biology" can be tied into lower concepts such as "sex" and then to "boy and girl." At the highest levels of abstraction, words like "justice" and "morality" can be defined only in terms of paradigms not readily reduced to simple engrams. Such paradigms are more readily expressed in other words. It is in these cases, where words can be defined only

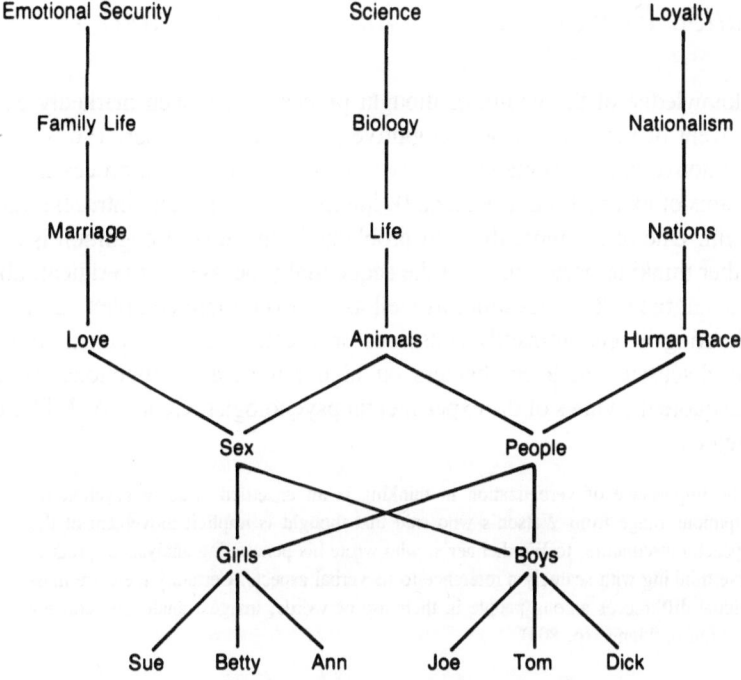

Figure 5-3 An abstraction ladder.

in terms of complex concepts and not in terms of simple images, that language adds not only extra complexity but also extra ambiguity to cognitive reasoning.

The functions of syntactics (syntax, grammar, logic), although more complex than those of semantics, presumably derive from the same underlying neurophysiological mechanisms. The meaning implicit in a word of given function, let us say a transitive verb, involves subsidiary meanings: for example, the transitive verb "to hit" implies an action "hitting," a subject "the bat," and an object "the ball." Thus, syntactically, if the words "hit," "the bat," and "the ball" must be joined in a sentence, the semantics of each word indicate that "the bat hit the ball" is a more meaningful sentence than alternatively "the ball hit the bat." Both sentences, however, are more meaningful than "hit the ball the bat." The concept of syntactical relationship as deriving from semantic abstractions is central to the neurophysiological construction of language.

These relationships are somewhat more difficult to comprehend in an uninflected language like English where word position in a sentence to a large degree defines the role of a word—subject, transitive verb, object. In highly inflected languages such as Latin and Russian where word endings completely designate the grammatical status of each word, the relationship between semantics and syntactics is much clearer.

Information Processing and Thinking (Cognition)

Our knowledge of the nature of thought processes has been markedly extended with the advent of the new science, cognitive psychology (Neisser, 1967). Thinking (verbal and nonverbal) presumably involves the logical sequential processing of cognitive engrams of external (environmental), internal (visceral), and intracerebral (ideational) origin. One of the more difficult problems in the area of cognition is to determine whether thinking occurs through the sequential processing of veridical, abstract, or symbolic engrams. This question, as well as the even more complex question as to whether thinking is predominantly conscious or unconscious, will constitute a major part of the discussion in later chapters on higher integrative functions. Here it is pertinent to quote the views of the experimental psychologist, George A. Miller (1951) on this subject:

> The importance of verbalization in thinking is an unsettled issue in psychology. Opinions range from Watson's who said that thought is implicit movement of the speech musculature, to Wertheimer's, who wrote his penetrating analysis of productive thinking with scarcely a reference to its verbal aspects. Certainly there are individual differences among people in their use of words, images, analogies, etc. for solving problems. (p. 804)

The implication of this statement, which more or less summarized the experimental work up to that time and remains equally valid now, is that thinking probably involves all three types of engrams in different combinations in different people, and probably in different combinations at different times in the same person. For example, Piaget has concluded that thinking begins in infants as veridical imagery and progresses to abstractions in early childhood. On the other hand, there is evidence that dreaming in adults occurs in the form of visual imagery of essentially primary veridical engrams, a throwback to a more primitive process. Although the participation of the various types of engrams—veridical, abstract, and symbolic—in thought processes presumably varies with the circumstances—more veridical and abstract in infancy, dreams and fantasizing—it appears that in adult human conscious thought, most activity is carried out through the systematic utilization of verbal, i.e., symbolic engrams. Stated in simpler terms, this means that most mature human communication both with oneself (thinking) and with others is carried out through the medium of language, albeit based always on the underlying abstract engrams.

The process of cognition may be viewed as a continuum beginning with the perception of external stimuli (iconic images), progressing to the development of short-term and then long-term memories, becoming more complex with the elaboration of abstract and symbolic engrams, and culminating in thought processes based on language with its underlying abstract engrams. The mechanics of these processes have only recently begun to be understood, largely through the contributions of cognitive psychologists and of researchers in computer models of "artificial intelligence." Lumsden and Wilson (1981) review the present conceptualization of the mechanics of conscious perceptual–cognitive activity; their summary view of the mechanisms involved is presented in diagrammatic form in Figure 5-4.

The Lumsden–Wilson model of human information processing summarizes many

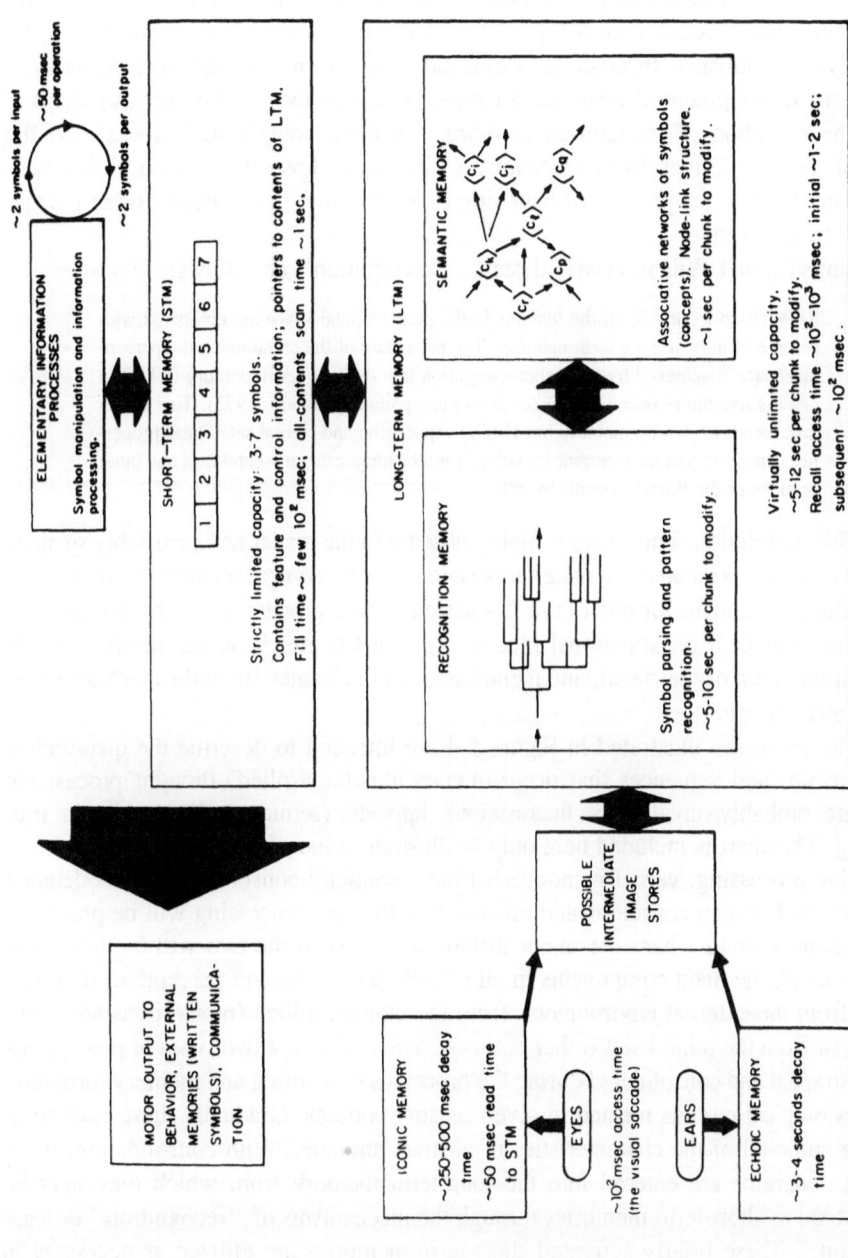

Figure 5-4 Human information processing. (From Lumsden and Wilson, 1981. Reprinted with permission.)

of the cognitive mechanisms described in this and the previous chapter. Iconic memory and intermediate image stores refer, respectively, to what we previously labeled iconic memory traces and short-term memory traces. Long-term memory stores are governed by two major operational modes, that controlling "semantic memory" and that controlling "recognition memory." Semantic memory functions largely through associational networks as illustrated in Figure 5-2. These associational connections are presumably accomplished through physiological mechanisms similar to those utilized during the development of associative pathways as described in the previous chapter.

The operation of recognition memory is a more complicated process. At the cortical level it derives from mechanisms similar to those that define abstraction. However, because the process of matching is active rather than passive, other mechanisms are involved.

Lumsden and Wilson (1981) describe "recognition" as follows:

> Recognition begins when the features in the preperceptual space are compared with perceptual units in long term memory. The placement of the stimulus on the perceptual space is achieved by its further integration into the long term memory (LTM), a process sometimes designated as secondary recognition (Massaro, 1975). This step is influenced not just by memory but also by expectation and mental set. These properties depend in part on reentrant signaling from the hippocampal–septal axis and other portions of the limbic system. (p. 60)

This description, I am sure, is highly obscure to the reader and justifiably so since we have not yet presented the material necessary for its comprehension. Nevertheless, it provides a roadmap for our future discussion. These processes will be described in detail in Chapter 8 on attentional mechanisms, in Chapter 9 on the mechanisms of recognition, memory retrieval, and mental set, and in Chapter 10 on the mechanisms of conscious cognition.

The processes illustrated in Figure 5-4 are intended to describe the quantitative relationships and sequences that occur in conscious (controlled) thought processing; they are probably invalid for unconscious episodic (semicontrolled) thought processing. The chart is included here only to illustrate some of the general principles of cognitive processing: verbal or nonverbal but essentially conscious. A more detailed comparison between conscious and unconscious thought processing will be presented in Chapters 9 to 12 where the major differences between the two will be described.

In brief, the main components in all thought processing are perceptions that may come from the external environment, from the internal milieu (motivations and emotions), or from the mind itself (other brain engrams). The first two types of perceptions are abstracted and consolidated during the processes of learning and memory formation in physiological circuits located in given sensory cortices. Gradually these configurations assume all of the characteristics of abstract engrams. With consolidation, these abstract engrams are entered into the long-term memory from which they may be reactivated as short-term memories through the mechanisms of "recognition" or "association." These briefly activated short-term memories are utilized as necessary in conscious processing and are then returned to long-term memory. The major cognitive principles influencing the flow of short-term memories are semantic (associational) and logical (syntactic). These latter dynamics, although established conceptually in linguistic studies, apply both in verbal and nonverbal thought processing since they derive essentially from the nature of the development and interaction of abstract engrams.

This description of the more complex operations of cognition is obviously incomplete and inadequate, as the Lumsden–Wilson model of conscious cognitive processing (Fig. 5-4) suggests only too strongly. However, these descriptions do serve to summarize the dynamics of cognitive process as they have been developed thus far in this volume. The reference in the Lumsden–Wilson Figure 5-4 to certain quantitative values (the unlimited capacity of long-term memory, the strictly limited capacity of short-term memory, the 50 msec period per operation for elementary information processing) obviously all need explanation. So also do the references in their excerpt to "preperceptual space," "expectation and mental set," and "re-entrant signaling from the hippocampal–septal axis." Greatest of all is the need for a definition of consciousness, since the operations described in Figure 5-4 are all assumed to be taking place at the conscious level.

These issues constitute the subject matter of Chapters 6 to 12 in the next section on "Mechanisms of Conscious and Unconscious Thought Processing." However, before leaving the area of cognition it is important to say something again about the relationship of motivational–emotional influences to cognitive process.

Association of Cognitive and Motivational–Emotional Influences

The description of strictly motivational–emotional mechanisms in Chapters 2 and 3 and of strictly cognitive mechanisms in Chapters 4 and 5 may have created the false impression that processes in these two systems occur independently and are ultimately associated only in some loose manner. It cannot be stressed too emphatically that that notion is completely erroneous. Such misconceptions arise from overly narrow approaches that concentrate on one behavioral system or another at the cost of excluding the total organism. Physiological psychology, for the sake of more accurate scientific analysis, tends to study each system independently of one another. Similarly, behavioral psychology prefers a simplified S → R paradigm where a given stimulus (S) results in a given response (R). A brief review of the mechanisms involved in learning quickly reveals the inadequacy of these two approaches.

Piaget (1978), in his work with cognitive development in children, early recognized that it was not the stimulus that led to a response in the classical behavioristic S → R formula but rather that stimulus as processed by the cognitive apparatus of the individual. Furthermore, Piaget and many other researchers in learning quickly recognized that cognitive processing was markedly influenced by motivational–emotional effects, both in perception and during subsequent abstractions and association. Finally, the type of response evoked by a given processed stimulus (PS) certainly depended greatly on motivational–emotional (ME) influences. Hence the paradigm of learning offered by Piaget and others looked more like the equation in Figure 5-5 than like the classical S → R:

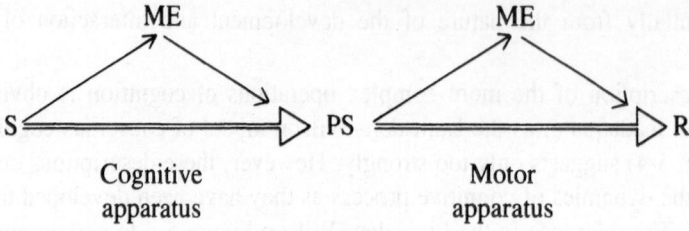

Figure 5-5 Interaction of cognitive and motivational–emotional (ME) influences in learning. R, response; S, stimulus; PS, processed stimulus.

However, even this improved formulation sets up a false distinction between cognitive elements (S + PS) and motivational–emotional elements. This is true because the latter must ultimately be expressed in terms of the former. Stated in other terms, motivational–emotional reactivities are expressed as sensory equivalents that, whether internal or external, are abstracted, associated, and appreciated (recognized) only as cognitive entities. Hence the motivational–emotional component of a cognitive experience, although deriving from a different behavioral system, is expressed cognitively through the same physiological mechanisms as are the purely cognitive elements.

This position has been most succinctly expressed in a letter by Lazarus (1981) in response to a letter by Zajonc (1980);

> . . . it is counterproductive to reify emotion and cognition as independent and merely interactive. In nature they are normally fused (Lazarus, Coyne, and Folkman, in press) as Zajonc acknowledges when he writes ''In nearly all cases however feeling is not free of thought nor is thought free of feelings.'' (p. 222)

This opinion is more than a statement of a general philosophy of psychology; it is a declaration of some essential biological truths. Learning cannot take place in the absence of adequately attuned motivational–emotional influences and these latter influences are themselves expressed as integral elements of every cognitive experience. Associated emotional influences must be described along both qualitative and quantitative parameters. They can be positive, neutral, or negative and in each of these qualitative categories they can be mild, moderate, or severe. There may even be mixed patterns in terms of these reactivities. The only thing there cannot be is complete absence of motivational–emotional charge.

The major anatomical locus for the interaction of motivational–emotional and cognitive engrams would appear, on the basis of neurophysiological evidence, to be most probably in the inferior temporal lobe and the entorhinal cortex. The higher levels of the motivational–emotional system converge on that area where the upper segments of the rhinencephalon (the amygdaloid–hippocampal complex, the septal region, and the cingulate gyrus) meet with the innermost areas of the cortex (the inferior and medial aspects of the temporal lobe). Similarly, the highest areas of abstraction for both the visual and auditory cognitive systems converge on the inferior temporal lobe. Thus anatomically the conjunction of these two systems at their highest levels (excluding for the moment the associational and higher processing systems of the cognitive system) occurs in the inferior temporal lobe. The experimental data that appear to confirm this interpretation stems from the previously described Klüver–Bucy experiment (see Chapter 3). In that study, monkeys in whom inferior and medial portions of the temporal lobe had been ablated completely lost their fear of specific objects (snakes, fire) of which they had previously been terrified.

Classical and Operant Conditioning

The equations of Figure 5-5 illustrate that not only are cognitive and motivational–emotional influences inevitably bound together but so also are the motor responses to those influences. Because our emphasis has been largely on mental functions, we have tended to ignore the entire area of motor activities. Yet behavior, animal or human, is largely defined by just such activities. In fact, behavioral psychology places as much importance on motor responses as determinants of animal and human behavior as it does on cognitive or motivational–emotional influences. This concept forms the basis of operant psychology (the general system based on operant conditioning) from which, in turn, learning theory psychology has evolved. Since learning theory psychology is one of the three legs on which the theoretical system of this volume rests (the other two being psychoanalysis and psychobiology), and since learning theory is itself an extension of operant psychology (the science of operant conditioning), it is incumbent on us to explore, at least superficially, the psychobiology of this latter mechanism.

Operant conditioning is itself a more complex development from a simpler mechanism, namely classical conditioning. In this simpler paradigm, an unconditioned stimulus (UCS) that evokes a given response (R) is paired with a neutral conditioned stimulus (CS). After a series of such exposures, the experimental subject (usually an animal) will respond to the CS in the absence of the UCS. For example, in Pavlov's famous experiment, a dog would salivate when given a plate of food to smell (the UCS). When the food was paired with the sound of a bell (the CS), after a series of such paired exposures, the dog would salivate with the sounding of the bell alone. Similarly, if the UCS is unpleasant, such as a shock to the hind leg, and the response (R) the lifting of the hind leg, then after conditioning to a red light (CS) the dog will ultimately lift its hind leg in response to the flash of the red light alone. These interactions are illustrated in Figure 5-6.

The physiology of the interactions among the various modalities in classical conditioning, although not completely determined, is not too difficult to conceptualize in terms of mechanisms already described in previous chapters or to be described in later chapters. There is first an interaction between a given perceived stimulus (P)UCS of a given motivational–emotional valence (positive in the case of food, negative in the case of shock), and a given efferent response (visceral in salivation, motor in lifting the hind leg). The pairing of the UCS with the CS results in the association of their perceived abstract engrams (P)UCS and (P)CS, much in the fashion of the association between other abstract engrams, as described in Chapter 4. Consequently, after repeated pairing of the stimuli, the exposure to CS alone will elicit the same response as that to the UCS (as illustrated in Fig. 5-6).

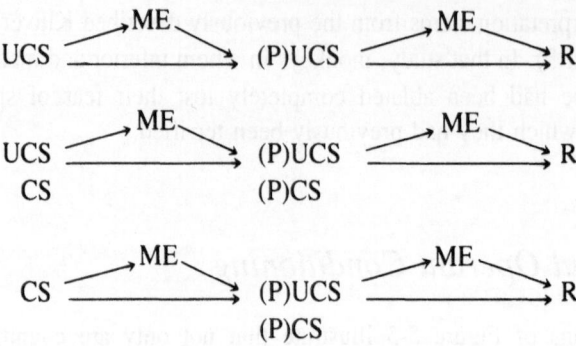

Figure 5-6 Mechanisms of classical conditioning. Abbreviations: CS, conditional stimulus; UCS, unconditional stimulus; ME, motivational–emotional; R, response; (P), perceived.

This mechanism is almost certainly further elaborated by an interaction between the (P)CS and the motor or visceral response itself. Motor and visceral responses are not simple R's as suggested in Figures 5-5 and 5-6 but are rather complex procedural processes at the unconscious level. (These processes will be described in some detail in Chapters 11, 17, and 20). Here it is enough to say that they themselves have representation in the brain both in their purely physiological form but also as cognitive constellations. It is in the latter form that they may become associated with the perceived conditioned stimulus so that the latter may take the place of the (P)UCS in driving the response.

Operant conditioning is an extension of classical conditioning. It is in operant conditioning that the major importance of motor reactivity in conditioning becomes evident. In this paradigm, an animal is taught to perform a certain motor function (most often, pressing a lever) in order to obtain a reward or to escape punishment. One example is the experiment by Old et al. (1972) described in Chapter 2 in which rats or monkeys learned to bar press in order to stimulate their own brain reward systems. After sufficient experience, these animals will continue to bar press even after the electrodes to their brains have been disconnected. In these instances, the motor activity itself has assumed the character of a stimulus that continues to excite persistent self-stimulation in a vicious cycle paradigm even when the reward is no longer present. However, if the response is not reinforced, at least sporadically, *extinction* will occur and the conditioned reactivity will slowly die out.

The concept of reinforcement, positive or negative, in operant conditioning is central both to its theory and practice. Positive reinforcement signifies continued reward for the proper performance of a required act. Negative reinforcement describes a paradigm in which the subject is required to learn to perform, or in certain instances, *not* to perform a certain act in order to avoid pain or discomfort. Thus negative reinforcement paradigms fall into two categories: *active avoidance* and *passive avoidance*. In active avoidance, the subject must learn to perform a specific act in order to avoid pain or discomfort. In passive avoidance, the subject must learn to abstain from a certain activity if he is to avoid pain or discomfort. Passive avoidance is also the mechanism through which extinction of a given operant response occurs, i.e., cessation of a response when responding is no longer rewarded.

These mechanisms are of great importance in explaining certain types of human behavior. They are particularly characteristic of certain processes that occur during the pathogenesis of the addictive disorders. The neurophysiology of these mechanisms is described in some detail in Chapter 19 (pp. 300–301) while their clinical significance in the addictive disorders will be elaborated upon in Volume 3 of this series. Operant conditioning exemplifies one of the areas where it is easiest to demonstrate the relevancy of psychobiologic mechanisms to clinical problems.

The examples of learning (Fig. 5-5), of classical conditioning (Fig. 5-6), and of operant conditioning given in this chapter are obviously most elementary and do not suggest the wide spectrum of experience that they can encompass. For example, the symbolic engrams of language can be utilized as stimuli for conditioning just as can veridical and abstract perceptions. Using just these three paradigms—learning, classical conditioning and operant conditioning—modern behavorist theory has attempted, not entirely without success, to explain human behavior. With some modifications, additions, and elaborations, learning theory has in my opinion been somewhat more successful. However, as stated in the preface, the absence within this theory of any real consideration of unconscious brain activity constitutes a serious shortcoming.

These descriptions of the motivational–emotional, motor, and cognitive parameters of behavior have roughly defined the mechanisms operating in each of these behavioral modalities as well as the interactions them. But these interactions between motivational–emotional, motor, and cognitive events occur at still another level of phenomenology, that in the area of consciousness or the unconsciouus. Affective–cognitive interactions may occur consciously, unconsciously, or indeed during modified states of consciousness. The preliminary descriptions of the three major behavioral systems permit us now to address the main area of interest in this volume, namely the nature and dynamics of conscious and unconscious behavior.

II

Mechanisms of Conscious and Unconscious Thought Processing

II

Functional Organization of the Consciousness System

The coordination of motivational–emotional, cognitive, and motor activities in different environmental settings is optimally accomplished through variations in the state of organization of brain function. One such state, "consciousness," has apparently evolved to deal most effectively with those demands in the internal and external milieus that require most immediate attention. Consciousness serves two functions: first, through mobilizing the sensory system to identify any urgent demands (internal drives, external threats, etc.) and second, through activation of the pertinent reactive systems (emotional, motor), to allow the organism to cope most effectively with significant events. The full spectrum of conscious activities constitutes a continuum leading from alertness to altered states of consciousness to deep sleep and REM sleep. Alert consciousness, the state of consciousness with which we are most familiar, results from the behavioral effects of the entire consciousness system raised to its highest level of activity. Other states of consciousness occur when different parts of the system are only partially activated.

Because alert consciousness is the dominant state in which man finds himself (16 hr out of a 24-hr day), because it encompasses the most vivid experiences (since it represents the focusing of all of the organism's resources upon specific limited events), because it actualizes the individual's most keen awareness of himself (cogito ergo sum), and because it is so thoroughly subjective, consciousness has always seemed to man as something not animalistic but rather distinctively human. It is still a question of philosophic discussion as to whether mammals below man possess any form of consciousness. The answer to that question must be that if they possess an equivalent neurophysiological awareness system in the brain, which all mammals do, then they should possess equivalent subjective consciousness. Certainly their consciousness may be of a different level of complexity than that of man, but that is true even among humans with various brain defects.*

---

*Of all vertebrates, only mammals show a P300 on the evoked potential (a sign of *conscious* attending) and θ activity in the hippocampus (a sign of *active* attending). These distinctions are expanded upon in Chapters 8, 17, and 22.

Nevertheless, the special characteristics of human consciousness—its subjectivity, its identification with personal existence, its ability to escape the limits of the real environment—often appear to endow it with qualities above and beyond the confines of neurophysiological activity. This is unwarranted. A brief re-examination of materials from the chapters on motivation, emotions, and cognition will reveal mechanisms that will at least begin to offer the basis for a purely biological view of conscious phenomenology.

In the chapters on motivations and emotions, we described the Papez–MacLean theory of emotions. That theory, based on much clinical and experimental evidence, concludes that the major critical area for "feeling" different emotional responses lies in various segments of the limbic system, most particularly in the thalamus. Evidence that still other types of feeling—sensations, feelings of self, and so forth—involve the thalamus, the limbic system, and other discrete areas of the brain (the self-awareness system) will be presented in this and the next chapter. The important point to be made is that consciousness is not a metaphysical concept; it is the subjective equivalent of neurophysiological activity in a given system of the brain produced by the simultaneous activation of the "alerting" and "awareness" neurophysiological subsystems.

It is well, at this point, to present an overview of the concepts to be described in this and the next chapter. Awareness itself is of two types: a general vague awareness of the environment and secondly a more specific awareness of oneself and of the relationship of that self to the environment. Recent experimental evidence suggests that the center for general awareness lies in the limbic area, more specifically in the thalamus and basal ganglia, while the centers for self-awareness lie in a system beginning in the basal ganglia and ending in the posterior inferior portions of the parietal lobe. This evidence will be presented in detail shortly.

The complete *consciousness* system consists of three components: an *activating system*, the *general awareness system*, and the *self-awareness system*. In normal consciousness, the activating system is the noradrenergic reticular activating system, producing normal alert conscious awareness. However, under certain circumstances, other activating centers will energize the awareness and self-awareness systems to produce different states of awareness. For example, in altered states of consciousness, activation of the self-awareness system comes from the thalamus, producing a relaxed hazy sense of the world. In dreaming, activation comes from cholinergic cells in the pons to produce still a different state of awareness.

In these terms, alert consciousness, i.e., the alert objective state of mind characterized by full awareness of oneself and of the outer world, occurs only when there is active stimulation of the noradrenergic reticular activating system with associated excitation of the general awareness system in the involved thalamic–basal gangliar nuclei and of the self-awareness system in the posterior inferior parietal lobe system. Less alert consciousness occurs with only partial excitation of the noradrenergic activating system as in stage 1 sleep. Impaired general awareness occurs with lesions of the thalamic–basal gangliar centers while impaired self-awareness occurs with lesions in the posterior inferior parietal lobes. Finally, in certain physiological states such as sleep, hypnosis, and so on, the entire awareness system—the thalamic–basal gangliar and posterior inferior parietal nuclei—may be activated by different activation systems, such as the cholinergic in the pons or the dopaminergic in the thalamus, to produce different states of consciousness.

Behavioral Parameters of Consciousness

Of all aspects of human behavior, consciousness is perhaps the most difficult to define. It has both an objective component (alertness) and a subjective element (awareness).* It is further characterized by a level of energy that has variously been labeled "arousal" or "activation." It also has a certain quality that we have described as "affect." Finally, the beam of awareness may be focused in one direction or another under the paradigm of "attention." These seven A's, alertness, attention, arousal, activation, affect, and the two awarenesses, represent different aspects of consciousness that because they are closely associated are frequently confused with one another. It will be the purpose of this chapter to suggest that the seven A's describe different dimensions of consciousness, each constituting a separate and discrete process and each under the control of a separate and discrete anatomical and physiological system in the brain. With different combinations of physiological activities, different objective and subjective states ensue.

If consciousness is truly as fragmented as here proposed, one may ask why it is usually experienced as a single integrated entity. This is a consequence of the modular organization of consciousness. The various systems of consciousness are so closely integrated in function and activity that changes in any one area are almost always associated with correlated changes in the other systems. For example, increases in arousal brought about by an increase in motivational excitation (affect) are usually associated on an almost one-to-one basis with comparable increases in activation, alertness, awareness, and attention. Usually, but not always, so that in every case instances of dissociation among the seven parameters of consciousness can be demonstrated. Consequently, one major thrust in this chapter will be directed toward those exceptions, i.e., the cases of dissociation, and toward the physiological and neurochemical mechanisms underlying them. Such an analysis, if successful, should support the multicomponent conceptualization of consciousness as opposed to a more unitary formulation.

If it is true, as we have postulated, that in the biological organization of life the energy that drives the organism derives from motivational influences, then it follows logically that in mammals the energies that drive the brain are first arousal and then activation, the electrophysiological equivalent of those motivational forces. Within this theoretical construct, motivational–emotional arousal produces electrophysiological activation of the brain, which is translated epiphenomenally into alertness and awareness. Finally, awareness is focused through attention onto the cognitively and motivationally significant events in the internal and external environments to determine the final sequence of drive-oriented behavioral responses.

In general, almost all increased emotional excitement and arousal is associated with increased alertness and activation. The reverse is also true; increased activation tends to be associated with increased arousal (Duffy, 1962). However, correlations are highly variable. The correlation among the various psychophysiological indices of arousal [e.g., heart rate, galvanic skin reflex (GSR), vasomotor reactions, catecholamine levels, and respirations] varies greatly and the correlation among the several

---

*Awareness in turn may be vague (general awareness) or specific (self-awareness).

electrophysiological indices o activation [e.g., electroencephalogram (EEG), evoked potential, and single nerve cell responses] is also fairly variable. In a series of experiments in which indices of emotional reactivity (arousal) and of brain activity (activation) were studied simultaneously under a variety of conditions, no significant correlations between signs of arousal and indices of activation were found (Sternbach, 1960). Apparently the two activities do derive from different although intimately related neurophysiological systems in the brain. Since the central and peripheral manifestations of the two activities are not infrequently dissociated, arousal and activation will continue to be treated as separate but related entities.

Electrophysiological Measures of Brain Activity

The general level of brain activation is related more or less directly to the behavioral level of alertness.* This latter parameter defines the general level of contact that the organism has with its environment. Where the level of alertness, i.e., degree of reactivity to the environment, is zero, the animal is said to be inert (unconscious?). As sensory and motor reactivities to external stimuli are increasingly greater than zero, the animal is said to be progressively stuporous, relaxed, alert, or agitated. The physiological level of energy in the brain can best be determined through a variety of electrophysiological indices, chief among which is the EEG. The behavioral level of energy is usually manifest in the observable states of the individual, e.g., the level of alertness, level of emotional arousal, and so forth.

The EEG is obtained through electrodes on the scalp that record the general level of electrophysiological activity in the brain. Under these conditions, a record of various types of brain activity is produced with different patterns more or less like the examples in Figure 6-1. Analysis of these patterns reveals that they differ mainly along two parameters: frequency (the number of wiggles per second) and amplitude (the general height of the wiggles). Frequency and amplitude are usually, but not always, inversely proportional. On the basis of these findings, five major types of wave forms have been differentiated. Gamma waves have the highest frequency (20–40/sec) and lowest amplitude, followed sequentially by β waves (12–20/sec), α waves (8–12/sec with moderate amplitude), θ waves (5–7/sec with rather high amplitude), and δ waves (2–4/sec with very high amplitude).

The EEG is the simplest and most direct technique for obtaining a rough indication of electrical activity in the brain. It is particularly valuable in diagnosing different states of consciousness since alert states are usually characterized by β and γ wave activity while coma is generally associated with δ wave activity. The EEG is of particular value in monitoring sleep activity, where the level of consciousness varies greatly from one stage to another. In general, α waves represent synchronized relaxing influences on the cortex (stemming from the thalamus); β and γ waves represent an alerting influence (stemming from the locus coeruleus and the reticular activating

---

*A notable exception is REM sleep where there is markedly impaired alertness and awareness associated with high arousal and high activation.

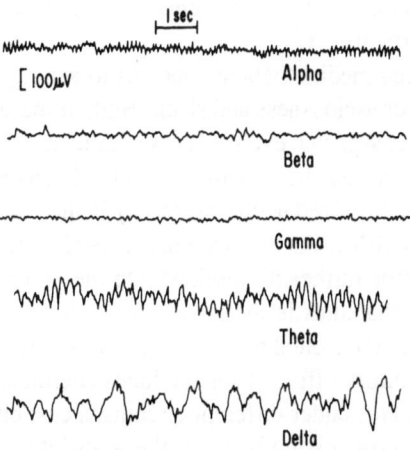

Figure 6-1 EEG wave forms.

system); and θ and δ waves represent a relative inactivity of the cortex (presumably secondary to reduced stimulatory locus coeruleus reticular activating system influences associated with increased inhibitory thalamic and septal–hippocampal impulses radiating upward to the cortex).*

Activating Systems of the Brain

The most primitive anatomical structure in the brain stem responsible for controlling energy levels in the brain is the ascending reticular activating system (RAS). The general distribution of the RAS was presented in Figure 1-1. It runs through the medial portion of the brain stem into the dorsal medial thalamus from which its impulses radiate to all portions of the basal ganglia, limbic system, and neocortex. Its central role in activation was established by Moruzzi and Magoun in 1949 by their demonstration that electrical stimulation of any portion of the brain stem RAS resulted in increased excitation of the entire brain. Its function in maintaining consciousness is demonstrated by the fact that total ablation of the system results in deep and irreversible coma. On the other hand, if the RAS is destroyed progressively in steps, consciousness may be retained albeit at a functionally lower level, indicating that other centers such as the medial thalamus and basal ganglia may take over if a sufficient period for compensatory reactivation is permitted (Hassler, 1978).

The control center for the RAS lies at its lower end in the locus coeruleus of the pons (Fig. 2-1). This center controls all noradrenergic (norepinephrine) activity in the brain through the radiations of two neuronal networks (the ventral and dorsal forebrain

*In some altered states of consciousness (ASC), there is θ-wave activity in the EEG, indicative of influences from the inhibitory septal–hippocampal circuit. The generation of θ waves from this circuit is discussed in Chapter 8, while θ-wave activity in certain ASCs is described in Chapter 21.

bundles). Its activity is reflected by the presence of β (high activity) or γ (very high activity) waves in the cortical EEG.

The relationship of the medial thalamic nucleus to activity in the locus coeruleus and the RAS is critical in consciousness and sleep. Both of these systems are centers of autonomous electrical discharge that exercise either stimulatory (RAS and thalamus) or inhibitory (thalamus) effects on the rest of the brain. It has been postulated that α rhythm which induces synchronized neuronal activity in the cortex (mildly stimulatory) stems from the thalamus (Morison and Dempsey, 1962; Andersen and Andersson, 1968) (see pp. 226–227 for further discussion). On the other hand, strong electrical stimulation of the medial thalamus in the intact cat produces 8–12 waves per second, similar to sleep spindles, in the frontal and temporal lobes of the cortex (Monnier et al., 1963), a specifically inhibitory effect. Thus the locus coeruleus is acutely stimulatory while the thalamic nuclei are, under different circumstances, either mildly stimulatory or actively inhibitory. Electrical stimulation of the RAS inhibits electrically produced medial thalamic spindling as well as naturally produced thalamic waves, a phenomenon known as "α blockade." Consequently, the locus coeruleus-driven RAS and the medial thalamus appear to have a reciprocal antagonist relationship where increased activity of the former inhibits activity of the latter and vice versa (Thompson, 1975).

The interaction between the locus coeruleus-driven RAS and the thalamus plays an important role in the control of consciousness. Although the RAS is the most primitive and essential brain structure involved in the maintenance of consciousness, the thalamus and basal ganglia also appear to play a key role. As previously described, if the RAS in animals is destroyed stepwise rather than all at once, a low-grade form of consciousness can be maintained providing that the thalamus and basal ganglia are left intact. Thus the influences of the thalamus appear to be of two kinds: one inhibitory upon the cortex as in sleep, the other mildly stimulatory and upward into the cortex in the form of activating α waves. The behavioral manifestations of α-wave activity are those of a rather low level of awareness, similar to that of twilight sleep or hypnagogic states. The median thalamus is also related in a feedforward–feedback circuit with the inhibitory septal–hippocampal complex which generates θ-wave activity, thus accounting for the close association between α- and θ-wave activity in sleep and in other altered states of consciousness (Fig. 6-2) (see Chapters 8 and 21 for a full discussion).

The Physiology of Sleep

Variations in the balance between locus coeruleus and medial thalamic activities result in different levels of consciousness that are best illustrated in studies of sleep (Snyder and Scott, 1972). The two major states of affected consciousness in sleep are normal sleep and REM sleep. Normal sleep (stages 1–4) is the consequence of the reciprocal relationship of the locus coeruleus-driven RAS and the medial thalamus, as previously described. The medial thalamus emits α waves but also sleep spindles, the latter leading to generalized inhibition, i.e., decreased activity of the cortex. The type of wave generated by the medial thalamus is thought to be a function of the level of the effective influence of the RAS upon it at any given time. If the RAS is only mildly active as in the so-called resting relaxed state, the medial thalamus gives off α waves and the individual is conscious but generally inattentive. As RAS activity gradually diminishes, α-wave activity increases in early stage 1 sleep (twilight sleep). In stage 2 it begins to diminish and is replaced by sleep spindles and θ waves (septal–hippocampal). In stages 3 and 4, as RAS activity becomes progressively less, the inhibitory influences from the medial thalamus and the septal–hippocampal complex gradually increase, resulting at first in slower spindling waves and then gradually increasing δ-wave activity (slow-wave sleep, SWS). Hence, most of the entire physiological process of normal sleep can be seen as one of gradually diminishing RAS influence and gradually increasing medial thalamic and septal–hippocampal influence.

Jouvet (1974) has postulated on the basis of available experimental evidence that the specific anatomical area that is responsible for inhibiting the locus coeruleus in sleep is the median raphe of the brain stem. This area, as illustrated in Figure 2-1, is the site of all serotonin neurotransmitter neurons in the brain stem, the fibers of which radiate upward into the hypothalamus, thalamus, basal ganglia, and cortex. Jouvet has demonstrated that destruction of the raphe system in cats results in an animal that is capable of the alert waking state and of REM sleep but not of normal SWS.

Rapid eye movement sleep has a number of unique characteristics that clearly differentiate it from any of the stages of normal sleep. Rapid eye movement sleep is also known as paradoxical sleep because of the dissociations in a variety of neurophysiological and behavioral activity that ordinarily are directly correlated. Most striking is the dissociation between the level of electrophysiological activity in the brain (activation) and the level of behavioral alertness. In REM sleep the EEG shows a pattern of predominantly β-wave activity, a pattern usually associated with objective alertness and subjective awareness. However, in REM sleep, the individual (animal or human) is in a state of behavioral inertness, objectively unconscious and most difficult to arouse. This phase of sleep is associated with a general state of marked muscular relaxation although there are visceral signs of excitement (increased pulse, blood pressure and respiration, penile erections, etc.). In addition, subjects awakened during REM sleep most frequently report that they were dreaming, suggesting a kind of internal consciousness at a time when there was no evidence of external consciousness.

There appears to be a close association between neurophysiological mechanisms of the RAS–medial thalamic consciousness control system and the behavioral manifestations of the progressive stages of normal sleep (stages 1–4). But the paradoxical dissociations that occur during REM sleep suggest the involvement of some different neurophysiological consciousness system. The nature of that system is not yet as well understood as is that of the normal sleep system, but recent anatomical and pharmacologic studies have shed some light on it.

Just as destruction of the raphe system in cats results in obliteration of SWS, so does destruction of the locus coeruleus result in obliteration of REM sleep with normal sleep activity remaining intact. On the other hand, it has been found that pharmacologic agents that reduce norepinephrine activity in the brain all result, contrary to expectations, in an increase in REM activity. This paradoxical and apparently contradictory finding suggests that there must be two control systems that are reciprocally inhibitory in the locus coeruleus. Recent studies have confirmed this expectation.

It has been found that two different types of neurons exist in the area of the locus coeruleus: giant reticular (FTG) neurons and typical norepinephrine neurotransmitter neurons. The giant reticular (FTG) neurons have their cell bodies close to the area of the locus coeruleus, but their fibers radiate extensively (McCarley and Hobson, 1974). These cells are ordinarily inactive during the waking state and in SWS, but become markedly active during REM periods at which time the noradrenergic activity of the locus coeruleus is shut down (Aston-Jones and Bloom, 1981). Rapid eye movement sleep in cats is associated with the production of PGO waves, large EEG spikes over the pons, lateral geniculate body, and occipital lobes (PGO is abbreviated from *pons*, lateral *geniculate* body, and *occipital* cortex). The occurrence of PGO waves in REM sleep suggests that that kind of sleep is activated from the lower brain stem as opposed to SWS which appears to be activated mainly from the thalamus and septal–hippocampal complex.

Clues as to the nature of the system opposing the noradrenergic come from pharmacologic studies. The cholinergic system is one of the oldest and most widespread neurotransmitter systems in all organisms so that it would be surprising if it were not involved in a function so vital as activation of the brain. Administration of cholinergic substances (acetylcholine, neostigmine etc.) is accompanied by intense activation of EEG as evidenced by the generation of marked desynchronization with resultant γ (rapid irregular wave) activity. However, these electrophysiological signs of hyperactivity are not necessarily associated with behavioral signs of hyperactivity; on the contrary, a comatose or SWS sleeping cat may remain comatose or in SWS, even though the EEG becomes that of an alert animal after the injection of a cholinergic activator. Similarly, the administration of the anticholinergic drug atropine to an alert awake animal will result in synchronization of EEG electrical activity with the production of hypersynchronized δ waves, but the cat will remain behaviorally alert and awake. This dissociation between the electrophysiological and behavioral effects of cholinergic and anticholinergic drugs has been called the "divorce" phenomenon and is reminiscent of the dissociation that occurs between electrophysiological and behavioral effects during REM sleep. The probable involvement of this system in the development of REM sleep is suggested by the fact that the intrathecal administration of cholinergic substances into the pontine area causes PGO spikes and REM sleep (Sitaram, 1976) while the administration of atropine abolishes PGO spikes and REM activity (Karczmar and Dun, 1978).

What is the significance of these complex experimental findings for our understanding of the various parameters of consciousness? It appears that there are at least two separate activation systems present in the lower brain stem: a noradrenergic system that controls both activation of the brain and levels of alertness and a cholinergic system that affects only activation of the brain. When the noradrenergic system has been suppressed by increased activity of the serotonergic system, activity of the RAS is diminished and the dopamine-driven thalamus takes over. The resulting behavioral states are progressively that of stage 2, stage 3, and then stage 4 (SWS) sleep. When increased cholinergic activity is superimposed on increased serotonergic inhibition, activation of the brain and increased arousal in the adaptative physiological systems occur but without any evidence of alertness. Thus a comatose cat will remain comatose after the injection of a cholinergic drug even though the brain becomes fully activated.

Consequently, the control of electrical activation in the brain may lie either with the noradrenergic or the cholinergic system, but the control of alertness (level of consciousness) apparently lies entirely with the noradrenergic system.

Recent evidence (Hobson et al., 1975; Sakai 1980) suggests that the various stages of sleep are modulated by the anterior hypothalamus (the parasympathetic nerve center) through its stimulatory effects sequentially, first on the raphe to induce deep sleep and second on the cholinergic FTG cells to produce REM. A diagrammatic illustration of the functional interrelationships of the various nerve centers in the brain stem is given in Figure 6-2. In the early stages of sleep the anterior hypothalamus is thought to stimulate the raphe, releasing serotonin which inhibits locus coeruleus activity. This decreases RAS activity and allows thalamic escape (α waves followed by θ and δ waves). Later in the sleep cycle, the anterior hypothalamus is thought further to stimulate the cholinergic FTG cells which excite the activating component of the RAS but not the alerting component. Here the pontine–geniculate–occipital system is also stimulated and REM sleep with dreams result. (For a more detailed discusssion of the mechanisms underlying dream production see Chapter 22, pp. 342–348.)

Whereas the anterior hypothalamus appears to modulate activities of the serotonergic raphe and of the cholinergic FTG cells, the posterior hypothalamus (the sympathetic nerve center) controls activity in the noradrenergic locus coeruleus (Fig. 6-2). Here lies the explanation for the usual close association between arousal and activa-

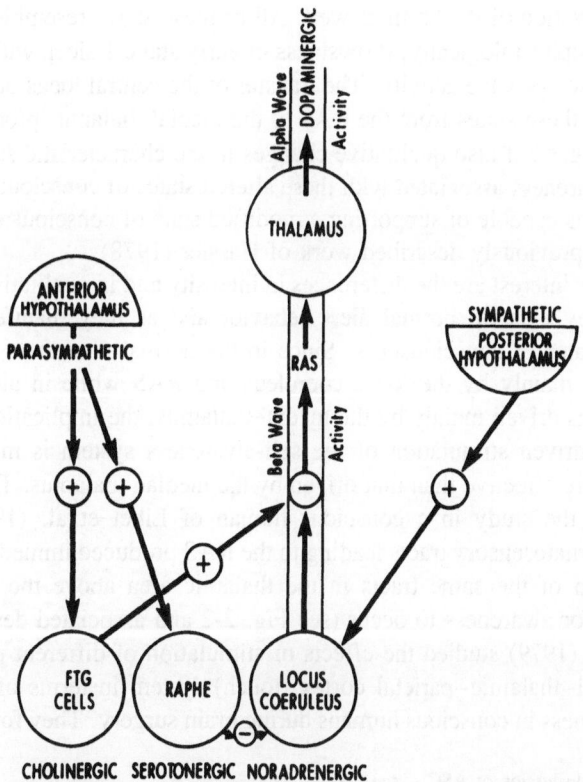

Figure 6-2 Nerve centers in brain stem associated with sleep.

tion, since arousal stems from the posterior hypothalamus and normal brain activation from the locus coeruleus. During SWS, if external stimulation is great enough, there is strong activation of the RAS and the individual wakes.

The apparent existence of two separate activating systems from the lower brain stem, one the norepinephrine locus coeruleus system which dominates normal behavior and the other the cholinergic FTG neuronal system of REM sleep, is a finding of great theoretical interest. The relationship of the cholinergic FTG system to psycho-biological concepts such as consciousness, awareness, self-awareness, attention, reality testing, and others remains obscure since our only access to that system is when it is functioning during REM sleep. In many respects dreaming, the major behavioral production of the FTG system, resembles hallucinations. One may speculate that the hallucinatory episodes in psychosis may possibly in some way involve the FTG system.

Altered States of Consciousness*

The physiology of altered states of consciousness such as twilight states, fugues, hypnotic states, biofeedback, alpha states, transcendental meditation, and so on appears to be related more to that of normal sleep than to that of REM sleep. All of these states are characterized by evidence not only of decreased behavioral consciousness but of decreased activation of the brain as well. All of these states resemble, both behaviorally and electrophysiologically, drowsiness or early stage 1 sleep with increased α-wave and decreased β-wave activity. The transfer of the central locus of activation for consciousness in these states from the RAS to the medial thalamus produces not only quantitative changes but also qualitative changes in the characteristic states of awareness and self-awareness associated with these altered states of consciousness. That the medial thalamus is capable of supporting a modified state of consciousness is strongly indicated by the previously described work of Hassler (1978).

Of particular interest are the differences in intensity and in qualitative character of awareness as they exist in normal alert behavior and as they manifest themselves during altered states of consciousness. Since in the normal alert state the awareness system is driven mainly by the locus coeruleus and RAS while in altered states of consciousness it is driven mainly by the medial thalamus, the implication follows that locus coeruleus-driven stimulation of the self-awareness system is more direct and consequently more effective than that driven by the median thalamus. This conclusion is supported by the study in a conscious human of Libet et al. (1979) in which stimulation of somatosensory tracts leading to the RAS produced immediate awareness while stimulation of the same tracts in the thalamic area above the RAS required additional time for awareness to occur (see Fig. 2-2 and associated description).

Libet et al. (1979) studied the effects of stimulation of different portions of the medial lemniscal–thalamic–parietal cortex (touch) system in terms of the effect on conscious awareness in conscious humans during brain surgery. They found that single

*For more detailed discussion of ASC's, see Chapter 21.

threshold stimuli from the peripheral end-organ and spinal cord were recorded in the parietal lobe as evoked potentials and were experienced subjectively almost immediately. However, even stronger stimuli delivered through electrodes implanted in the medial lemniscus of the upper brain stem in the thalamus or in the primary receiving area of the parietal lobe of conscious surgical volunteers, although they produced evoked potentials, were not experienced subjectively by these individuals. Furthermore, Libet and his group (1979) demonstrated that only after continual direct supraliminal stimulation of the thalamus and parietal lobe in humans was there any subjective awareness of sensation and then only after about 0.5 sec, a delay that did not occur with skin or spinal cord stimulation. These workers postulated that peripheral and spinal cord stimulations produce activation of the RAS which permits immediate subjective experience of the sensation while direct stimulation of the specific somatosensory tract in the thalamus or parietal lobe, by circumventing brain stem mechanisms, necessitates longer periods of stronger stimulation to achieve awareness. This evidence indicates that the entire awareness system is activated most efficiently by stimulation of lower nerve tracts ending in the RAS and less efficiently through direct stimulation of the thalamus (Fig. 2-2).

It appears then that consciousness may be driven by one or another of three different activation centers: the norepinephrine RAS (emanating from the locus coeruleus), the cholinergic FTG cell system in the pons, and the dopaminergic alpha rhythm system radiating upward from the thalamus (Fig. 6-2). Brain activation by each of these centers is associated with a different state of awareness. One can explain the marked variation in general level of awareness in different states of consciousness either by postulating activation of different awareness systems by the different neural centers (locus coeruleus, median thalamus, and cholinergic FTG cells of the pons) or alternatively by invoking a single awareness system which is differentially activated by each of these neural centers. The study by Libet et al. (1979) described above appears more consistent with the second formulation since it indicates that excitation of the awareness tract is most effective when stimulation is directly to the noradrenergic RAS low down in a sensory system (peripheral end-organ and spinal cord) rather than to the thalamic radiations (median thalamus and parietal lobe). The different subjective descriptions of the various kinds of awareness present in the alert condition, in altered states of consciousness, and in REM sleep suggest a qualitative difference in states of awareness as well as a quantitative one. Apparently, even though there is only one awareness system, stimulation of different neural centers within it produces different kinds of awareness. Consequently, the state of awareness is determined by the interaction of a particular activating system (locus coeruleus, medial thalamus, or FTG cells) with a particular pattern of activation of the awareness system.

Although each of the subcortical activating centers can and does drive the general awareness system, only when that system is activated through the RAS does true consciousness with total awareness occur. The sense of awareness in altered states of consciousness is similar to that in alert consciousness but less intense and less distinct. The sense of awareness in REM state dreams is of course of another order altogether since it lacks entirely the kind of conscious awareness characteristic of alert conscious activity.

Anatomy of the General Awareness System

The general awareness system has its major focal centers in the area of the medial thalamus and basal ganglia. Specific lesions of some of these neural centers produce behavioral deficits that suggest the nature of the role played by those neural centers in establishing consciousness and awareness. Evidence for the role of different neural centers for promoting the sense of self-awareness comes predominantly from the study of humans with pathological defects in various areas of the brain.

The first brain stem centers involved in the phenomenology of general awareness appear to be the thalamus and posterior hypothalamus. Lesions of these areas in humans (where the RAS is intact) results in the syndrome known as akinetic mutism. This has been described by Girvin (1975) as follows:

> Akinetic mutism is a peculiar alteration in consciousness characterized by the appearance of seeming wakefulness but the absence of any evidence of the expected human content of consciousness; there is absence of any but rudimentary movement, emotional expression, response to commands, or other evidence of mental activity.

The dissociation in akinetic mutism characterized by some level of alertness combined with the absence of awareness suggests that functionally these two reactivities are not identical. The thalamus and posterior hypothalamus appear to contribute a general level of awareness in what has been called the state of vigilance (level of wakefulness) associated with RAS activity. Other clinical evidence suggests that the thalamus is at least a major center in generating the sense of feeling that is involved in translating physiological events into subjective experience. In an associated thalamic syndrome (Dejerine–Roussy), the feelings connected with various sensory stimuli, particularly touch and pain, are distorted rather than obliterated; they are either grossly exaggerated or diminished depending on the type of location of the lesion involving the thalamus. In these individuals, level of consciousness is not significantly disturbed but their reports of even strong emotional reactions often seem devoid of feeling. It is for this and other reasons that the thalamus and posterior hypothalamus together with parts of the contiguous basal ganglia (Hassler, 1978) are considered the seat of subjective motivational and emotional experience as described in Chapters 2 and 3 (Papez–MacLean).

It appears that specific areas of the basal ganglia are especially critical in certain elements of consciousness phenomenology, especially those comprising the affective components of awareness. Hassler has described patients with large lesions in the basal ganglia who showed many of the deficits characteristic of akinetic mutism. The areas involved include the globus pallidus and the putamen nuclei which apparently have consciousness and attentional functions rather than the motor control reactivities more characteristic of the rest of the basal ganglia (see Fig. 2-2).

Still another element in the general awareness neural system is the nucleus basalis of Meynart, a center in the substantia innominata serving a cholingergic activating function for the neocortex similar to that of the FTG cells for the brain stem. The nucleus basalis is a vital connecting link between the general awareness system and the self-awareness system and is particularly important in attentional and memory retrieval activities. As such it will be described in greater detail in Chapters 8 and 9.

Thus the general awareness neural system consists of the posterior hypothalamus, the dorsal median and anterior nuclei of the thalamus, the globus pallidus and putamen of the basal ganglia, and the nucleus basalis of Meynart in the substantia innominata. The individual units of this sytem, although anatomically disparate, operate in an integrated fashion to provide all of the primitive elements of consciousness and attentional activities. Indeed, when this system and the noradrenergic RAS are intact and functioning, consciousness may seem quite normal even when other vital structures in the limbic system (e.g., the hippocampus) have been surgically removed, On the other hand, damage to the general awareness system, depending on its extent and location, results in a variety of serious syndromes ranging from intractable coma, to akinetic mutism, to the Dejerine–Roussy syndrome, to the amnesia of Korsakoff's syndrome (see Chapter 9). Accordingly, the general awareness system provides the major elements of consciousness and attentional activities. Other systems, for example those for self-awareness (Chapter 7), for attention (Chapter 8), and for recognition, memory retrieval, and mental set (Chapter 9), merely refine the more basic and primitive functions of the general awareness system.

The anatomical arrangement of the general awareness system proves to be quite similar if not identical to that part of the motivational–emotional system illustrated in Figures 2-2 and 2-3. The concordance between these two systems is not too surprising when one considers that motivational–emotional feelings comprise a large part of conscious experience. Even more interesting is the fact that this same complex has major responsibility for directing attention and for accomplishing recognition and memory retrieval as will be described in Chapters 8 and 9. On the other hand, it is also clear that this system alone is unable to provide the total experience of conscious awareness. For that, neural structures and functions which reflect the internal representation of the self are essential. The nature of these will be presented in the next chapter.

7

Self-Awareness and the Anatomy of the Subjective Self

Activity at the three levels of the consciousness system as described in the last chapter—the RAS, the general awareness system, and the self-awareness system—is reflected in three behavioral levels of consciousness: alertness (RAS), general awareness (thalamic–basal gangliar complex), and focused self-awareness (the cortical component of the self-awareness system). Operationally, each level depends upon the integrity of the level below it so that a lesion at a lower level will obliterate the functional reactivity at any level above it. Lesions in the locus coeruleus or the RAS result in total behavioral inertness, those in the thalamic–basal gangliar nucleus produce an awake state without any evidence of awareness (akinetic mutism), while those in the posterior parietal lobe complex (the cortical component) result in an unfocused state of general awareness.

The behavioral reactivities controlled by the cortical component of the self-awareness system are of extreme importance because in large part those reactivities represent the core of the self-concept. The total sense of self stems from a variety of experiences (thinking, perceiving, planning, etc.), but the most primitive elements derive from feelings from the body itself. This psychobiological concept differs from psychoanalytic theory in which the newborn infant goes through a period of massive confusion during which it cannot differentiate between the environment and itself. According to psychobiological theory, the primitive sense of self is a built-in mechanism that begins to operate at birth. It is very primitive and becomes better elaborated only with development and experience so that the psychoanalytic view of a developing self-concept, although different, is still compatible with psychobiological theory.

Of the various functional characteristics of the self-concept, that associated specifically with the cortical component of the consciousness system is self-awareness. Although self-awareness means literally only awareness of oneself, its implications for consciousness phenomena go far beyond that limited significance. As will be described, the absence of self-awareness is associated with the absence of the ability to focus on specific items in the environment as a result of which the environment remains unobserved and to some extent unobservable. It appears that in the functioning mammalian organism, the obliteration of self-awareness is associated with a marked diminution in the *significance* of objects in the environment, since significance is measured in terms of the self. Consequently a monkey with ablation of the cortical self-awareness system will have intact sensory functions (seeing, hearing, etc.), but will evince no interest whatsoever in the environment surrounding him (Mountcastle, 1978).

This half physiological, half psychological introduction to the phenomenology of the self-concept is necessary to place it in proper perspective. The cortical self-awareness system to be described has as its central effect just that: self-awareness. The anatomical structures providing that effect represent the core, but only the core, of the self-concept system. Additional functions of the self-system are elaborated on that core to generate the subjective sense of personal existence which represents the essence of the sense of existing as a specific individual, separate and distinct from other individuals and from all other physical objects in the world. But that sense of self, so important in defining the parameters of motivational–emotional behavior (as in the instinct of self-preservation), is equally important in defining the boundaries of the cognitive and physical worlds surrounding the individual.

The last section of this chapter will deal in an introductory fashion with other aspects of the self-system, above and beyond that of self-awareness. The introduction of the concept of the total self in this section of our presentation is a necessary digression from the specific subject at hand of consciousness and the unconscious. As will be seen, how material is absorbed into consciousness and how material shifts back and forth between consciousness and the unconscious can be understood only in terms of the concept of a larger self-system overlooking the entire operation. Consequently, throughout this and the following sections, different elements of the self-system and their effects on subsidiary activities will be introduced, described, and analyzed at various points in the narrative.

Anatomy of the Cortical Self-Awareness System

Higher centers of the consciousness system are responsible for processing more cognitive elements of awareness than the general awareness system would be capable of. On the basis of extensive clinical observations and experimental studies in monkeys, Mesulam and Geschwind (1978) have developed a hypothesis that provides evidence for the involvement of the basal ganglia, other parts of the limbic system, and the cortex in the phenomenology of self-awareness. These authors postulate that the self-awareness system extension from the RAS and the thalamic–basal gangliar complex has its diencephalic site in the nucleus accumbens septi (a nerve center intermediate between the septal area of the limbic system, the hypothalamus, and the basal ganglia) and its major paleocortical focus in the substantia innominata (a diffuse area contiguous to the basal ganglia). From these brain stem and paleocortical centers, Mesulam and Geschwind have been able to trace projections to the posterior inferior

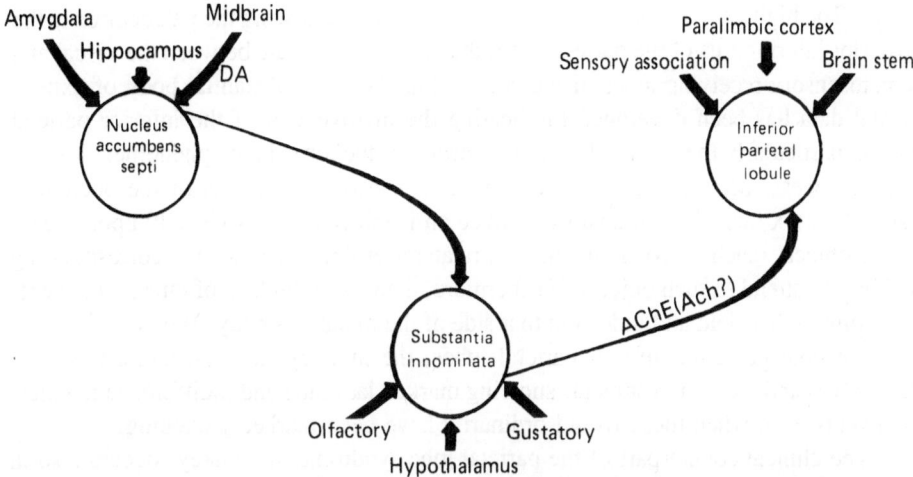

Figure 7-1 Neural tracts converging on the posterior inferior parietal lobe. Abbreviations: ACh, acetylcholine; AChE, acetylcholinesterase; DA, dopamine. (From Mesulam and Geschwind, 1978. Reproduced with permission.)

parietal lobes on both sides (Fig. 7-1). They have further tentatively determined the nature of the neurotransmitters that activate this system, dopamine on the brain stem component and probably acetylcholine on the projections from the paleocortex to the inferior parietal lobe (see Fig. 7-1).

With the introduction of the neocortical extension to the basic general awareness system, a new type of cognitive and personal quality is added. The involvement of the posterior inferior parietal lobe where the major proprioceptive neural tracts from the body converge initiates a sense of self that was not necessarily present in the sense of general awareness stemming from the median thalamic–basal gangliar complex. This feeling of self-awareness, together with the general sense of cognitive enrichment contributed by neocortical activities, makes the sense of self-awareness associated with activation of the total awareness system (RAS, thalamic–basal gangliar complex, and nucleus accumbens, substantia innominata, posterior inferior parietal lobe) qualitatively and quantitatively different from that associated with activation of the general awareness system alone.

The lower elements of the self-awareness system in the nucleus accumbens septi and in the substantia innominata play important roles in tying specific engrammatic material that has been raised by the attentional system (see Chapter 8) into the self-awareness system. The important role played by the hippocampus and the amygdala (the key control centers for attentional activities) in facilitating passage of material into the self-awareness system through the nucleus accumbens septi is illustrated in Figure 7-1. So also is the role of the mesencephalic (reticular) activating system in connecting the general awareness system to the self-awareness system. The interconnections among these various systems as illustrated in Figure 7-1 represent the patterns of structure and function underlying the neurophysiology of consciousness and awareness.

From the basal ganglia and limbic system, the self-awareness system rises to the cortex. The highest center in the self-awareness system following the paleocortex is the posterior inferior area of the parietal lobe, that area intermediate between the visual and somatosensory receiving areas of the cortex (Fig. 7-1). A substantial body of experimental data has been developed implicating the involvement of the inferior parietal cortex (particularly the occipital–parietal portion of the lobe) in the phenomenology of self-awareness. Mountcastle et al. (1975) have shown that lesions of the occipital–parietal cortex (area 7) in monkeys produce an inability to focus visually upon meaningful objects (such as food) in the contralateral environment with a corresponding inability to attend to such objects. Furthermore, there is a total lack of interest in events occurring in that field and indeed in that side of the monkey's body. Where lesions are made in both posterior inferior parietal lobes, the monkeys lose all interest both in themselves and their environment, showing marked lassitude and indifference to external events even when these would ordinarily have been markedly exciting.

The clinical counterpart of the parietal lobe syndrome in monkeys occurs also in man when destruction of the inferior parietal lobe results as the consequence of either strokes or tumors. In man, this results in a rather remarkable condition known as the unilateral neglect syndrome in which the individual often behaves as though one half of the world did not exist at all. Mesulam and Geschwind (1978) describe characteristic behavior in patients with this syndrome as follows:

> One patient may shave only one half of his face; another may only dress half of his body; still another may read only half of each sentence on a page. Indeed, we have seen an alcoholic patient who suffered such a stroke and was admitted to the hospital with florid withdrawal hallucinations in addition to severe unilateral neglect; the striking feature of this case was that all of the hallucinations were located in one half of the sensory space and no hallucinations were reported in the neglected sensory space!

As previously described, the bilateral destruction of these areas in both parietal lobes in monkeys produces a syndrome of marked indifference to the environment, even though there is no obvious impairment of any specific sensory modality. Mountcastle (1978b) writes of such animals that even though they are sensorily intact, they seem to have completely lost interest, both in themselves and in the surrounding environment. The exaggeration of the syndrome when both inferior parietal lobes are destroyed suggests the bilateral involvement of these areas in the self-awareness system. On the other hand, many clinicians have observed that the unilateral neglect syndrome occurs much more frequently in man with lesions of the right inferoparietal lobe than with those of the left. Indeed, Mesulam and Geschwind (1978) report three cases with right inferoparietal lobe lesions associated with generalized attentional difficulties in both left and right sensory fields similar to those found in monkeys with bilateral inferoparietal lesions. Mesulam and Geschwind, arguing both from the greater prevalence of the unilateral neglect syndrome with right inferoparietal lesions than with left and from their three cases of generalized defects in attention in patients with right-sided lesions, conclude that self-awareness may be localized more in the right brain than in the left. This position has been challenged by those who not infrequently find unilateral neglect syndromes in patients with left-sided lesions where the syndromes tend to be obscured by the associated aphasia. The position taken in this volume based on an evaluation of both sets of evidence is that the self-awareness system is represented in both hemispheres but probably more actively in the right hemisphere because of the nature of its function. This position will be elaborated upon further in Chapter 14 which discusses cerebral hemisphericity.

Heilman and Watson (1977) have observed that in the unilateral neglect syndrome the unawareness of events on one side is characteristic only of the unmotivated state, i.e., in the neutral condition where attention has not been actively drawn to the affected side. When attention is actively directed to the affected side, the individual does become aware of the existence of objects and activity in that area. Apparently, in the neglect syndrome due to damage of the Mesulam–Geschwind system there is impaired awareness but not total absence of awareness. Consequently one must assume that the retained limited awareness is the product of the activity of the more primitive centers such as the RAS, the hypothalamus, the thalamus, and the basal ganglia, i.e., of the general awareness system. These observations only reinforce the more critical significance of the general awareness centers in all consciousness phenomena; the cortical self-awareness system merely elaborates on those more basic activities.

Mechanisms Underlying Activities in the Posterior Inferior Parietal Lobe Complex

The inability to focus on significant objects in the contralateral field in these cases may be related to a functional deficiency in saccadic visual scanning of the environment, a mechanism that is apparently necessary for registering elements in the visual scene upon consciousness (Mountcastle, 1978b). That such saccadic scanning is an essential element in producing awareness of retinal images is indicated by the work of Riggs et al. (1953). These investigators, through an ingenious arrangement of prisms, were able to develop an experimental setting in humans where saccadic movements of the eyes were compensated for so that fixation of perception on a given object caused the image of that object to fall on a fixed area of the retina. Under these circumstances, the image of the object disappeared, i.e., the subject reported that he no longer saw it. This finding was subsequently confirmed by Pritchard et al. (1960).

It would seem that the images generated by saccadic movements are an essential element in the conscious perception of visual events. The reception area for such activity lies in area 7 of the brain, i.e., the area subtending perceptions that have both visual and somatosensory components (Mountcastle, 1978b), and coincidentally the critical area in the posterior inferior parietal lobe. Ablation of area 7 in monkeys produces a defect, not in ordinary saccadic scanning which is controlled at the brain stem collicular level, but in attentional saccadic scanning. Thus the phenomenology of attention, the subject matter of the next chapter, appears to involve the posterior inferior parietal lobe in a very direct way.

Even though the posterior inferior parietal lobe is involved in visual activities which include sensory motor input (e.g., saccadic scanning), most of its critical functions lie in the reception and analysis of sensory stimuli from the internal milieu. These stimuli fall into two major categories: somatosensory impulses from the body, skin, and musculature and motivational–emotional stimuli from the viscera.

The thalamic–basal gangliar complex, beside being a major center for emotional reception, is the most important relay station in the brain stem for somatosensory transmission (Fig. 2-2). Similarly, the parietal lobe, which is predominantly responsible for somatic sensory reception, is also the major cortical receiving area for the somatosensory elements of emotional experience, an important component of these effects. At first thought, it might seem strange that the neural system for self-awareness should center in the thalamus and the parietal lobe, the major seats of the somatosensory system, but on further reflection this arrangement appears to be biologically reasonable. Feeling must be central to self-awareness. The axiom reads, "I think therefore I am," but as previously noted, a better paradigm might be, "I feel therefore I am." In addition to the strong sense of feeling associated with emotional experience (as registered in the thalamus and parietal lobe), the sense of feeling that accompanies somatosensory impulses—touch, pain, heat, cold, and proprioception—comes closer to the sense of being than that which accompanies any other experience. It is probably no accident that the word "feeling" is used in the same way in most languages to express a sense of existence, of emotions, of touch, and of pain. Affective and somatosensory stimuli, which are constant and persistent even though we are unaware of them most of the time, produce the sense of one's body which is the most basic element in the "sense of self." It is difficult to conceive how an individual can be aware of his environment if he is not aware of his own body. This concept is not contradicted by those episodes of amnesia where the individual may forget who he is; in those instances he still knows that he is. It is most probable that a major component of the sense of self is produced by the constant barrage of affective and somatosensory stimuli converging from all parts of the body; the majority of these stimuli may not reach consciousness most of the time but they must register a sense of feeling in the thalamus and parietal cortex even though the individual may be unconscious of it.

Mountcastle (1978b) has summarized the evidence for the involvement of the parietal system in cognitive self-awareness as follows:

> I suggest that the internal construct of the image of self and self-in-the-world which centers in the parietal lobe is one of the many neural mechanisms important for conscious awareness and conscious action. A patient with parietal lobe lesion has a defect of conscious awareness, for he no longer has the capacity to attend to the contralateral world; for him it no longer exists. And, the withdrawn self-isolation of a monkey after bilateral parietal lobe lesions suggests a reduction in his level of conscious awareness. He has lost to a remarkable degree that direction, information-seeking behavior characteristic of attending primates. (p. 48)

As stated by Mountcastle, the cortical self-awareness center in the inferoparietal lobe together with the more primitive diencephalic system previously described appear to act as the core of a self-image or self-concept system which probably encompasses the activities of the entire brain. Mesulam and Geschwind have described the various tracts that lead from the other major cortical control centers into the self-awareness centers of the inferoparietal lobe. These are illustrated in Figure 7-2. The convergence of all cognitive and motivational–emotional impulses on the self-awareness center in the inferoparietal lobe contributes to the total concept of self. This is not to suggest that

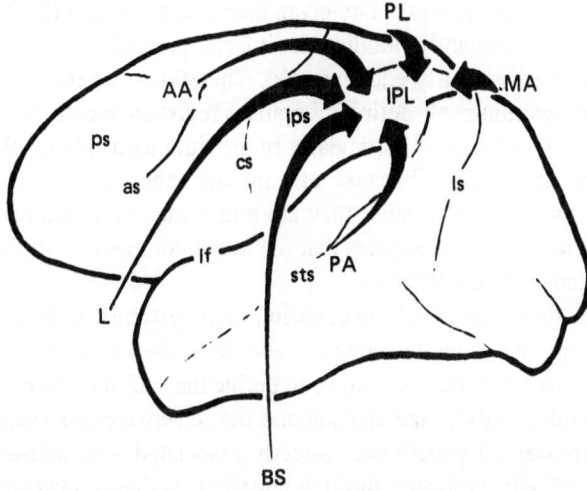

Figure 7-2 Neural pathways connecting limbic system with the posterior inferior parietal lobe. Abbreviations: AA, anterior association cortex: as, arcuate sulcus; BS, brain stem; cs, central suleus: IPL, inferior parietal lobule; ips, intraparietal sulcus: L, limbic areas in the basal forebrain; lf, lateral fissure: ls, lunate sulcus: MA, medial association cortex; PA, posterior association cortex; PL, paralimbic cortex, ps, principal sulcus; sts, superior temporal sulcus. (From Mesulam and Geschwind, 1978. Reproduced with permission.)

the self-concept is limited in any way to the self-awareness system; indeed, like every other abstract engram, the self-concept must encompass activity in the entire brain. However, the evidence does seem to indicate that the inferoparietal lobe, and particularly that on the right side, may play an especially important role in the phenomenology of self.

The Anatomy of the Self

On the surface, the most compelling definition of the self would appear to involve consciousness for it is only when some element of acute awareness is present that the sense of self is pervasive. Even during dreams the sense of self is associated with awareness of self albeit in an altered form. But only in the full awareness of the alert conscious state when the noradrenergic alerting system is fully active can the total sense of selfness be fully appreciated. Since the noradrenergic RAS is the initiator of conscious activity, it might appear that activity involving the alerting system and the self-awareness system provide the most important physiological mechanism in the representation of the self-function.

From a psychobiological point of view, however, it is apparent that the sense of self does not derive solely from conscious experience but that, on the contrary, it stems more basically from the steady stream of unconscious stimulation. As will be described in Chapter 10, consciousness has a kinematic quality where only a relatively few elements are brought to awareness at any given moment; consequently the vast input of somatosensory stimuli constantly flooding the inferior parietal lobes to constitute self-awareness cannot be consciously encompassed. Therefore, one must assume that the constant stream of incoming self-defining impulses registers unconsciously, mainly in the inferoparietal lobes and more particularly in the right hemisphere. Whether sense-of-self stimuli are unconscious because of constant habituation (see Chapter 8) or whether they are unconscious because they are transmitted predominantly to the right hemisphere (see Chapter 15), it appears that the major components of the self-concept are unconscious rather than conscious.

The tentative identification of the conscious self-system with three physiological systems, the alerting, the general awareness, and the self-awareness, is still somewhat simplistic. More correct probably would be to define the self in terms of a *self* structure that is based physiologically in the alerting and the self-awareness systems but which ultimately encompasses all experiences directly associated with self-awareness. The momentary sense of self, activated through attention, is determined by that which is momentarily significant to the self, where significance is defined in either cognitive or motivational–emotional terms. The permanent sense of self derives from persistent unconscious sensory activities. In these terms, the self possesses a physiological core but its total operation is defined equally by the sum total of all experiences that have become associated with that core (see Fig. 7-2).

Even the acutely self-aware component of the self-concept, by definition conscious, varies markedly in different altered states of consciousness. The conscious awareness of oneself in the alert condition is different from (1) that in the twilight state, (2) that in dreams, (3) that in hypnosis, (4) that under the influence of alcohol, (5) that under the influence of other sedatives, (6) that under the influence of stimulants, and (7) that under the influence of hallucinogens. In that sense the acute sense of self is a function of the momentary chemical and physiological state of the brain. The first four of the above-listed states of consciousness comprise more or less normal physiological conditions; the last four are those imposed chemically by drugs. Still other states associated with psychopathology such as in schizophrenia, mania, or depression undoubtedly produce still different "senses of self." Hence the concept of the self must be broad enough to encompass all of the various "senses of self" that are possible in the psychobiological system.

In general, except in severe psychopathology associated with depersonalization, the unconscious sense of self is probably more monolithic and relatively invariable than the conscious. However, even this more constant image varies considerably over the space of a lifetime. In these terms the conscious component of self-awareness may be seen as the *phase* condition while the unconscious component represents the long-term *state* condition.

These descriptions of the self-concept address mainly the subjective elements of the entity. Equally important are the efferent decisional operations on the basis of which behavior is determined. As will be described in Chapter 9, the decision-making apparatus of the brain is lodged largely in a consortium of neocortical centers including the prefrontal lobes (integration), the posterior inferior temporal lobes (motivation and emotion), the anterior and posterior associational areas (cognition), the posterior inferior parietal lobes (self-awareness), the left-hemispheric language centers (language), and the percentral frontal lobe motor area (motor). Within the context of this integrated cortical complex, self-awareness functions are somewhat stronger on the right hemisphere while language and decisional activities are somewhat stronger on the left (see Chapter 14).

In this way, the self-concept encompasses three major components: the subjective, lodged in the thalamic–basal gangliar complex and extending upward to the posterior inferior parietal lobe (Fig. 7-1); the executive, centered in the cortical consortium as just described and illustrated in Figure 9-3; and the substantive, consisting of the influx of all experience represented in neural engrams impinging on the self-center (Fig. 7-2). The full consciousness of normal alert awareness is experienced only when this entire system is fully activated by the noradrenergic-driven RAS. A vaguer, less distinct sense of awareness occurs in altered states of consciousness when the locus coeruleus is only partially active and the major alpha-driven rhythm derives from the thalamus. Still more bizarre is the sense of self in REM dreams where, because of the inactivity of the locus coeruleus, there is no conscious sense of self but where there is nevertheless a strong unconscious awareness of one's own identity. It is this last unconscious awareness that represents the unconscious self-concept that permeates all levels of the consciousness–unconscious spectrum. As will be described in Chapters 12 and 22, the special sense of self in REM dreams probably stems from an atypical cholinergic activation of the self-system in the absence of noradrenergic activation of the consciousness system.

Although the basic anatomies and functions of the self-awareness system in man, apes, and lower mammals are not significantly different, the qualities of self-awareness and consequently of consciousness in these various species almost certainly are. This is due to the kind of ego material that is transmitted from the rest of the cortex to the posterior inferior parietal lobe as illustrated in Figure 7-2. If, as we have postulated, the richness of conscious experience depends upon the strength of the self-concept and that, in turn, depends upon the ability to conceptualize the abstraction of self, then only in the highest mammal, man, do complete self-awareness and complete consciousness occur. The richness of conscious experience also varies with the level of complexity of the cognitive material fed into it; this also correlates with evolutionary level. Thus in mammals, the quality of general awareness is probably equal across all species. However, the quality of self-awareness varies strongly, from little or none at the lowest levels to highest in man, since the quality of conscious self-awareness varies concordantly with that of the cognitive content.

The introduction of the self-concept into our considerations at this point has been somewhat gratuitous, since this section is concerned essentially with the nature of conscious and unconscious thought processing. However, the critical role played by the self-awareness system in consciousness phenomena made that introduction here necessary. In the next chapter, which deals with "attention" (the mechanism by which the consciousness stream is focused onto the significant cognitive and motivational–emotional events in the external environment and internal milieus), it will be seen that the self-concept plays an equally critical role. Indeed, the entire thrust of the attentional process is first to identify those experiences that are of greatest cognitive and affective significance to the self and secondly to bring the vast resources of the self-structure to bear upon them.

The opposite side of the coin is that there is great difficulty in defining the structure and function of the self except in terms of conscious and unconscious thought processing. The nature of self-awareness differs markedly in the conscious and unconscious states. Hence it is critical that we define those states as we define the operation of the self within them. But those states themselves are markedly influenced by the actions of the self-structure. This produces a kind of feedback interaction where it is difficult to define either entity without simultaneously defining the other.

One of the more interesting implications of this dilemma is its similarity to that existing in psychoanalytic theory on the functional role and topographic position of the "ego," the Freudian analogue to the psychobiological self-system. In his earliest formulations, Freud conceptualized the ego as existing topographically largely in the conscious and preconscious realms, but gradually he came to feel that there was a major unconscious component within it as well. Such similarities in the psychoanalytic and the psychobiological conceptualizations of the ego and self systems, respectively, recur continually and will be commented on as they occur throughout this volume.

8

Attention as Directed Consciousness

In Chapter 6, consciousness was defined as an epiphenomenon of the functioning consciousness system. Activation of the locus coeruleus-driven reticular activating system (RAS), of the thalamic–basal gangliar brain stem *awareness* system, and of the nucleus accumbens, substantia innominata, and posterior inferior parietal lobe *self-awareness* system produces a generalized state of alertness and awareness. However, this condition if not further directed would be without sufficient specificity or concentration to cope with critical events in the environment. To enhance the effectiveness of consciousness activity, higher organisms are endowed with a complex consciousness-directing mechanism known as the attentional apparatus. This apparatus evaluates environmental events that are deemed biologically significant, directs consciousness more specifically onto those events, ties those events directly into the activated self-concept system, and mobilizes all resources to deal most effectively with them.

Also implied in the function of *attending*, i.e., of directing consciousness specifically onto the pertinent events in the environment, is the function of *nonattending*, i.e., of diverting consciousness from insignificant events. It is apparent that the act of attending must involve a vast active effort of reducing the impact of insignificant stimuli. Consequently, the functions of the attentional mechanisms are first to discriminate between the significant and the insignificant and second to simultaneously direct the attentional beam toward the significant and away from the insignificant.

Through the focusing at any given moment on the relationship of the preeminent motivational and emotional needs of the organism to the perceived realities of the external environment, attention is able to extract the essential ingredients in that interaction and to prepare the animal for appropriate responses. Not only does attention define the problem, it alerts the appropriate response systems and even provides the general energy necessary for the response. Perhaps most important of all, attention brings the total of these coordinated perceptions, motivations, and adaptations into contact with the self through the mechanism of attending, so as to enable the organism to mobilize all of its resources to cope with the particular situation attended.

The Phases of Attention—Early and Late

Using psychological and behavioral parameters of perception, Broadbent (1977) studied the process of attention and the various stages through which it passes. Through experimentation, he developed evidence that the attentive processes occur in two phases: the first, a passive one, in which stimuli are scanned globally for physical properties and the second, an active one, in which stimuli are searched specifically for meaning and total organismic significance. In the first phase, general cognitive features (e.g., verbal versus nonverbal) and general emotional features (i.e., the type and intensity of emotional charge) are evaluated and the further course to be taken by that stimulus determined. In this preattentive process (i.e., the process that determines which of several stimuli are to be attended to and which are to be ignored), several other parameters are also evaluated: physical properties (intensity, spatial arrangement, novelty, etc.), semantic characteristics (word frequency, letter order, etc.), association of meaning (doctor–nurse, black–white, etc.), and emotionality (pleasant or unpleasant). On the basis of these determinations specific stimuli in the environment are selected for further processing while the rest of the environment remains unperceived.

In the second phase of attention, recognition is accomplished through the matching of stimuli of given characteristics (i.e., physical properties, semantic properties, meaning, and emotionality) against engrams of similar characteristics that have been reactivated in the brain. However, the early passive global scanning phase of the preattentive process does this superficially while more specific evaluative processes are carried on in this second phase. Navon (1977) has presented a similar version of the attentive process. He has used the term *suggestion* to describe the early global flow of information from stimuli into the perceptual system and the term *inquiry* for the later detailed probing of the environment by the system to test a hypothesis brought up by suggestion. Lumsden and Wilson (1981) in the passage quoted in Chapter 5 refer to the two phases of attention respectively as the *preperceptual* and the *perceptual*.

Most experimental studies suggest that the first phase of the attentive process is generally an unconscious one while the second phase is often acutely conscious. For example, in Broadbent's first passive phase of the preattentive process where the direction of attention is determined by the physical properties of the stimulus, the observer is usually unaware at first as to what those physical characteristics are. Only in the later stage of attention when significance is attached to those physical properties, does he become aware of them.

These early behavioral interpretations of the two stages of attention were soon supported by a number of electrophysiological studies. Particularly interesting are those studies of evoked potential equivalents of different stages of attention. Hillyard and his group (Hink and Hillyard, 1978) have done much of the experimental work on which these hypotheses are based. Following Broadbent's division of the attentive process into the early *stimulus set* phase and the later *response set*, Hillyard found that the N_1-P_2 (N_{100}-P_{150}) component of the *auditory* evoked potential correlated highly with behavioral activity of the first type, while the P_3 (P_{300}) component correlated highly with behavioral activity of the second. These findings were subsequently confirmed with *visual* evoked potentials. Parasuraman and Beatty (1980), in an experiment using visual stimuli of gradually increasing intensities, demonstrated that *percep-*

tion of an indistinct stimulus occurred simultaneously with the development of a significant N_1-P_2 wave while delayed *recognition* was associated with the development of a significant P_3 (P_{300}) wave. Physiologically this suggests that a flashing word stimulus, so indistinct as to be illegible, does not carry sufficient valence to maintain attention. Once recognition of the word stimulus occurs, i.e., matching up with an established engram in long-term memory, interest is maintained, attention is held, and a significant P_3 occurs.

The concept that the two stages of attention reflect activities at different levels of sensory processing in the central nervous system seems eminently plausible. Primary sensory tracts ascend in the brain stem to the thalamus which has important relays to the contiguous hypothalamus and basal ganglia. Since these areas have been shown to have significant primitive activities of motivational–emotional, cognitive, and consciousness dimensions, functional considerations suggest that they constitute the major lower center for information processing. From here the normal flow is to the particular sensory cortex for cognitive processing and to the inferior temporal lobe for motivational–emotional evaluation. From these control centers integrated information flows to the prefrontal area which controls the attention-directing activities of the amygdaloid–hippocampal complex. Finally, from the amygdaloid–hippocampal complex, the stimulus train is directed both downwards to the thalamic–basal gangliar nucleus to assume the qualities of general consciousness and upward to the posterior inferior parietal lobe to become fully endowed with the qualities of self-awareness.

This sequence of cognitive and affective informational processing is well established neurologically. It is only necessary here to consider the mechanisms through which the determination for different types of processing is made during the passage of the stimulus wave train up the brain stem, through the neocortex, and back to the amygdaloid–hippocampal complex. For convenience we will label the first component in the brain stem the upstream phase of information processing and the second, in the cortex and amygdaloid–hippocampal complex, the downstream.

Anatomy and Physiology of the Early Upstream Phase of Attention

The upstream phase of information processing, that characteristic of the early transit of the stimulus sensory train through the brain stem, is obviously not uneventful since during that passage the variety of effects characteristic of the early phase of attention are accomplished. Among these effects are a general categorization along various motivational–emotional dimensions (pleasant–unpleasant, significant–nonsignificant) and also along various cognitive dimensions (verbal–spatial, analytic–holistic, and so on). These categorizations result not only in relaying the incoming stimuli to specific tracts for specific operational treatment, i.e., conscious-unconscious, and emotion arousing or not arousing, but also as we shall see in Chapter 14 they determine whether processing will be predominantly in one hemisphere or the other.

The anatomical site for the early general scanning function of the attentional process appears to be in the area of the thalamus, hypothalamus, and basal ganglia. It is extremely interesting, yet not surprising, that the same area responsible for experiencing the subjective feelings of emotions and consciousness should serve a similar function in perception. The motivational–emotional activities of the hypothalamus, thalamus, and basal ganglia are indeed the primitive elements from which all motivational–emotional functions evolve. The interaction of motivational–emotional and cognitive influences in this area has been well established; evidence for diencephalic interactions of this type has been provided by Old's (1973) demonstration of increased unit cell activity in the hypothalamus and thalamus associated with specific sensory stimuli to which the animal has been affectively conditioned (see Chapter 13).

There is also substantial evidence that the thalamus possesses a cognitive organization sufficiently complex to accomplish the early rough scanning function hypothesized for this area. For example, in rats ablation of the entire visual cortex does not result in total blindness but rather only in markedly impaired function, implying some residual visual capacity at the thalamic level. Even in humans with lesions of area 17, there is an effect known as "blind sight" where the ability to guess at the location of objects in the environment remains intact even though the individual is effectively blind. Whether this is due to thalamic activity or to parallel processing around the lesion is not definitely known but present evidence suggests that both may be true.

Equally significant is the active involvement of thalamic nuclei in directing appropriately evaluated perceptual stimuli into the appropriate sensory channels. One of the most important functions of the early scanning phase of attention is to enhance sensory signals coming from the significant event while inhibiting sensory stimuli from other less significant events. At a primitive level, this is most easily accomplished by enhancing stimuli in the particular sensory modality (visual, auditory, tactile, etc.) in which the significant event is couched and in reducing the intensity of all of the other sensory modalities.

The neurophysiological process through which attention is concentrated in a given sensory modality is thought to be accomplished through a prefrontal lobe–thalamic feedback arrangement which inhibits electrical activity in the unattended sensory channels. One of the neurophysiological mechanisms through which the frontal lobes specifically direct the attentional beam by inhibiting the activities of irrelevant sensory systems has been worked out for rats by Skinner and Yingling (1977). These mechanisms are illustrated diagrammatically in Figure 8-1. When the mesencephalic reticular formation (another name for the upper reticular activating system) is stimulated by somatosensory stimuli, a reflex circuit is activated from the frontal cortex to the reticular thalamic nucleus which in turn inhibits the medial and lateral thalamic geniculate bodies, the transfer centers for auditory and visual stimuli, respectively. In this way, attention is withdrawn from the irrelevant sensory systems and directed to the somatosensory. Similar neurophysiological interactions exist between the hippocampus and the several thalamic nuclei so that the hippocampus may constitute an additional mechanism for the inhibitory action of the frontal lobe upon the thalamus (Swanson and Cowan, 1976). This latter important interaction is elaborated upon later in this chapter and again in Chapter 19.

There is strong evidence that nuclei in the basal ganglia are also involved in the early scanning phase of attention. Hassler (1978) has provided perhaps the most convincing evidence to implicate the basal ganglia in basic attentional processes. He

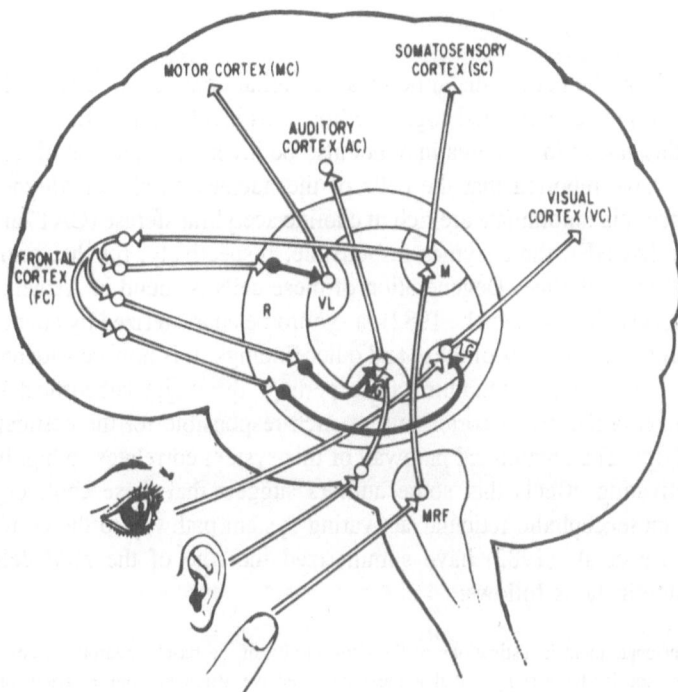

Figure 8-1 Model of prefrontal–reticular thalamic inhibitory system in humans. Abbreviations: FC, frontal cortex; MRF, mesencephalic reticular formation; R, reticular thalamic nucleus; LG, lateral geniculate; MG, medial geniculate; AC, Auditory cortex; MC, motor cortex; M, medial thalamus; VC, visual cortex; VL, nucleus ventralis lateralis. (Adapted from Skinner and Yingling, 1977.)

has reported that both in animals and in humans damage to the globus pallidus (a segment of the basal ganglia) results in severe deficits both in attentional reactivities and in consciousness phenomena. The attentional deficits resulting in humans from massive damage to this area are of a much more extreme nature than those associated with bilateral amygdalectomy and hippocampectomy so that the upstream attentional reactivities governed by basal ganglia function are more primitive and basic than are those of downstream processing. In addition, Hassler (1978) implicates strong interacting neural connections between the thalamus and the basal ganglia as accounting for the intimate involvement of both of these systems in attentional and consciousness phenomena (Fig. 2-2). These data together with those presented in Chapter 6 for the thalamic–basal gangliar seat of general consciousness establish the thalamic–basal gangliar system as the major switch center in the upstream processing of perceptive stimuli. Further evidence for the designation of the thalamic–basal gangliar system as a major subcortical center for differential hemispheric channeling of perceptual stimuli will be provided in Chapter 14 on hemispheric differentiation. (See studies by Riklan and Cooper, 1977: Glick et al., 1977; Butler, 1979; and Wood, 1975.)

Anatomy and Physiology of the Late Upstream Phase of Attention

It is not clear whether the thalamic–basal gangliar complex is sufficiently sophisticated to perform the complicated cognitive functions involved in upstream processing or whether other nuclei in that area may not also be involved. Parent et al. (1979) and Kuhar (1976) have reported that the cells of the nucleus basalis of Meynert (nbM) within the substantia innominata are rich in choline acetyltransferase (CAT) and acetylcholinesterase (ACHE), the enzymes responsible, respectively, for the synthesis and breakdown of acetylcholine. Degeneration of these cells is found in Alzheimer's disease in humans (Whitehouse et al., 1982), a syndrome characterized by attentional and memory deficits. On the basis of these and other findings, it is now considered that the nbM cells in the substantia innominata are perhaps the major subcortical source of cholinergic innervation of the cortex and as such responsible for the cortical level of electrical activity. The anatomical pathway of this system correlates so highly with its functional activating effects that some authors suggest that these cholinergic tracts represent the mesencephalic reticular activating system pathway to the cortex.

Whitehouse et al. (1982) have summarized the role of the nbM cells of the substantia innominata as follows:

> Recent anatomical investigations of the connectivity of the basalis neurons in non-human species have suggested that these cells receive afferents from a variety of sources, including the amygdala, hypothalamus, peripeduncular nucleus, midbrain, and other brain stem nuclei (Jones et al., 1976; Krettek and Price, 1978) and that, in turn, nbM neurons project to the amygdala, thalamus, hypothalamus, brain stem, olfactory bulbs, hippocampus, entorhinal cortex, and neocortex (Divac, 1975; Otterson, 1980). Hence, the nbM is in a critical position to integrate information from a variety of subcortical sources and to directly influence the cerebral cortex. The roles of the nbM in behavior and cognition remain to be defined. Psychopharmacological studies and experimental lesions suggest that the basal forebrain cholinergic pathways, particularly those projecting to the hippocampal formation (Segal and Landis, 1974) play an important role in memory processes (Smith and Swash, 1978). (p. 1238)

Coyle et al. (1983) have expanded on these interrelationships as follows:

> Studies of the activity of nbM neurons in the primate indicate that many cells exhibit rapid changes in firing in relation to different stimuli and behaviors (Rolls et al., 1979). Some neurons in particular respond to the sight of food or to delivery of a food reward, suggesting a role of this structure in feeding behavior. More generally these nuclei may contribute to reward, learning, and attentional mechanisms. (p. 1188)

The close association of the nbM neurons in the substantia innominata with the control centers in the thalamus and the amygdaloid–hippocampal complex provides a network of interaction in several areas: electrical activation, consciousness, and analysis of incoming perceptions. Early consciousness effects are further activated through stimulation of the nbM in the substantia innominata and thence onto the cortical self-awareness system. In all, the evidence appears to be strongly suggestive of a subcortical network consisting mainly of thalamic and basal gangliar nuclei that screen perceptions on their way to the cortex (upstream processing) and may again be involved with the amygdaloid–hippoccampal complex after the stimulus train has passed through the cortex (downstream processing). The role of the nbM in this process would presumably be facilitory both during upstream and downstream processing.

This interpretation fits with Broadbent's two-phase behavioral formulation of the attentional process, with the first phase vague, diffuse, and unconscious, usually insufficient to activate the substantia innominata–inferoparietal lobe axis (Fig. 7-1) and the second phase after cortical processing and downstream processing in the hippocampus sufficient to activate the self-awareness system. On the other hand, when the stimulus is cognitively or emotionally strong enough as with highly emotionally charged stimuli, it may activate awareness through the nbM cells of the substantia innominata even in the first phase. (See discussion on p. 112 on the orienting response.) The concept of the upstream and downstream processing of perception, first through the thalamic–basal gangliar complex and later after cortical processing through the amygdaloid–hippocampal complex, with the nbM facilitating transmission at both levels, appears to provide a reasonable context for the two-phase formulation of attention.

This formulation does not rule out the possibility that the hippocampus may also be involved in the upstream processing of perceptions. The work of Segal and Landis (1974) and of Smith and Swash (1978) as described by Whitehouse et al. (1982) on p. 110 is highly suggestive. Current wisdom holds that hippocampal input occurs after processing in the associative and entorhinal cortical areas has taken place; such downstream activity is certainly the predominant and perhaps even the sole manifestation of hippocampal function in perception (Moscovitch, 1979). There appears to be sufficient capacity during upsteam processing of perception in the surrounding subcortical structures such as the hypothalamus, thalamus, and basal ganglia for at least some rough cognitive and affective analysis of the impulse to be made with or without input from the amygdaloid–hippocampal complex. Edelman and Mountcastle (1978) found *recognizer* cells in the basal ganglia (not to be confused with the behavioral act of recognition) to have primitive cognitive functions that would be compatible with discriminatory activity during Broadbent's passive phase of attention. On the other hand, Wickelgren (1979), in his study of recognizer functions of the hippocampus, reported that these cell groups performed the more complex tasks of *chunking,* which is more characteristic of the later aspects of matching and relating engrams. This further supports the thesis that early simple upstream processing occurs mainly in the thalamic–basal gangliar complex while more complicated downstream processing is accomplished in the amygdaloid–hippocampal complex after passage through the cortex.

Attentional Functions of the Thalamic–Basal Gangliar Complex

The primitive scanning mechanisms of the thalamic–basal gangliar complex operating during the upstream phase of information processing support an important biological function. That function, as defined in Broadbent's study of attention, is to scan the environment generally for clues of events of motivational–emotional and cognitive significance. This first critical evaluation is followed up through other mechanisms that allow the organism to deal appropriately with the evaluated data.

On the basis of the original evaluation, specific events in the environment are judged to be of great, moderate, little, or no cognitive–affective significance. The description of each category of event and of its appropriate management follows:

1. Events of very high cognitive–affective valence. Some events are too urgent to permit more leisurely evaluation at higher cognitive–affective centers. Consequently they directly activate both the energy and directive elements of the consciousness system. Such direct activation of attention without previous full processing through the neocortex is characteristic of the "orienting response," to be described shortly.
2. Events of moderate but not urgent cognitive–affective valence. Such events are channeled into the regular tracts in the neocortex for full evaluation and then onto the amygdaloid–hippocampal complex where the subjective and objective parameters of attentional awareness are defined.
3. Events of slight cognitive–affective valence. These events are not considered sufficiently significant to warrant attentional consideration and are processed through unconscious (semicontrolled) mechanisms (to be described in Chapters 11 and 12).
4. Events of no cognitive–affective significance. These events are not processed at all and are essentially obliterated.

The Orienting Response

The orienting response represents a situation in which a perceived external event, because of its very high cognitive–affective valence, is considered to be too urgent to permit routine processing. The attentional system is thus immediately activated. Because of the acuteness of the event, the orienting response lends itself readily to experimental exploration so that many attentional mechanisms have been discovered through its study.

Studies on the orienting response are characteristically made on subjects in the relaxed state. The relaxed human or animal at rest is physiologically in an altered state of consciousness, more similar to the first stage of sleep than to the state of alertness characteristic of true consciousness. An EEG in this situation shows mainly α rhythm indicating a relatively low level of locus coeruleus and RAS activity; the individual is functioning predominantly under medial thalamic control. Nevertheless, the locus coeruleus-driven RAS is not inactivated but continues to scan the environment drowsily for significant events which may command its attention.

If an unexpected stimulus occurs, the animal responds with a stereotypical reaction known as orienting. The orienting response is a primitive reactivity common to all mammals, characterized by an overall alerting of the organism in response to a novel stimulus. For example, if a dog is lying quietly in a soundproof room, the sounding of a noise at the dog's left side will characteristically evoke the following responses: the head will be lifted and turned to the left, the ears will pick up, and the eyes will turn toward the sound; there will be increased sweating, increased GSR activity, pupillary dilation, and increased cardiovascular (pulse rate and blood pressure) responses. In addition, there will be increased activation of the EEG (β waves) and an increase in the amplitude of the late components of evoked responses, i.e., P_{300} but over the frontal cortex as much as over the parietal lobe. This overall response is nonspecific; it will be the same whether the novel stimulus is a sound, a flash of light, a touch, or an odor. Within limits, it will not vary quantitatively with the intensity of the stimulus (Sokolov, 1963).

There are two other characteristics of the orienting response that require description. For one thing, a stimulus is defined by any sudden physical change in the sensory environment; it may be caused as well by the cessation of a constant noise or of a constant light in the environment to which the animal (or human) has become adapted (habituated). The second characteristic is that of habituation itself which is the adaptation of the orienting response to the constantly repeated stimulus. For example, if a repetitious but irrelevant sound is introduced into the environment, following the initial orienting response the animal rapidly habituates to the noise and gradually returns physiologically to the baseline state. Habituation occurs when the organism concludes (consciously or unconsciously) that the stimulus is no longer relevant. The phenomenology of habituation suggests the operation of inhibitory influences* that are biologically just as important as excitatory ones.

Biologically, the orienting response serves a purpose similar to that of the early scanning phase of attention in that it identifies some element in the environment that demands further attention. However, where the scanning apparatus evaluates the entire environment for elements of interest in a relatively relaxed fashion, the orienting response, because it is activated by an implied threat, involves the second phase of the attentional process more immediately. Normally, the early and late phase of the attentional process, i.e., scanning and full attention, are represented by different mechanisms, but not unexpectedly the orienting responds involves partial elements of both mechanisms.

In electrophysiological studies, the orienting response shows a pattern intermediate between that of the early upstream processing and that of the full attentional response of downstream processing. Evoked potential studies of the orienting response show the normal N_1-P_2 configuration of upstream processing; however, the irregular P_{300} of the orienting response is earlier (250–300 msec) and over the frontal lobe rather than, as in normal downstream processing, later (350–400 msec) and over the parietal lobe. This suggests a more direct activation of the thalamic–frontal cortical circuit and of the amygdaloid–hippocampal complex in orienting than in the downstream phase of normal attention. It also suggests a somewhat lesser level of self-awareness than in normal attention since here the P_{300} is experienced mainly over the frontal rather than over the parietal lobe.

*Presumably from the thalamic–frontal cortical inhibitory circuit or from the septal–hippocampal complex.

Anatomy and Physiology of the Downstream Phase of Attention

The second phase of attention, i.e., full attention, is activated when either the orienting response or the scanning phase of attention determine, in their brief evaluation of the environmental event, that it is of sufficient interest (in either a positive or negative sense) to warrant further investigation. Under these circumstances, the attentional system is fully activated, beginning with an immediate and marked increase in RAS activity and rapidly involving the mobilization of the rest of the attentional system. Essentially this means first arousing the entire consciousness system (RAS, general awareness, and self-awareness) and secondly concentrating the total resources of that system (evaluative and responsive) in the specific direction of the given significant event.

In downstream processing, the stimulus wave train passes from the thalamic–basal gangliar complex through the nbM, up into and through the neocortex, and from there back onto the amygdaloid–hippocampal complex where the final leg of the attentional circuit is completed. The influences generated in the various neocortical systems during this passage are transmitted onto the amygdaloid–hippocampal complex to determine its management of the event: either to exercise attention and tie the event into the awareness system or alternatively not to. The final action of the amygdaloid–hippocampal center not only determines the level of consciousness for any given experience, it also controls the direction of attention and through its control of the anterior and posterior hypothalamic nuclei, the level of arousal as well.

Passage through the neocortex of course constitutes the most complicated phase of information management. It occurs for all events that have been scanned by the lower thalamic–basal gangliar complex and passed on for further processing. A complete determination of the level of significance is made during passage through the several systems that control the various behavioral modalities. Through parallel processing the wave train passes simultaneously through the inferotemporal lobe for motivational–emotional evaluation; through the involved sensory association areas for cognitive processing; through the postcentral frontal lobe for motor responses; through the prefrontal lobe for decisional input; and through the posterior inferior parietal lobe to involve the self-awareness and self-concept systems. The sum total of these evaluations are then exercised upon the amygdaloid–hippocampal system to determine the attentional behavior of that complex. However, these processes are too important and too complex to be merely interjected here since they involve such complicated procedures as recognition, memory retrieval, mental set, and other decisional operations. Accordingly, even though these processes occur physiologically at this point, their consideration will be postponed until the next chapter.

The final step in the attentional process is that in which the amygdaloid–hippocampal complex, under the influence of the various neocortical centers, directs attention and ties the event into the consciousness system. Because of the anatomical position of the amygdaloid–hippocampal complex intermediate between the brain stem and the neocortex, there is a natural tendency to assume that the complex serves a similar intermediate sequential role in the processing of perception and behavior.

However, the evidence does not appear to support that simple interpretation. The sequence of activities for sensory processing predicates previous cortical processing of the impulse train before reaching the amygdaloid–hippocampal complex; it is through such interactions that frontal cortical and inferotemporal cortical influences presumably make themselves felt.

Two pieces of evidence speak for the late involvement of the amygdaloid–hippocampal complex. The first is the complexity of matching and chunking cognitive activities in the cellular constellations of the hippocampus as reported by Wickelgren (1979). It seems unlikely though not impossible that such sophisticated maneuvers would be possible with the relatively unstructured stimuli existing in the brain stem. More importantly, the P_{300} wave characteristic of amygdaloid–hippocampal attentional activity (see Fig. 8-2) occurs rather late in the passage of the stimulus train (i.e., at 300–400 msec) at which time at least a first pass through the cortex must have occurred. It seems reasonable to speculate that although some of the activities of the amygdaloid–hippocampal complex described in this chapter may be upstream, i.e., prior to cortical processing, most are certainly downstream, i.e., secondary to cortical processing (Moscovitch, 1979).

The Role of the Amygdaloid–Hippocampal Complex in the Orienting Response and in Attention

In animals, ablation of the hippocampus results in a marked decrease in orienting reactivity (Isaacson, 1974). A similar reduction in orienting responsivity occurs in animals with ablation of the amygdala. Thus it appears that the major impulse for the orienting response is implemented through the amygdaloid–hippocampal complex. Further evidence for this interpretation stems from the finding that with isolated damage to either the prefrontal or inferior temporal lobes (both cortical areas that tend to suppress subsequent amygdaloid–hippocampal function), but with the amygdaloid–hippocampal complex intact, there is increased orienting responsivity (Isaacson, 1974).

Primary support for the thesis that the orienting response is activated through the amygdaloid–hippocampal complex comes from electrophysiological research with evoked potentials. As described in Chapter 4 and as depicted in Figure 4-5, the P_{300} wave, the final major positive deflection in the curve, occurs only when a stimulus is being most actively attended. Although the P_{300} wave of the evoked potential has been variously attributed to a variety of motivational and behavioral influences, the generally accepted position is that it is largely a function of the intensity of attention (directed consciousness) being leveled (Donchin et al., 1981). Within the context of this paradigm and of the Mesulam–Geschwind model (Fig. 7-1), with attentional activity electrical impulses (the P_{300}) would rise from the hippocampus and amygdala to impinge on the nucleus accumbens septi to activate the awareness system. Under these conditions the awareness system should reflect the P_{300} throughout its length.

Recent investigations of evoked potentials with deep intracerebral electrical probes in conscious humans have provided substantial evidence that the P_{300} apparently does originate in the hippocampus or amygdala, i.e., the rhinencephalon, and radiates up through the posterior association area and the parietal lobe. Studies by Halgren et al. (1980), in a conscious epileptic patient being tested for intracerebral foci of hyperirritability, strongly support this interpretation. An illustration of the comparative response to unattended (dark line) and attended (light line) stimuli at the cortex, amygdala, hippocampal gyrus, and hippocampus is given in Figure 8-2, where the difference between the two curves in the P_3 range represents the P_{300} wave. As can be seen this is greatest in the amygdala and both hippocampal regions. Similar results were found in a study by Wood et al. (1979) where the deepest electrodes in the area of the hippocampus and amygdala showed the largest P_{300} waves. Another finding of interest in both studies was the greater radiation of these reactivities up toward the parietal lobe (the central electrodes) as opposed to the occipital lobes. Even more provocative was the finding that the right central electrode showed significantly greater P_{300} responses throughout than did the left central electrode in both studies, although both patients tested had epileptic foci of irritability in the left hemisphere.*

Thus from the evidence of ablation studies and of the EEG patterns of response, it appears that orienting reactivity, the most elemental form of conscious attention, derives largely from the amygdaloid–hippocampal complex. In this paradigm the orienting response is a warning mechanism to alert the organism that a significant event

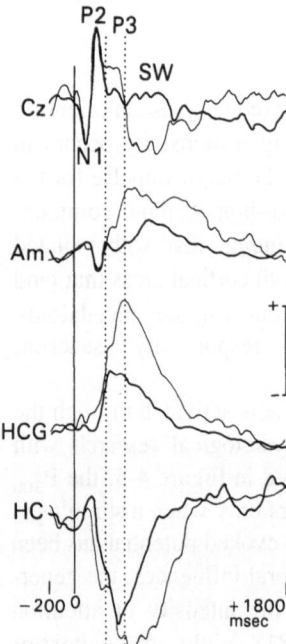

Figure 8-2 Evoked potentials from intracranial electrodes to attended and unattended stimuli. Abbreviations: Cz, cortex; Am, amygdala; HCG, hippocampal gyrus; HC, hippocampus. (From Halgren et al., 1980. Reproduced by permission.)

*The possible significance of this lies in the evidence that the self-awareness system may be more strongly represented in the right than in the left hemisphere (see Chapter 7). It is of further interest in that damage to the right inferior parietal lobe produces greater impairment of the orienting response than does similar damage in the left hemisphere (Heilman and Watson, 1977).

either in the external or internal environments is occurring, and that an additional level of organismic involvement is required. That additional level is achieved first through increased stimulation of the thalamic–basal gangliar complex and second through activation of the second stage of attention which brings into readiness the entire self-awareness system with all of the resources that system may have at its disposal.

To further increase the biological effectiveness of the orienting response, the arousal system is simultaneously activated to elicit the necessary motivational–emotional response appropriate to the situation. Increased energy reserves associated with changes in body physiology are also activated in this response. The anatomical and physiological innervation of the arousal system by the amygdaloid–hippocampal complex has been described by Isaacson (1972). He has presented a hypothesis based on experimental data that the relative balance between the emergency and the vegetative response systems is determined in the hypothalamus under the direct control of the amygdaloid–hippocampal complex. Electrical stimulation of the amygdala produces excitation in both the posterior and anterior hypothalamic areas with greater effect on the former; hence the overall effect is to stimulate emergency reactivities. Electrical stimulation of the septum and hippocampus essentially produces inhibition of the posterior hypothalamic center with predominantly vegetative consequences. Similarly, ablation of the amygdala results in an excess of activity in the neurons of the anterior hypothalamic vegetative system while ablation of the hippocampus or septum results in overactivity in the posterior hypothalamic emergency system. Presumably, these anatomicophysiological connections account for the arousal and activation effects that accompany the orienting response.

Directional Activities of the Amygdaloid–Hippocampal Complex

One of the most unique cognitive characteristics of attention is its selective directional quality. The orienting response as previously described involves not only a generalized alerting of attentional mechanisms but a focusing of perceptive and motor reactivities in the specific direction of the activating influences. The ability of the hippocampus to direct a beam of attention into a three-dimensional external environment is apparently facilitated by the geometric arrangement of spatial representation within it. In this respect, the hippocampus is closest in structure and spatial transformation to the parietal lobe. O'Keefe and Black (1978) have offered the so-called hippocampal cognitive map theory which postulates that in the hippocampus a three-dimensional map of the surrounding environment is reconstructed on the basis of which sensory input from that environment can be analyzed directionally. Once the location of the significant stimulus has been identified, appropriate mechanisms are activated to focus the attentional beam through inhibition of attention directed in all other directions.

It appears that both the previously described thalamic–frontal cortical feedback circuit (Fig. 8-1) and a directionally defined activity of the hippocampal–amygdaloid complex constitute the mechanisms through which the efferent response of appropriately directing the beam is accomplished. Apparently this effect occurs not only through stimulation of the pertinent sensory channels, but equally significantly through the simultaneous inhibition of access to awareness by all other sensory channels. For example, the selection of vision as the critical channel involves the simultaneous inhibition of auditory, somatosensory, and other sensory channels. The focusing of attention on a given area in the visual field may involve the relative inhibition of stimuli coming from elsewhere in the visual field. Many experiments illustrate these principles. If evoked potentials are being simultaneously elicited to flashes and clicks, attention focused on either will result in a reduction in the amplitude of the evoked potential response to the other. Similarly, Posner et al. (1980) showed that in a given visual field reaction times to stimuli in a peripheral area being attended are significantly lower than for those in the central area even when the attended area is distant from the central one subtended by the fovea.

There is experimental evidence to suggest that the amygdaloid–hippocampal complex may carry out its attentional–directing functions through cognitive excitatory–inhibitory mechanisms similar to those previously described for the effects of this complex on arousal. The putative *inhibitory role of the hippocampus* and the *stimulatory role of the amygdala* have been described by several eminent neurobiologists including Gray (1972), Douglas (1972), and Isaacson and Pribram (1975). These two neural centers, anatomically adjacent to one another, exercise antagonistic effects on the arousal system through excitatory or inhibitory effects on the anterior and posterior hypothalamic nuclei; it is postulated that they exercise similar excitatory–inhibitory control over brain stem transmission of sensory impulses (Swanson and Cowan, 1976). In this paradigm, the hippocampal–amygdaloid complex represents one major control center for the control of excitatory–inhibitory balance in the brain, while the thalamic–frontal feedback circuit constitutes another. In all probability, the activities of these two centers are closely coordinated.

Several features in the representation of attention as a directed beam are to be emphasized. First, the beam of attention may be mild or intense depending upon the level of cognitive or motivational–emotional significance and on the corresponding level of arousal and activation. Second, the diameter of the beam may be narrow (focused) or wide (diffuse). Third, there is a central beam of attention in which contact with the consciousness system is most complete and a fringe of awareness in which contact with the consciousness system is less complete. Events in the environment are either acutely attended to and rate highly in individual's awareness (focused attention), partially attended to and having only a slight level of awareness (fringe), or unattended to (unconscious). Events are brought into acute awareness from the environment as are memories from the unconscious and both are returned to unconsciousness as the sweep of the attentional beam passes on (see Fig. 22-1).

Stimulatory Activity of the Amygdala

It appears from this description that the amygdaloid–hippocampal complex has a variety of active excitatory functions, but many of its activities also contain inhibitory elements. The excitatory activities include (1) generation of the orienting response, (2) locating of the orienting stimulus in space and directing the beam of attention appropriately, (3) activating the arousal system during the orienting response, and (4) connecting attended engrams to the self-awareness system. Several of these activities, e.g., generation of the orienting response and activating the arousal system, apparently are integrated in both the hippocampus and amygdala; however, the hippocampus appears to be the more important functional center in those processes where inhibitory influences are the greatest.

As opposed to the hippocampus, the amygdala tends to play a more active role both in emotional and cognitive functions. The active role of the amygdala in the expression of aggressive behavior was described in Chapter 3. Other work has indicated that the amygdala is the center in which sensory and emotional stimuli are actively integrated to induce emotional responses (Kaada, 1982). The amygdala is also intimately involved in attentional mechanisms as indicated by the origin of the P_{300} equally in amygdala and hippocampus (Fig. 8-2).

A recent paper by Murray and Mishkin (1985) suggests that the amygdala plays an important integrative role in cognitive performance. These investigators taught monkeys unimodal (visual *or* tactual) and crossed bimodal (visual *and* tactual) associational recognition tasks. They found, in their own words that "Amygdalectomized monkeys, like their controls, accurately recognized objects both visually and tactually; yet, unlike their controls they failed to recognize by vision an object they had just examined by touch" (p. 604). Hippocampectomized monkeys, on the other hand, had very little impairment on either unimodal or bimodal tasks.

This evidence supports the concept that in attention and cognition the amygdala and hippocampus function as an integrated unit with amygdala responsible for more stimulatory influences and the hippocampus for the more inhibitory. In emotional reactivities, the amygdala also appears to play an active role in integrating sensory and emotional stimuli (Kaada, 1982; Mishkin, 1982). The role of the hippocampus in these latter reactivities, although more obscure, may again be inhibitory (see Chapter 19).

Hippocampal θ Rhythm and Hippocampal Inhibition

A finding of great interest in all mammals (possibly excepting primates and man) is the presence of a slow θ rhythm (4–8/sec) in the hippocampus during periods of intensely attended activity (Winson, 1985). This activity occurs during highly motivated events such as predatory, escape, and searching activities in the alert stage. Paradoxically it occurs also in REM sleep. The activation of θ rhythms in the hippocampus is accomplished through the neurotransmitter norepinephrine so that disruption of the activity of that neurotransmitter in the hippocampus results in an obliteration of θ rhythm (Dahl et al., 1983). Since norepinephrine drives alert consciousness as well as EEG β rhythm, its direct relationship to θ activity in the hippocampus during periods of attended activity is highly consistent.*

---

*Hippocampal θ activity during REM sleep when norepinephrine activity is low is apparently driven by cholinergic influences. See Chapter 22.

Further evidence of the significant role of the hippocampus in the attentional process has been presented by Bennett (1975). He found θ-wave activity in the frequency range of 4–7/sec to emanate from electrodes in the hippocampus under a variety of conditions that appeared to indicate intense attentional activity. Bennett refers to the work of Arastyan et al. (1959) who observed that θ activity in the cat's hippocampus appeared regularly in association with the orienting response, while at other times hippocampal electrical activity was characteristically β or γ, i.e., fast desynchronized. Bennett performed a variety of further studies and concluded that "the occurence of dorsal hippocampal θ in the cat is related to specific processes of attention to environmental stimuli" (p. 96). A similar effect in the hippocampi of rabbits when acutely attending to an environmental stimulus was first reported by Green and Arduini (1954). Cats, on the other hand, showed maximum θ rhythm in the hippocampus during predatory activities, events certainly calling for the most intense attention (Robinson, 1980).

What is the significance of hippocampal θ activity during directed alert activity? Winson (1985) postulates that such activity constitutes a mechanism for cognitive processing of material that comes in during the day. This process is apparently continued in mammals during REM sleep as, in computer terminology, a kind of "off-lined processing." This view was first advanced by Jouvet (1974) and has recently been supported, although in a somewhat different form, by Crick and Mitcheson (1983).

Presuming for the moment that this formulation is correct, and there seems to be substantial evidence to support it, what is the nature of θ activity in the hippocampus? The origin of the θ wave has been traced back to the septum, a generally inhibitory structure in the limbic system, most important in repressing spontaneous rage reactions (Chapter 3). In view of the fact that most hippocampal functions are inhibitory (Gray, 1970), it seems reasonable to hypothesize that θ activity in the hippocampus is associated with inhibitory activity. This interpretation is supported by the work of Winson and Abzug (1977) who found that stimulatory impulses were able to pass directly through the hippocampus without "gating" (i.e., blocking) only during deep slow-wave sleep when there was no θ wave present in the hippocampus; contrariwise, such impulses were "gated" during directed alert activity and during REM sleep when there was β activity in the EEG and θ activity in the hippocampus.

The fact that the hippocampus should play a predominantly inhibitory role in the attentional and particularly in the memory retrieval process should not be surprising. Attention and memory retrieval are by definition selective mechanisms utilizing processes of trial and error in which rejection of inappropriate matches rather than mere random matching is the key element.

Relationship of the Thalamic–Basal Gangliar Complex and the Amygdaloid–Hippocampal Complex in Attentional Activities

The two centers, the thalamic–basal gangliar and the amygdaloid–hippocampal, operating in tandem control all of the intricate mechanisms associated with attentional activities. The functions of the thalamic–basal gangliar complex, although more primitive and less complex, are also more critical. Indeed, where major damage occurs in this complex (usually due to strokes), consciousness and attentional activities in humans become severely impaired. If damage is extensive enough, total coma ensues. Where it is more localized to the thalamic and hypothalamic areas, akinetic mutism with impaired consciousness and loss of attentional responses results.

Conversely, as will be described in detail in the next chapter, total surgical ablation of both amygdalae and hippocampi may be performed in humans (for the treatment of intractable epilepsy) without significant effects on consciousness or attentional capacities. Obviously, major control for these latter activities lies in the thalamic–basal gangliar complex. On the other hand, more subtle reactivities such as the ability to recognize relatively recent experiences or to learn new ones are essentially lost. Thus with amygdaloid–hippocampal ablation, primitive consciousness and attentional capacities are retained but more refined ones are missing.

Mishkin (1982) has suggested an arrangement similar to ours for the interactions between the thalamus and the amygdaloid–hippocampal complex. He writes (as reported in Reiser, 1984):

> . . . a neural model is presented, based largely on evidence from studies in monkeys, postulating that coded representations of stimuli are stored in the higher-order sensory (i.e., association) areas of the cortex whenever stimulus activation of these areas also triggers a cortico-limbo-thalamo-cortical circuit. This circuit, which could act as either an imprinting or rehearsal mechanism, may actually consist of two parallel circuits, one involving the amygdala and dorsomedial nucleus of the thalamus, and the other the hippocampus and anterior nuclei. The stimulus representation stored in cortex by action of these circuits is seen as mediating three different memory processes: recognition, which occurs when the stored representation is reactivated via the original sensory pathway; recall, when it is reactivated via any other pathway; and association, when it activates other stored representations (sensory, affective, spatial, motor) via the outputs of the higher-order sensory areas to the relevant structures. (p. 85)

This formulation is not inconsistent with that presented in this volume but in addition invokes thalamic activation as arising subsequent to that of the amygdaloid–hippocampal complex in the processes of active recognition and awareness. Perhaps the most plausible theorem would postulate the existence of a circuit in which the thalamic–basal gangliar complex would act both initially as a screening device in upstream processing and would also be reactivated subsequently as the core of the consciousness system in downstream processing. Mishkin's proposal is also compatible with our previous theorizing on the balancing effects of the two circuits, the stimulatory amygdala and dorsalmedial thalamus complex and the inhibitory hippocampal–anterior thalamus complex. However, Mishkin's formulation is, to my mind, less complete because it does not stress the two-phase nature of attentional activities.

Expanding further on Mishkin's work, Reiser (1984) writes:

> More recently his group has uncovered evidence that leads them to postulate a second system, in which stimulus representations stored in the cortex are connected to the striatal complex or basal ganglia. This cortico-striatal system appears to function independently of and in parallel with the cortico-limbic memory system just described. Mishkin calls this cortico-striatal system a *habit* system, since it involves

noncognitive links to subcortical structures. He tentatively proposes that since the striatal complex is older than the limbic system and cortex (i.e., precedes them in phylogenesis), it would be reasonable to assume that it precedes them in ontogenesis as well. This proposal is indeed supported by developmental studies of infant monkeys. Speculating further, Mishkin (1982) asks if the learning process is actually shared by the two systems—the one for what he terms "habit memory" (referring to learned motor responses that occur without stimulus recognition) and the other for cognitive memory as we know it.

This second system postulated by Mishkin (1982) would be somewhat analogous to upstream processing as described in this chapter but even more comparable to the unconscious processing of procedural data as described in Chapter 11 and 12. As will be further elaborated in those chapters, unconscious processing of both episodic and procedural material is accomplished mainly at the level of the thalamic-basal gangliar complex. Episodic (substantive) material is processed largely through thalamic and possibly early hippocampal activities, while procedural material is processed largely through basal gangliar activities. The interaction of these two activities, as illustrated in the diagram of the thalamic–basal gangliar complex (Fig. 2-2) accounts for many of the effects of unconscious upstream processing for both episodic (substantive) and procedural (structural) data.

Experimental Demonstration of Upstream and Downstream Processing

The integrated operation of upstream and downstream processing in the normal intact human can be demonstrated experimentally. The thesis that both unconscious upstream and conscious downstream processing occur simultaneously during normal perception is supported in experimental studies examining reaction times and evoked potential patterns to different cognitive elements of a single visual stimulus. For example, word stimuli may be utilized as tests for more primitive responses to physical characteristics (color, position of a letter in the word, etc.) or for more cognitive characteristics (meaning). Posner and Wilkinson (1969) have shown that differentiation of the physical properties of a stimulus occurs with the N_1-P_2 wave at about 100 msec, while processing for meaning occurs with the P_{300} wave at 300–400 msec (Fig. 8-3). Thus it appears that processing for the physical characteristics of a stimulus occurs early during upstream passage (100 msec) but that processing for cognitive characteristics occurs later during downstream passage of the stimulus (at 400 msec). These data suggest that different mechanisms are involved in the processing of physical and cognitive elements of the same stimulus.

Posner (1980) has postulated that the most plausible explanation for the early dual processing of the same stimulus as shown in Figure 8-3 would be parallel processing through different channels for different analyses. If that occurs no later than 100 msec after stimulation and perhaps as early as 60–80 msec, it appears unlikely that channeling takes place in the cortex. Rather the occurrence of such an early reaction at 60–80 msec provides an example of upstream processing in the thalamic–basal gangliar

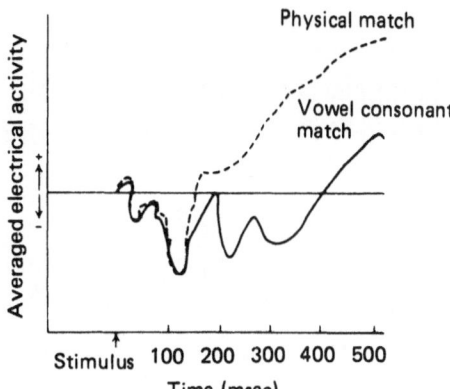

Figure 8-3 Evoked potential to letter stimuli evaluated for physical and semantic characteristics. From Posner, 1978. Reproduced with permission.)

complex as well as an example of parallel processing. Presumably, the early 60- to 80-msec event takes place in the thalamic–basal gangliar complex and the late 350-msec event in the amygdaloid–hippocampal complex.

The interaction of these two circuits, important as it is in attentional activities, is equally important in the processes of recognition and memory retrieval (to be reviewed in the next chapter) and in the processes of conscious and unconscious cognition (to be reviewed in Chapter 12). The exact mode of interaction of these neural entities is not presently known, although the hypothesis offered by Mishkin (1982) seems eminently plausible.

The most significant step in the downstream processing of information, that occurring in the neocortex intermediate in the passage of the stimulus train from the thalamic–basal gangliar complex to the amygdaloid–hippocampal complex, was deliberately omitted from the discussion in this chapter. As previously stated that was done not because that step was not important enough to be considered, but rather because it was too important to be considered superficially. Accordingly, the next chapter will be devoted to the discussion of that most important intermediate stage of information processing.

Recognition, Memory Retrieval, Mental Set, and Other Decisional Operations of the Neocortex

In the last chapter, the attentional process was presented somewhat mechanically as a two-phase evaluating process—upstream and downstream—with the two phases activated, respectively, at the subcortical thalamic–basal gangliar complex and after substantial processing in the cortex, in the amygdaloid–hippocampal complex. Subject to influences impinging on them from the surrounding behavioral systems, these centers either (1) activate or fail to activate the consciousness system, (2) excite or inhibit arousal and brain activation, (3) tie positively evaluated events into the consciousness system, and (4) appropriately direct the beam of attention.

This description of the attentional process provides mechanisms for the tying into consciousness of significant events from the external and internal (visceral) environments, but it neglects other major processes involved in this operation. For example, the evaluative process through which significance is determined (the "recognition" process) is only vaguely suggested. The mechanisms through which consolidated mental engrams are brought into awareness (memory retrieval) have also not really been described. The nature of continuous conscious mentation (thinking) is patently different from the artificially isolated single attentional events described in the last chapter. Finally, the entire issue of "mental set," which to a large extent monitors the thinking process, has been generally ignored. Even though attentional mechanisms do establish the general course of conscious mentation, these other processes strongly affect the manner in which those attentional mechanisms operate.

Cognitive Processing during Attention (Perception versus Recognition)

Earlier, the Parasuraman and Beatty (1980) study was described in which perception of an external event was shown to occur early in processing, coincident with the

N_1-P_2 wave at about 100 msec, while recognition was shown to occur later, coincident with the P_3 wave at 350–400 msec. An important parameter in the distinction between "perception" and "recognition" in the Parasuraman and Beatty experiment appears to be the matching of the external sensory pattern with some internal sensory engram and the bringing of this to awareness. Some matching presumably occurs in the early passive phase of attention, but apparently not of sufficient significance to warrant recognition (i.e., activation into the self-awareness system). Perception without recognition is a passive process in which the vague outlines are perceived with little interest; perception with recognition is the consequence of an active process of matching externally perceived engrams against internal engrams which allows a full evaluation of the cognitive, motivational, and emotional significance of the event to the entire self-concept. The evidence seems clear that perception without recognition is characteristic of the first stage of attention while recognition and identification of significance are functions of the second stage.

The mechanisms governing the operation of recognition are only now being uncovered. On the basis of evidence deduced from electrophyiological responses to various illusions, Gregory (1975) concludes that the brain actively processes perceptions in terms of both innate mechanisms and past experiences, thus imposing order and meaning upon engrams derived from either within or without the brain. Gregory uses the paradigm of object identification by computers as a model for types of brain mechanisms presumably involved in processing perceptions. He writes:

> . . . lines, corner, edges, and so on may be informational units, like phonemes; scenes (sets of objects viewed from a given position) may be "parsed" like sentences. The corollary notion is that we derive meaning from retinal images rather as we derive meaning from sentences, and that both work by following the rules of a "generative grammar" much as described by Chomsky for language. But the current view is that, for both language and scene analysis, far more stored information of object characteristics (data base) is required than was supposed necessary by Chomsky and the first enthusiasts of generative grammars. The rules and forms of sentences are not sufficient: the meanings of words as based on experience of object situations are important also. This direction of thought can lead to regarding perceptions (and sentences), entertained and tested by perceptual processes, as like hypotheses in science.

As Gregory describes it, the visual parsing of objects is like verbal parsing except that here spatial outlines constitute the elements on the basis of which matching takes place. The difference between the upstream parsing process in the thalamic–basal gangliar complex and the downstream matching process in the amygdaloid–hippocampal complex is reflected in the functions of the corresponding cells in the two areas. The "recognizer" cells in the basal ganglia described by Edelman and Mountcastle (1978) respond only to relatively primitive cognitive qualities (shape, color, etc.) while the recognizer cells in the hippocampus described by Wicklegren (1979) respond to complex chunks of cognitive information. Consequently, identification at the thalamic–basal gangliar center is vague and general (perception) while that at the amygdaloid–hippocampal center is highly specific (recognition).

The definition of recognition as the process of matching external perceptions against existing internal correlates, implies a second level of activity. That is "memory," the reservoir of all such internal neural constellations against which external perceptions are matched. The process of fitting certain perceptual patterns to existing memory patterns is usually unconscious and differs in that respect from the end product of memory retrieval. Recognition involves running a given percept through long term memory (LTM) till a suitable match occurs, at which time recognition is established, with or without conscious retrieval of the initial memory. In memory retrieval, a pertinent perception or thought, activated by proper motivation, induces a search through long-term memory to bring the sought for recollection to awareness. The two mechanisms are obviously related, but in the case of recognition, the function of memory is passive while in memory retrieval, it is more active.

"Matching" is presumably accomplished through closeness of the neural configuration of the percept to that of the related long term memory. The more points the two configurations have in common, the more apt the memory constellation is to be reactivated, albeit at the unconscious level, and the more readily recognition is completed. Matching may be done against veridical engrams in long term memory, as in recognizing another person; against abstract engrams in LTM, as in identifying an unknown species of animal as a dog; and against symbolic engrams in LTM, as in recognizing a long forgotten name.

A parenthetical note here about the mental mode of matching as opposed to the computer mode. Mental matching is done through a series of approximations through the cognitive abstraction apparatus (Oden and Massaro, 1978). Perceptions are run through different abstraction channels until the engram with the closest fit is uncovered (see recognition memory in Lumsden–Wilson chart, Fig. 5-4). Computers thus far are unable to completely abstract the essence of a given concept; for example, they cannot identify the letter "A" in all of its multiple configurations. Animal memory is immeasurably larger than computer memory so that the number of existing engrams against which a given perception may be matched is vast. It is in the very looseness of matching, both in recognition (mental approximation versus computer identification) and in association (mental loose associations versus computer absolute associations) that the superiority of brain cognition over computer cognition lies. This constitutes the so-called fuzzy logic of brain function, which despite its title, is actually advantageous.

Affective Processing during Attention

Just as all perceptual stimuli receive cognitive evaluation both early during upstream processing at the thalamic–basal gangliar complex and later during downstream processing in the neocortex, so also do they receive motivational–emotional evaluation. The mechanisms through which such evaluations are accomplished are presumably similar to those involving cognitive processing, namely a matching of the cognitive elements and then the assumption of the affective valence of the existing related engrams. However, new affective valence may also be contributed by the specific motivational–emotional influences being exercised in a particular situation. These affective charges would be generated in the motivational–emotional system and would be superimposed on the identified cognitive perception in the manner described in Chapter 5. The exact mechanisms by which emotional valence is either established or superimposed are unknown; presumably identification would be through the recognition apparatus while superimposition of emotional valence would be through association.

Most significant is the fact that some sort of unconscious recognition of the emotional component of an event occurs earlier than cognitive recognition of the same event. Indeed recognition of the emotional valence of a percept may occur in the absence of conscious cognitive recognition of the stimulus itself. Kunst-Wilson and Zajonc (1980), using a paradigm based on the established preference of subjects for familiar over nonfamiliar stimuli, tested thresholds for recognition at the cognitive level versus that at the affective level (like–dislike). They found that their subjects were able to express their affective preference correctly for familiar objects at exposures below those necessary for conscious cognitive recognition. They concluded that affective processing of stimuli was achieved at a lower neural level in the brain than was cognitive processing. This study is supportive of the concept of the differential upstream processing of emotional and cognitive stimuli at the subcortical level with the first more specific and the second more diffuse.

The Kunst-Wilson and Zajonc study suggests that *major affective evaluation may occur at the subcortical level in the thalamic–basal gangliar complex.* There is substantial evidence to support this position, evidence that will be presented in Chapter 13 and 14. However, affective screening also occurs during the downstream phase of processing in the neocortex. This is exercised mainly under the paradigm of mental set, to be discussed later in this chapter.

The Neurophysiology of Memory Retrieval

The processes of memory retrieval are closely allied to those of recognition except that the former are implemented largely through the associational apparatus while the latter are activated largely through the abstraction apparatus. Behaviorally, memory retrieval is best considered as the function of a given mental set, systematically probing long-term memory stores to select the desired engram and bring it to awareness. The entities involved in this process comprise at least the self-concept system (ending in the inferoparietal lobe), the motivational system (ending in the inferotemporal lobe), and the executive system (the prefrontal lobe), all acting in an integrated fashion upon the thalamic–basal gangliar centers and the amygdaloid–hippocampal complex. Anderson (1983) has described the probing operation of memory retrieval as a systematic scanning along associational lines (see Figs. 5-2 and 5-4). Although these descriptions are somewhat vague, they loosely define the neurophysiological parameters of the process.

Memory retrieval may start at the inner end of the cognitive apparatus with a given thought activating a desired memory or it may begin as in recognition with a particular perception activating a hidden memory. In either event, since memory retrieval is a true attentional process, it is necessary to postulate the involvement of both attentional centers, the brain stem thalamic–basal gangliar and the rhinencephalic amygdaloid–hippocampal. Furthermore, it must be assumed that regardless of the origin of the memory retrieval impulse (internal from thought processes or external from perception), the order of retrieval must originate in the thalamic–basal gangliar complex (upstream) and terminate in the amygdaloid–hippocampal (downstream).

Evidence for the thesis that both the dorsal median thalamus and the hippocampi are involved in memory retrieval comes from anatomical studies of patients with amnesia. Much of the work on the human amnesic syndrome has been done in subjects with Korsakoff's syndrome, a condition where the dorsal medial thalamus and mammillary bodies are more characteristically implicated than is the hippocampus (Victor et al., 1971). Since both the dorsal medial thalamus and the mammillary bodies are in close neural connection with the hippocampus by way of the septum (Swanson and Cowan, 1976), there is anatomical evidence to suggest an interaction. Consequently, there is every reason to consider the dorsal medial thalamic nucleus as the early component of the frontal lobe–hippocampal attentional and memory retrieval systems.

A different amnesic syndrome develops with damage to the amygdaloid–hippocampal complex. The classic case of bilateral hippocampal damage was described by Milner (1966) in a patient H.M. who had a bilateral amygdalectomy and hippocampectomy for intractable epilepsy. After surgery, H.M. developed what appeared to be an essentially total inability to establish new memories although old preoperative ones remained intact. Neither was there any difficulty in establishing brief or short-term memories; the deficit appeared to be in the process of consolidation. Subsequent work with similarly operated upon individuals has established this type of amnesic syndrome as characteristic of hippocampal dysfunction.

The original interpretation of the findings in both of these amnesic syndromes was that of a deficit in encoding of short-term memories into intermediate and long-term ones. This interpretation is apparently valid and will be discussed shortly. However, subsequent work by Weiskrantz and Warrington (1970) indicated that the problem was not only one of consolidation of such memories but also one of retrieval.

Deficits in Memory Retrieval and Recall

Weiskrantz and Warrington demonstrated in amnesic patients that some memories were formed more or less normally but that the subjects were unable to retrieve them without assistance. On the other hand, when adequate cues were offered, memory retrieval but not conscious recall was essentially normal.*

Although Weiskrantz (1978) never specifically designates this aspect of the amnesic syndrome as an inability to bring unconscious memories to awareness, his descriptions suggest that this is at least part of the mechanism involved. He writes:

> By now it is known that amnesic subjects can learn and remember a variety of tasks when they are tested in particular ways. The only person who remains unconvinced about this is the amnesic subject himself, who persists in failing to acknowledge that his performance is based on specific past experience, or may occasionally confabulate about such a basis. (p. 382)

Weiskrantz (1978) concludes:

*The entire question of the differences in the processing of factual (episodic) data as opposed to that of instrumental (procedural) skills will be discussed in Chapter 10.

> . . . it appears that the patients themselves on one level do not have access to their memories; nor is it necessary as a practical requirement that they have such access in order for their memories to be tested and demonstrated objectively. None of the current theories of the amnesic syndrome appear to have focused on the striking dissociation between the subjects' commentaries and their objective performance, which suggests a dissociation between levels of processing rather than a failure on any particular level. (p. 385)

The deficit described is clearly at least in part an inability to bring long-term memories to awareness. It appears probable that the retrieval of memories involves a process similar to that of attention during recognition. One can conceptualize memory retrieval as a several-step process beginning with (1) the identification of a long-term memory engram in the unconscious reservoir with a short-term engram of perception or thought, followed by (2) the reactivation of the long-term memory engram through the direction of the energizing beam of attention, and finally (3) the connection of the long-term memory engram with the awareness system through the tying-in function of the hippocampus. As will be seen, the amygdaloid–hippocampal complex is essential only for retrieval of factual (episodic) data. Certain types of automatic activities and behaviors (procedural) can be functionally retrieved (although not to consciousness) even in the absence of hippocampal function.

In hippocampal amnesia, where the anatomical deficit is acutely imposed through surgical intervention, the inability to retrieve episodic material covers the period of three years prior to surgery; older memories remain retrievable (Milner et al., 1968). This finding suggests that after three years memories become sufficiently consolidated to be retrievable to full consciousness through the thalamic–basal gangliar component of the memory retrieval system even without the involvement of the amygdaloid–hippocampal complex. Mishkin's (1982) model hypothesizes an intimate interaction of the two systems which would explain the compensatory activities of each in the absence of the other. This theory was discussed in Chapter 8.

Deficiencies in Consolidation (the Inability to Learn)

The second major deficit in both diencephalic and bitemporal amnesia lies in the area of establishing new memories (the inability to learn). This learning disability is particularly marked for episodic data (i.e., memories dealing with specific people, places, and events) and less true for procedural data (i.e., memories of particular procedures).

The physiological deficit represented here apparently derives from some deficiency in the consolidating process. That process was described in Chapter 5 as one in which synaptic connections were strengthened, first physiologically and then anatomically, through the repetition of similar impulses by way of abstraction or association mechanisms onto the same neurons. The identical nature of the deficits in learning in both types of amnesia suggests similar defects in this physiological function in the two syndromes.

Extrapolating from the roles of the thalamic–basal gangliar complex and of the amygdaloid–hippocampal complex in attentional, recognition, and memory retrieval processes, it would seem that the defect must be at the level of the matching process in the abstraction and associational networks. Matching mechanisms in abstraction and association are critical processes in recognition and memory retrieval; they are equally critical in learning. Learning takes place only when a new experience is superimposed on an old partially learned experience and becomes better consolidated with repeated experiences. But to accomplish this, each new experience must be directed into the same general network as the old experiences, otherwise each new experience remains just that. Thus the two attentional centers provide directing and matching mechanisms for the formation of new consolidated engrams as well as for reactivation of established engrams.

The previous description explains more than just the inability to learn new material in the mesencephalic and bitemporal amnesic syndromes. It also explains why closely attended learning of episodic material in the intact individual is immeasurably more effective than only slightly attended or unattended learning. The mechanisms of attention, acting through the mechanisms of recognition, provide the basis for all conscious cognitive operations and facilitate the process of consolidation through repeated activation of the same neural connections.

Given the upstream–downstream formulation of the attentional process, one would expect some differences in the memory deficit syndromes represented, respectively, by damage to the upstream thalamic–basal gangliar mechanism (mesencephalic amnesia) and damage to the amygdaloid–hippocampal complex (bitemporal amnesia). Several pieces of evidence support this interpretation. First is a study of the neuropsychology of amnesia by Squire (1982) in which he distinguishes between those amnesic states of the Korsakoff type and those associated with hippocampal lesions. As Squire writes, "Recent studies of forgetting provide strong evidence that there are at least two distinct amnesic syndromes and that diencephalic amnesia and bitemporal amnesia are fundamentally different" (p. 241). The diencephalic syndrome of Korsakoff's disease is characteristically associated with major difficulties in encoding and consolidating new cognitive material; the hippocampal deficits involve more of a difficulty in memory retrieval.

Whereas damage to either system is sufficient to produce serious memory deficits, damage to the hippocampus alone is not sufficient to produce attentional difficulties. When the thalamic–basal gangliar system is destroyed as in the previously described akinetic mutism (Chapter 6), then the capacity for attending is completely lost. These findings are in keeping with the experimental evidence that demonstrates direct involvement of the thalamic–basal gangliar nuclei in generating the general state of consciousness and awareness. The amygdaloid–hippocampal complex is more directly involved in the process of recognition and in tying recent events into the self-concept system than it is in the basic phenomena of general consciousness.

These discussions also illuminate the functional differences between the thalamic–basal gangliar complex and the amygdaloid–hippocampal complexes in consciousness phenomena. The level of consciousness associated with perception and attention stem largely from the thalamic–basal gangliar nuclei. The patient H.M., despite the absence of both amygdaloid–hippocampal complexes, had no deficits in perceptual or attentional awareness but he did have severe deficits in recognition and in recent memory retrieval. It appears that the thalamic–basal gangliar complex ties perceptions directly into awareness while the amygdaloid–hippocampal complexes tie memories indirectly into awareness but directly into the self-concept. This interpretation is consistent with the previously described findings of Libet et al. (1979) which showed peripheral sensory stimulation to be experienced consciously almost immediately while cortical stimulation took about 0.5 sec longer to achieve the same effect. That would be about the time necessary for complete cortical and hippocampal processing and for transmission back to the thalamic–basal gangliar consciousness complex (Mishkin, 1982).

The Diencephalic–Rhinencephalic Memory Retrieval System

The structures involved in the diencephalic amnesic syndrome are obviously not the same as those of consciousness and attention, since neither of these latter functions are significantly impaired in that syndrome. In Korsakoff's amnesia, the prototypical diencephalic syndrome, the pathologically involved brain stem structures are the dorsal median thalamic nucleus and the mammillary bodies (Brion, 1969). These centers constitute only a small portion of the major thalamic–basal gangliar complex responsible for the control of consciousness and upstream attentional processing (Fig. 2-2). Apparently the remaining intact elements of the thalamic–basal gangliar complex are sufficiently functional to permit relatively normal consciousness and attentional activities. Similarly, the total ablation of the amygdaloid–hippocampal complex appears to have little effect on consciousness and attentional activities.

Although the diencephalic and rhinencephalic (bitemporal) amnesic syndromes do show some differences, the similarities between them are more remarkable considering the differences in the anatomical structures involved. In both instances there is a loss of memory for recent events with retention of old long-term memories. In the case of the bitemporal syndrome where there is an immediate acute onset coincident with surgery, memories of events that occurred more than three years earlier appear to be intact and retrievable. This time span, i.e., three years, is apparently the period necessary for permanent consolidation of long-term memories to occur, a finding corroborated by Squire and Cohen (1979) on patients treated with electroconvulsive therapy. The fact that retention of long-term memories occurs in both the diencephalic and the bitemporal amnesic syndromes suggests that both the dorsal median thalamic–mammillary body circuit and the amygdaloid–hippocampal complex are necessary for short-term recognition, learning, and retrieval but that either alone can accomplish the retrieval of three year or older long-term memories (Squire et al., 1982).

The interaction of the dorsal median thalamic–mammillary body circuit and the amygdaloid–hippocampal complex postulated here as essential for the processes of recognition, learning of episodic data, memory consolidation, and memory retrieval appears consistent with experimental evidence (Mishkin, 1982). It also seems eminently consistent with the close interaction of the thalamic–basal gangliar complex and the amygdaloid–hippocampal complex in attentional activities as postulated in the last chapter.

The Phenomenology of Mental Set

Mental set may be defined as the specific cognitive and emotional orientation of the organism in a given situation. As such, it is determined generally by the entire previous cognitive and emotional history of the organism and more specifically by the immediate situational setting. The latter in turn may be defined internally or externally: internally by the personality and experience of the individual (the self) and externally by the specific demands of a given situation. In experimental studies, a specific mental set is established through direct instructions from the investigator on how the subject is to react in a given experimental situation. The phenomenology of mental set as studied experimentally is extremely variable depending upon the particular behavioral modality being studied and upon the particular experimental situation.

An example of the cognitive effects of mental set was presented in the previously described experiment by Teyler et al. (Fig. 4-6) in which the verb "to rock" and the noun "rock" produced different evoked potentials. It appears that a given word may elicit entirely different abstract engrams and evoked potentials depending upon the specific meaning of a given stimulus under different circumstances. Specific interpretations and ultimate responses are in turn determined by the mental set at a given moment, a state that is evidently controlled by influences emanating from higher hierarchical control centers in the brain. The Teyler et al. (1973) experiment illustrated in Figure 4-6 provides supportive evidence for the existence of some such control center to establish the set which in turn determines the meaning of ambiguous stimuli, as in this case, for the word "rock." It is very difficult to explain the data of this experiment in terms of a behavioristic S → R paradigm since here there is rather a situation of

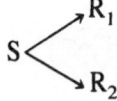

where the choice between R_1 and R_2 is determined by a cognitive set. Nor need this set have been established by the experimenter; when the subject was instructed to select one or the other meaning on his own, the resulting evoked potentials were similar to those produced under the instructed conditions.

In this case, the effects of mental set are predominantly cognitive since they determine the selection of a given meaning of a word. Other influences bearing upon the amygdaloid–hippocampal complex to determine the direction of attention and the subsequent generation or nongeneration of a P_{300} wave are of two types: motivational, presumably stemming from the inferotemporal lobe, and those of expectancy, probably stemming largely from the prefrontal lobe. Two experiments illustrate the relationship of these effects to the initiation of the P_{300} wave, i.e., the wave of attention. For motivation, a demonstration of the differences in the P_{300} response to more and less meaningful stimuli is offered in a study of Begleiter et al. (1983). Subjects were presented two visual stimuli of equal size and intensity, a 0 and a 1. They were instructed to press one button whenever the 1 flashed and another when the 0 flashed.

They were also told that they would be given a dollar for each correct identification of the 1 stimulus. Subjects' attention on each stimulus was thus equal but the motivational significance of the 1 was greater than that for the 0. Evoked potentials were recorded over the frontal, central, parietal, and occipital areas. The P_{300} was significantly greater over the parietal area for the target stimulus (1) than for the relatively neutral stimulus (0). Begleiter et al. (1983) interpreted this finding as indicative of the activating effects of greater motivation upon the generation of the P_{300} wave. This interpretation is undoubtedly correct, but a more general conclusion might be that the greater P_{300} wave is the consequence of more intense attentional activity generated by high motivation.

The P_{300} of attention can be activated even in the absence of an actual stimulus if the expectancy for such a stimulus is high enough. Picton and Hillyard (1974) exposed subjects to a repeated visual stimulus presented at regular intervals with the stimulus presention omitted infrequently and randomly. They then recorded the evoked potential produced during the period of the expected but unpresented stimulus. The results are shown in Figure 9-1. The response to the expected but absent stimulus showed no N_1-P_2 wave but a high P_{300} wave suggesting that hippocampal activation had occurred even in the absence of a stimulus. This experiment provides further evidence that the N_1-P_2 wave represents essentially exogenous influences while the P_{300} wave represents essentially endogenous ones.

The occurrence of electrical activation of the brain in the absence of any external stimulus in the Picton experiment is an explicit demonstration of mental set. It is similar to that referred to in Chapter 4 in the Teyler experiment where the same word "rock" produced two different evoked potentials (Fig. 4-6). The Picton experiment

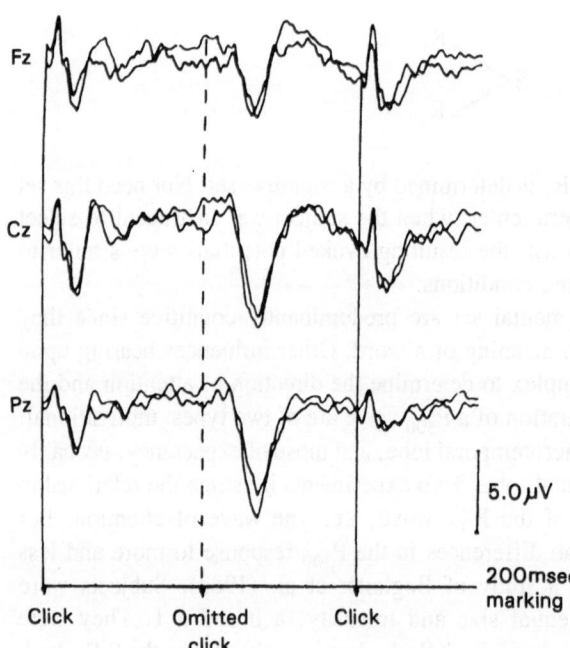

Figure 9-1 Evoked potentials to expected but unpresented stimuli. (From Picton and Hillyard, 1974. Reprinted with permission.)

(Fig. 9-1) suggests that the hippocampus might be the control center for mental set, but biologically the paleocortex is probably too primitive a structure for so advanced a function. Mental set appears to be a high-level decision-making operation that one would expect to be located at the highest level of brain function, that is, the prefrontal cortex.

On the other hand, the Begleiter and co-worker experiment suggests a different kind of situation where motivational influences rather than expectation determine the mental set. Here the motivational–emotional complex (the inferior temporal lobe, etc.) would appear to have greater input. Experimental evidence suggests that the decision-making capacity of the brain may be shared by the prefrontal and inferotemporal cerebral complexes with the frontal complex activated more by cognitive factors while the inferotemporal complex is activated more by motivational–emotional influences (Pribram, 1980).

The Neurophysiology of Mental Set

Phenomenologically, mental set appears to act as a feedforward mechanism that can affect perceptual activity in a variety of ways. In the Picton and Hillyard paradigm (Fig. 9-1), expectation of a stimulus produces a large P_{300} even where no stimulus appears. This evidently illustrates mental set as a stimulatory influence. In the study of Teyler and co-workers, (Fig. 4-6), mental set apparently determines the selection of one pathway of word processing as against another. In the studies of Begleiter and co-workers, (1983) positive motivational effects influence physiological response. Some insights into the neurophysiological mechanisms underlying these phenomena may be provided by the following studies.

An example of feedforward effects on the transduction of perceptions into neurophysiological equivalents is illustrated in studies by Begleiter et al. (1973) on evoked potential correlates of visual stimuli under a variety of mental set conditions. These investigators ran a series of experiments in which bright and dim flashes were randomly presented; bright flashes were preceded by a high-pitched tone, dim flashes by a low-pitched tone. Visual evoked potentials were correspondingly of larger or lesser amplitude depending on the intensity of the stimulus. Subjects were then presented with only intermediate flashes of medium intensity preceded by either the high-pitched or low-pitched tones. Visual evoked potentials associated with high-pitched tones showed significantly greater amplitude of the vertex P_{200} wave than did those associated with low-pitched tones, indicating that anticipation of a bright or dim flash affected the evoked potential response even when the stimulus was a constant medium-intensity flash (Fig. 9-2). Changes in the P_{200} complex of the evoked potential suggest that the cognitive effect occurs during processing in the associative cortices. This interpretation is supported by the fact that significant P_{200} differences for the medium flash under the two different conditions were found for potentials obtained over the vertex (association cortex) but not for those obtained over the occipital lobes (the primary receiving area) (Fig. 9-2). The increase in amplitude of this wave with bright-light expectancy and the slight decrease with dim-light expectancy over the association

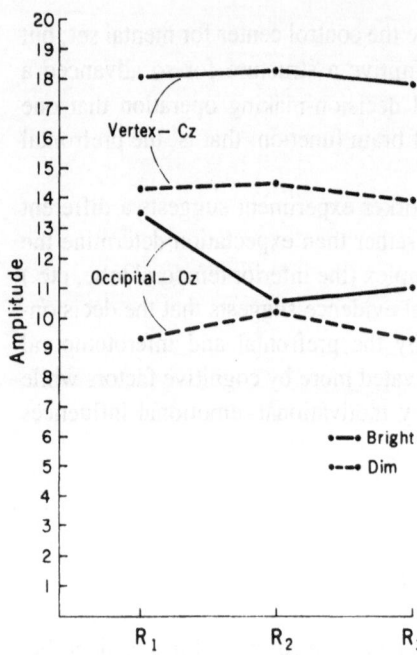

Figure 9-2 Evoked potential amplitude (N_{200}) to bright, dim, and intermediate flashes under conditioning. (From Begleiter et al., 1973. Reprinted with permission.)

areas suggest that both excitatory and inhibitory influences may be operative, although the excitatory effects seem larger.

Begleiter et al. (1973) suggest that the occurrence of either the "brightlike" or "dimlike" evoked potential to a flash of medium intensity is due to the reactivation of previous memories. This interpretation seems quite probable despite appropriate evoked responses obtained at the occipital electrodes (Fig. 9-2). An alternative and perhaps equally likely interpretation might be that excitatory or inhibitory influences are being brought to bear on the associative processing cortices to either enhance or impair physiological transduction. However, no known neurophysiological mechanism operating directly onto specific areas in the cortex is known to exist. But inhibitory influences from the prefrontal cortex onto relay stations in the brain stem, possibly similar to the frontal–thalamic mechanisms described by Skinner and Yingling (1977) and illustrated in Figure 8-1, might explain some of these effects. The inhibitory effects might also be upon the superior colliculi where parallel visual pathways leading directly to the associative areas originate and where such inhibitory effects from the prefrontal cortex have been demonstrated (Meredith and Stein, 1983).

The general characteristics of mental set phenomena in these studies suggest either a cognitive or emotional presetting in the brain at some higher level which feeds onto lower levels to affect their function during perceptions. The two highest brain areas where emotional and cognitive activities interdigitate most actively are the inferior temporal lobe and the prefrontal lobe. We have already described how in the Klüver–Bucy syndrome where both inferior temporal lobes have been resected the animals' motivational behavior becomes bizarre. The aberrations in those behaviors are of course of a different order than those connoted in the term, mental set, since they involve marked changes in motivational and emotional attitudes. Nevertheless, mental set can certainly significantly influence emotional reactivities as illustrated in the Begleiter et al. (1983) study. Specifically cognitive effects are probably activated through prefrontal lobe mechanisms as in the Picton and Hillyard study (Fig. 9-1).

Role of the Prefrontal Lobe in Attention and Mental Set

The prefrontal lobe is the most characteristically human portion of the brain, but we have not discussed its functions until now. This has been true because the prefrontal lobe is involved in activities that are most peculiar to primates and humans, while previous descriptions have applied to almost all mammals. The functions of the prefrontal lobe are also more difficult to define because they are so ephemeral. With destruction of the prefrontal lobe due to damage or surgery, the individual functions more or less normally; there are none of the obvious disruptions that one finds after destruction of any of the other lobes of the cortex. More sensitive tests of intellectual and attentional function do reveal significant behavioral changes with prefrontal lobe damage, changes which when extrapolated back to normal provide insight into the important role that the lobe does have in normal behavior.

Lesions of the prefrontal lobe result in three major types of dysfunction: an increase in orienting response behavior, perseveration, and an inability to establish temporal relationships. On the surface, these may seem to be relatively insignificant defects, but further analyses reveal that each of these represent the loss of an extremely important function, particularly in the intricate control mechanisms of attentional activity and mental set.

Damage to the prefrontal lobe in humans (and in primates as well) results in significant changes in orienting response behavior. For one thing, there is a significant increase in such behavior; it is as though there was an increased sensitivity to novel stimuli in the environment. Second, there is a decreased tendency to habituate, further exacerbating the orienting activity. Finally, there is an inability of the prefrontal lobe patient to fix his attention (to establish a mental set) on any given stimulus, despite verbal instructions from the examiner. These functional deficits are translated into a variety of behavioral incapacities. First, the individual is highly distractible, unable to focus his attention on any given task. Second, he appears to lack motivation just because he cannot fix his attention. Finally, as a consequence of this last deficit, the patient no longer shows a P_{300} on his evoked responses, despite his efforts to focus attention.

The attentional deficits that arise in the absence of adequate prefrontal lobe function tend to delineate its normal role in that activity. The prefrontal lobe acts as a filter for incoming stimuli, selecting those that are pertinent and rejecting (inhibiting) those that are not. Pertinence is defined in cognitive and motivational–emotional terms; the information on which these decisions rest derive from the major cognitive associational areas and from the motivational inferotemporal lobe. Information of a more verbal type may flow directly from the language complex in the left hemisphere to the prefrontal lobe. Neural tracts from the self-awareness system in the inferoparietal lobe to the prefrontal lobe transmit information in both directions. Through mechanisms not presently understood, the prefrontal lobe appears to integrate all of this information and on that basis makes the decision as to which of the innumerable stimuli in the environment will be attended to. Once made, the decision is relayed to the amygdaloid–hippocampal complex that under prefrontal lobe influence either directs the appropriate attentional beam or conversely habituates (i.e., loses interest) (Fig. 9-3).

The predominantly inhibitory role of the frontal lobe as illustrated in its repression of irrelevant stimuli is more clearly delineated in the second deficiency characteristic of frontal lobe dysfunction, namely perseveration. This behavioral deficit manifests itself as the inability to inhibit a learned reaction pattern, once that response is no longer appropriate. This so-called deficit in passive avoidance conditioning is translated behaviorally into perseveration, i.e., the inability to inhibit incorrect responses despite their immediate inappropriateness, once they have been well learned in previous settings (Iversen, 1973).

The third deficit associated with frontal lobe lesions, the inability to establish temporal relations, is less obviously involved in attentional mechanisms and more intimately involved in determining mental set. The frontal lobe monkey and also the frontal lobe patient have difficulty in performing sequential tasks, particularly if there are significant time lapses between those tasks. Frontal lobe monkeys have great difficulty functioning in delayed response situations, e.g., tasks where a lever must be pressed 15–20 sec after a light is flashed if a reward is to be obtained. The ability to conceptualize time is considered one of the most advanced characteristics of human thinking. With it one plans ahead and projects one's activity into the future. In the absence of this faculty, intellectual function is markedly limited (Iversen, 1973).

All three of these frontal lobe functions are involved in the processes of mental set. The increased orienting responsivity in frontal lobe damage secondary to decreased ability to habituate leads to easy distractibility; normal frontal lobe activity is necessary for concentrated attention. The deficit of inhibitory activity implicit in perseveration explains the frontal lobe patient's inability to learn new tasks. Finally, mental set is predominantly a temporally determined mechanism since it projects action into the future.

There is reason to believe that mental set effects are implemented through impulses from the frontal lobe to brain stem centers [as in the Skinner–Yingling (1970) frontal–thalamic feedback circuit] and to the amygdaloid–hippocampal complex. The mechanisms of these putative feedforward mechanisms are not well understood. Specific frontal–hypothalamic anatomical tracts have been demonstrated and these presumably might account for some of the affective manifestations of mental set. The Skinner–Yingling mechanisms may account for a variety of cognitive effects. Still other frontal-brain stem feedforward mechanisms may exist, such as the previously postulated tracts from the prefrontal area to the superior colliculi (Meredith and Stein, 1983), to the hypothalamus, and to various elements of the limbic system. Most important of all are of course the excitatory–inhibitory influences of the prefrontal area upon the activities of the amygdaloid–hippocampal complex.

Attention, recognition, memory retrieval, and mental set are all activities that involve specific decisional processes. In each instance, there is the selection of pertinent material and the concomitant neglect of masses of irrelevant material. Once the decision is made, the mechanisms for implementation are largely those described for the processes of recognition and memory retrieval. The manner in which decisions are reached and the mechanisms by which these decisions are channeled to the implementing machinery present an interesting theoretical problem.

A Theoretical Model for the Decision-Making Function in Attention, Recognition, Memory Retrieval, and Mental Set

A theoretical model of the hierarchical relationships among the various brain centers controlling the programs for attention, recognition, memory retrieval, and mental set is illustrated diagrammatically in Figure 9-3. Most but not all of the subcortical and cortical centers involved in each of these activities are shown. The specific

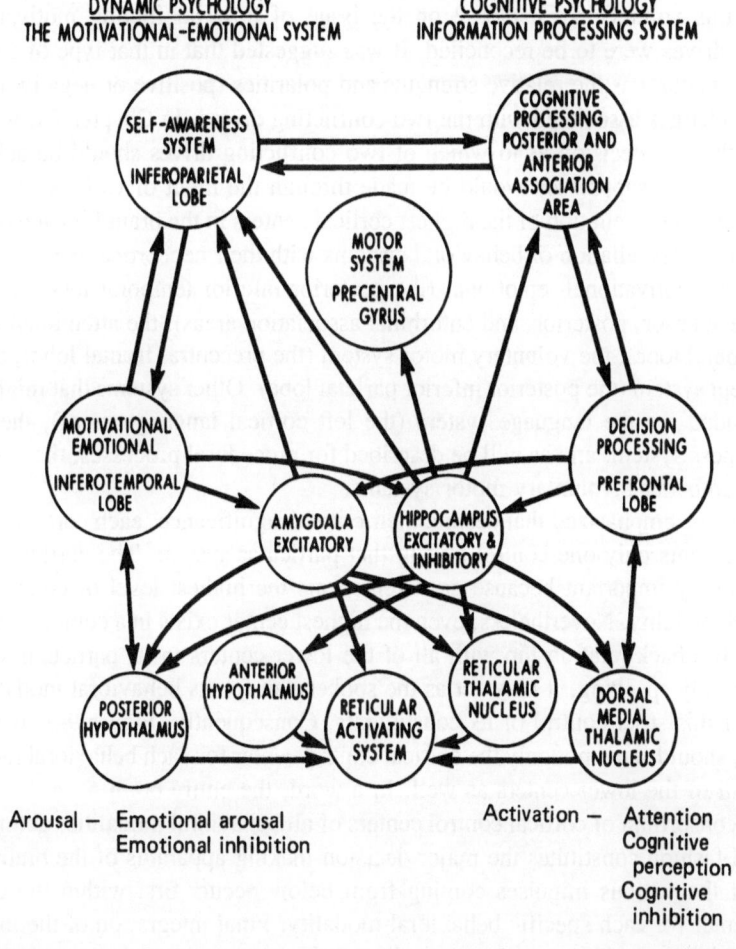

Figure 9-3 A theoretical model of the hierarchical control system of the brain.

interactions among centers for each of the different functions have been described in this and the last chapter. Even though the mechanisms for the various functions differ somewhat, they are sufficiently similar to permit all of them to be incorporated under the single rubric of Figure 9-3.

Figure 9-3 offers a diagrammatic anatomical model of the structures involved in decision making (mainly cortical centers) and in decision implementation (mainly subcortical centers). However, it does not provide much understanding of the functional interactions among the various centers on the basis of which decisions are made. One might possibly utilize the computer model of various systems, each with its own system control center (the various cortical processing areas), converging onto a central executive control center (the prefrontal lobe) where final decisions are made. But this model does not seem completely applicable to humans since the component elements can function even in the absence of the prefrontal lobe. The executive control center in human mental activity appears to exist rather in the totality of cortical control centers so that in the absence of any one of them the others can continue to function, however inadequately.

The question of decision making as a critical psychological function was first raised in this volume in Chapter 2 on the issue of how conflicting motivational–emotional drives were to be reconciled. It was suggested that in that type of conflict, the critical factor was the relative strengths and polarities (positive or negative) of the emotional charges associated with the two conflicting drives. In Chapter 2 it was also indicated that the decision as to which of two conflicting drives should be acknowledged and which suppressed would be made through the input of various behavioral systems onto a constellation of the highest cortical centers in the brain for each of these systems. The constellation of behavioral systems with their neocortical control centers included the motivational–emotional (the posterior inferior temporal lobe), the cognitive (the anterior, posterior, and entorhinal association areas), the attentional system (the prefrontal lobe), the voluntary motor system (the precentral frontal lobe), and the self-concept system (the posterior inferior parietal lobe). Other systems that might have been included are the language system (the left cortical language areas), the entire consciousness system, and as will be described for procedural processes, the nigrostriatal and cerebellar involuntary motor systems.

It must be emphasized that despite their critical significance, each cortical control center represents only one control unit in that particular system. The cortical centers are particularly important because each represents the highest level of control in its behavioral modality. Nevertheless, even the highest center exists in a complex feedforward and feedback relationship with all of the lower centers in its particular system. Metaphorically speaking, it may act as the spokesman for its behavioral modality but only under this strict control of its constituents. Consequently, Figure 9-3, if it were complete, should show not only the cortical control center for each behavioral modality but also all of the lower centers as well. In a word, the entire brain.

The consortium of cortical control centers of all behavioral modalities acting in an integrated fashion constitutes the major decision-making apparatus of the brain. Integration of the various impulses coming from below occurs first within the cortical control center for each specific behavioral modality. Final integration of the information channeled through the various cortical control centers is normally carried out in the prefrontal lobe. From there feedforward stimuli are directed to the cognitive apparatus through the amygdaloid–hippocampal complex and to the motivational–emotional system through the hypothalamus and limbic system. However, in the absence of the prefrontal cortex, coordination of the various cortical control centers is effectuated through some more democratic decision-making process.

From an organismic point of view, the cortical decisional-making apparatus may be seen as the executive behavioral component of the self-system, much as the self-concept anchored in the self-awareness system constitutes the subjective component. The two components, although at times operationally discrete,* must be conceptualized as the efferent and afferent components, respectively, of a single self-system. Although it is difficult to prove this experimentally, the two components must interact at all levels since, at least in theory, the self-concept subjective element is an integral part of the cortical consortium (the executive self) that controls behavior. The nature of these interactions apparently varies in the disparate conditions of conscious and unconscious mental activity, an issue to be addressed in later chapters.

Attention, recognition, memory retrieval, and mental set represent the mechanisms through which the flow of mental ideas is accomplished in the ongoing stream of conscious thought. They are the influences that shape and control that flow. But the stream of consciousness is an entity in itself with phenomenological and physiological characteristics of its own, separate and distinct from those influences mentioned above. The dynamics of conscious thought processing (perceiving and thinking) provide the subject matter for the next chapter.

---

*For example during periods of some altered states of conciousness and in dreams.

The Alert Conscious State: Controlled Processing of Episodic and Affective Data

The descriptions presented thus far in this volume have emphasized the separate individual elements of consciousness but have not really addressed the single integrated quality of awareness as we know it. In this chapter those processes that bring together those disparate elements into a single unified whole will be discussed.

The dynamics of attention, perceptual recognition, memory retrieval, and mental set define the mechanisms by which a given event, positively evaluated, is admitted to awareness. This is a somewhat artificial exposition since, except in experimental situations, events are not channeled singly into consciousness. Rather there is a continuum of events, each tied in some meaningful fashion to the one before and to the one following, so that the entire sequence has cognitive coherence and emotional significance. The sum total of a prolonged sequence of perceptual and mental events where each event as well as the entire sequence is influenced by attentional, memory retrieval, and mental set factors constitutes conscious brain activity.

The term conscious brain activity contains in itself certain fundamental assumptions. For one, it is assumed that each event in the sequence has been cleared by the combined system of attentional, perceptual recognition, memory retrieval, and mental set mechanisms. It is also clear that there are different modes of conscious mental activity ranging from that of essentially external origin (conscious perception) to that involving both the external and the internal (conscious recognition) to the predominantly internal (conscious thought). In each case the individual is aware of his thoughts and as a result of the involvement of his entire self-system is in control of them.

Other qualities of conscious thought processing derive from the nature of cognitive processing. As shown in the Lumsden–Wilson diagram of such processing (Fig. 5-4), perceptions or thoughts coming in at the left lower border are matched with engrams in the long-term memory through recognition (abstraction) and associative mechanisms. On the basis of these processes, certain engrams are momentarily brought into awareness (short-term memories). It is these momentary flashes of remembered engrams, brought into awareness, that constitute the substantive material of consciousness. These activated short-term memories are extremely short-lived; they decay rapidly and return to long-term memory. However, they are rapidly replaced by other activated short-term memories to continue the flow of consciousness.

This flow of consciousness—the literary "stream of consciousness"—characterizes our subjective appreciation of the state of awareness. In the writings of James Joyce, one idea follows another at intervals of several seconds to constitute a river of thoughts. But in conscious perception, each picture follows the next at the rate of probably 20–25 frames/sec, somewhat above the rate of 16 frames/sec necessary to maintain a sense of continuous awareness.

The thesis that consciousness is discontinuous and composed of frames changing at the rapid rate of about 20–25/sec is an extremely important one since it defines both the subjective quality and functional operation of the phenomenon. The best evidence for this interpretation comes from various physiological and psychological studies that deal with the rapidity with which sensory stimuli can be processed, with the decay times (i.e., persistence) of different neural processes, and with the number of frames/sec necessary to maintain a sense of continuity. Most of these data are summarized on the Lumsden–Wilson chart illustrated in Figure 5-4, but a quick review of some of the experimental evidence from which these figures are derived may be helpful.

Two items on the Lumsden–Wilson chart are of particular note here: the first, the approximately 50 msec read time to short-term memory for visual iconic memories and the second, the approximately 50 msec per operation time for elementary information processing. Each of these dimensions establishes a rate of 20–30/sec for their individual operations, namely, visualization and thinking. The rate of separate operations for tactile processing has been established by evoked potential evidence using the recovery function paradigm. In these studies, two somatosensory stimuli given sequentially at very short time intervals are treated by the brain as one until the interval reaches 20–30 msec at which time the stimuli are successfully separated. Apparently this is the time it takes for brain function to recover its capacity to accept and process new stimuli, i.e., at the rate of 35–50 new stimuli/sec. This figure is supported by psychological studies with the flicker–fusion test where a rapidly flickering light fuses perceptually into a single continuous light at about the rate of 50–60 flashes/sec. The rate for fusion of auditory stimuli is even higher at about 80–100 clicks/sec.

Simon (1979) describes a psychological study that not only establishes the time of 50 msec as that necessary for perception but also illustrates the limited capacity of consciousness. He writes:

> The stimulus for all the experiments to be described is a rectangular array of English letters, selected at random and displayed in three rows of four letters each. The stimulus is displayed in three rows of four letters each. The stimulus is displayed for 50 msec, and it is of such size and intensity that there is no question of visual confusion. In the first experimental paradigm (Immediate recall experiment), the subject is instructed to repeat back the sequence of stimulus letters as soon as he has

seen them. Typically, a subject will recall an average of about four to six letters correctly. (p. 667)

Simon's study involved the complex process of semantic recognition during the up-stream phase of perception and established that that could be accomplished with only a 50 msec exposure. Sagi and Julesz (1985) studied the dynamics of the preattentive or upstream phase of perception and found that physical characteristics of geometric stimuli could be identified after as little as 5 msec of exposure. Moreover, several different physical properties could so be identified. Sagi and Julesz (1985) concluded that the preattentive phase is characterized by parallel processing of different mechanisms while the attentive phase of recognition is accomplished more slowly through controlled serial processing.

These studies indicate that iconic images can be assimilated consciously at the rate of about 20–25/sec, but that only four to six individual letters can be so handled simultaneously. These experiments thus establish the capacity of short-term memory for perceptual stimuli at about 5-7 perceptual images per moment.* Other studies establish the fact that iconic images persist for a period of about 200 msec contributing further to the sense of continuity (Sperling, 1960).

In these terms, perceptual awareness is best conceptualized as picture frames projected on a kinescope or film projector, each frame static and different from the others but each sufficiently similar to the one before it and the one after to permit a sense of continuous action. Although each frame lasts only about 40 msec, iconic images constituting the elements of each frame last up to 200 msec (0.2 sec) providing a continuity of substance that is reflected in the continuous sense of awareness.

The substantive content of consciousness and its particular sense of continuity stem mainly from the brain's mode of processing cognitive material. Conscious thought processing is illustrated in the Lumsden–Wilson diagram (Fig. 5-4) as a process in which only about 6–8 short-term memory chunks may be brought to awareness at any given time. New elements are brought from long-term memory to short term-memory at an unknown rate but presumably many times a second. The average duration of attended short-term memories is said to be about 0.2 sec but the average time for processing each "frame" is only about 40 msec. The persistence of short-term memories for about 0.2 sec assures a smooth transition from each cognitive frame to the next. The pattern of images is constantly changing but retains continuity during that 1-sec period. Consequently, the flow of conscious processing, the so-called stream of consciousness, is an ever changing river of interacting perceptions and memories, which like Heraclitus' river of existence is constant but always different. The richness of human consciousness lies not in any special physiological arrangement but in the richness of the cognitive data that flood in to constitute its substance.

This kinematic description of the nature of conscious activity appears at first inspection to be contrary to common human experience which insists that conscious awareness is a constant continuous phenomenon and not an intermittent discontinuous one. However, experience with motion pictures shows that projections of separate pictures at a rate of 16 frames/sec or faster are seen as continuous rather than, as they

---

*A "moment" is defined as the period of a single frame varying in length from 1/25 to 1/40 of a second.

really are, intermittent. Consequently, there is no real conflict between the kinematic description of conscious activity and behavioral experience.

Quantitative Aspects of Consciousness

An important characteristic of conscious experience is its apparently limited capacity. In the Lumsden–Wilson model of cognitive functioning (Fig. 5-4) the total capacity of short-term memory is given as six to eight chunks of information. These statistics come from memory experiments that show that an extremely limited number of stimuli can be perceived and kept in awareness at any given moment, namely six to eight (Simon, 1979). However, subjective experience reveals that one can consciously perceive a greater number and variety of stimuli in one's environment at any given moment than six to eight. Some more specific definitions of what constitute pieces of information is obviously needed. A formulation by Jung (1978), even though it has some substantial errors in it, helps at least to define the problem. The formulation is illustrated in Figure 10-1.

Jung has reviewed, on the basis of the estimated number of neurons active at any given time in the human brain, the approximate number of possible connections and

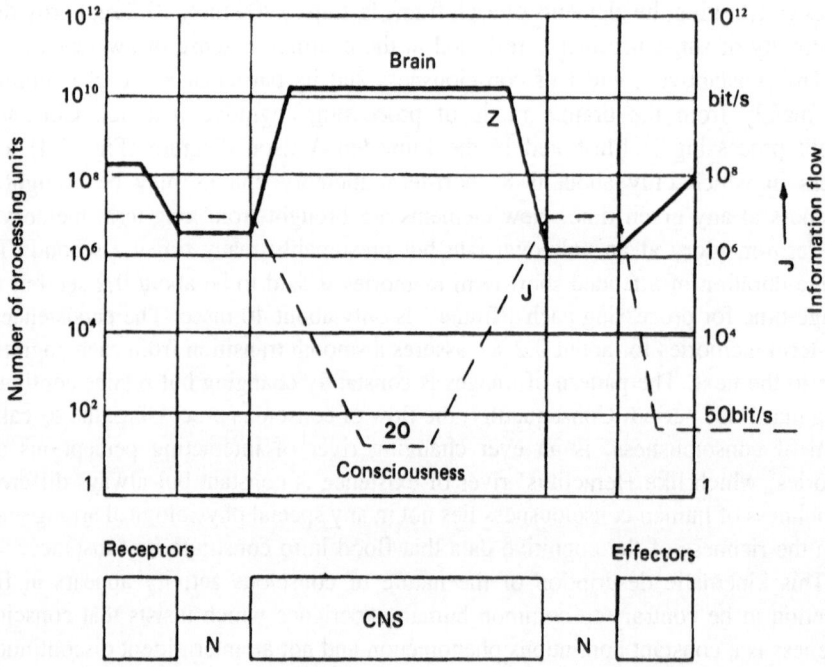

Figure 10-1 Information flow in the central nervous system. Information is selected in consciousness to represent the actual essentials with an extreme reduction from 10^7 to about 200 bits/sec for conscious perception and to about 50 bits/sec for voluntary action (broken line J). (From Jung, 1978. Reprinted with permission.)

the maximum number of bits of information that can be maintained in directed consciousness (attended to) or acted on at any given moment. On the basis of the evidence in the literature, Jung calculated that at any given moment in the relaxed individual, approximately 10^7 or 10 million bits of information are being generated by all external and internal receptors as well as by the brain itself (thought, feelings), and that these 10^7 bits are being processed by 10^8 or 100 million processing units (receptors and neurons).

A "bit" of information is assumed by Jung, on the basis of computer terminology, to require a constellation of about 10 different neurons (10 diodes in computers) to establish a specific configuration. But in perception as in memory, individual elements are represented not as bits but as configurations of bits or "chunks" (Simon, 1979). A given percept or memory (a chunk), depending on its complexity, may comprise anywhere from 100 to 1000 bits involving somewhere between 1000 to 10,000 neurons. Elements in consciousness or memory are represented as chunks so that it is six to eight chunks of information and not bits which may be maintained in memory at any given split second. Jung errs in his calculations in confusing bits of information with chunks and on the time parameter by confusing seconds with the split seconds of frames, probably 40 to 50 msec in duration (Simon, 1979).

Jung errs again in restricting the content of conscious cognitive activity to 20 bits per second and of conscious behavioral reactivity to 50 bits/sec. Instead these should read 6–8 chunks/frame and 50 chunks/frame, respectively. As Simon (1979) writes, "The chunking hypothesis asserts that human short-term memory is limited in the number of symbols (or chunks) it can hold, not in the number of bits of information it can hold" (p. 294). Consequently, a word of 10 letters represents a single chunk, even though each letter may involve as many as 100 bits of information, for a total of 1000 bits. If we arbitrarily assign a value of 1000 bits of information per chunk, a holding capacity in short-term memory of 7 chunks/frame, a persistence period of about 0.2 sec for each short-term memory, and a kinematic rate of 20–25 frames/sec, we achieve a total of about 140 chunks/sec or about 140,000 bits/sec. This is certainly of a different order of magnitude than that postulated in Jung's calculations. Nevertheless, in comparison with the total capacity of the brain of ten billion bits, conscious activity represents a very small proportion of the total.

The focusing of attention, in Jung's formulation of different states of mental function, activates the brain, raising the number of active brain units involved to 10^{11} or 100 billion neurons, i.e., the total capacity of the brain; the number of bits of information available rises correspondingly to 10^{10} or ten billion. Electrophysiologically speaking, the quietly resting individual is considered to be in α rhythm where, according to Jung, probably no more than 1% of all brain cells are actively functioning.* In attention, i.e., in full consciousness, the brain is in γ rhythm and all neurons are actively functioning. The total number of units of information of which a person can be aware of at any given moment is thus calculated to be about 140 chunks/second or 140,000 bits out of a presumed total of 10 million chunks (ten billion bits) that are flooding into the system each moment, the rest remaining at some level of

---

*This is also incorrect. As will be seen in the next chapter, even in deep slow wave sleep, about one third of the neurons in the brain remain active.

unconscious activity. In terms of behavioral responsivity, Jung calculates that one utilizes up to 50 chunks of information (50,000 bits) as efferent motor concomitants to the 6–8 chunks of sensory information being processed consciously in each 50-msec frame, or approximately 1 million bits/sec.

The physiological formulation presented here for attention is in all ways theoretically compatible with the pattern of psychological characteristics described for conscious perception and information processing as shown in the Lumsden–Wilson model in Figure 5-4. Of particular interest are the characteristics of short-term memory as capable of holding a limited number of complex engrams (chunks) in awareness at a given moment (6–8) and capable only of utilizing these materials sequentially (i.e., serial processing) over time. Both of these characteristics speak for a localized bottleneck type of operation as opposed to one involving the free flow of material throughout the brain. In the anatomical model of conscious information processing presented in Figure 9-3, the hippocampal–amygdaloid complex represents the critical rate-limiting bottleneck through which all "recognized" material flows into awareness. The finding by Wickelgren (1979) of constellations of cells in the hippocampus capable of receiving engrammatic patterns of stimulation as chunks from the cortex supports the thesis that the hippocampus is equipped to play the critical cognitive role previously attributed to it. Similarly, the work of Bennett (1975), showing that the hippocampus goes from a rapid β-wave type of electrical activity during behavioral inactivity to a slow θ-wave rhythm (4–7 sec) during attention, is also consistent with a relatively slow processing of material in the hippocampus. Finally, the limited area capacity of the hippocampal–amygdaloid complex in comparison with the rest of the brain is compatible with the limited holding capacity of short-term memory.

In these terms, consciousness consists substantively of all of those perceptions and short-term memories that are held in awareness at any given moment, where each moment is measured as $\frac{1}{25}$ to $\frac{1}{40}$ of a second. The summoning up of short-term memories (from the long-term memory store) to awareness at an extremely rapid rate (25–40 sec) through the limiting funnel-like amygdaloid–hippocampal complex produces the movie-camera-like effect of the stream of consciousness. The nature of cognitive information processing as described in the Lumsden–Wilson model (Fig. 5-4) also contributes to the sequential structure of conscious thought because the dominant mechanism for raising successive frames operates through the associational and the abstraction networks, both sequential operations. Thus, according to this theoretical formulation, conscious thinking would have to be limited, strictly sequential, and predominantly associational. In part these qualities derive from the critical role played by the amygdaloid–hippocampal "funnel," but in part they derive also from the type of material, now to be described, which is processed by the attentional system.

The Substantive Nature of Conscious and Unconscious Material—Episodic and Procedural Data

Perhaps the most unique characteristic of conscious processing is the kind of cognitive and emotional material that can effectively be brought to awareness. There are many different types of information that are processed in the brain but only a few of the existing varieties are able to be consciously realized. Consequently, conscious and unconscious cognition are distinguished not only by certain functional characteristics but equally by the nature of their content.

Briefly stated, the most ubiquitous cognitive material in consciousness is designated "episodic." Because it is the main stuff of which consciousness and awareness consist, it is what we all think of as the material of everyday experience. Operationally, it is defined by all of the cognitive events and episodes as well as by all of the affective reactivities that occur during our waking or dreaming hours. Physiologically, as Posner (1978) suggests, these cognitive elements appear to be defined by sensory impulses that are perceived and processed through the classical sensory tracts rather than through parallel pathways.

At the opposite extreme, unconscious material may be divided into two categories; that which can achieve awareness (episodic) and that which cannot (procedural). In the latter category are visceral engrams, somatosensory engrams belonging to involuntary motor activity, and vestibular engrams belonging to equilibrial activity. In these major activities, afferent information is fed largely into the basal ganglia and the cerebellum and efferent response patterns derive from those organs. As previously described, the cerebellum is a brain unto itself with about 50 billion neurons, equal in complexity to the cerebrum but lacking entirely in the quality of consciousness. Not only does the cerebellum lack an awareness system of its own, but it also does not generally connect with the awareness system of the main brain. On the other hand, in certain unusual conditions such as vertigo or learning a golf swing, mechanisms of equilibrium and/or involuntary motor activity are brought into awareness through activation of normal brain stem and cerebral mechanisms. Normal cerebellar activity constitutes true unconscious material that biologically cannot be brought into awareness. Similarly, the mechanisms that control visceral homeostasis (blood pressure, temperature, etc.) also operate under normal conditions outside of consciousness.

Squire (1982) has reviewed the literature on the types of learning that either are or are not impaired in individuals (human or primate) with bilateral resection of the hippocampi and amygdalae. These findings are summarized in Table 10-1 (courtesy of J. Ranck).

Table 10-1 Types of Memory Impairment in Individuals with Resected Hippocampi[a]

Functions Impaired	Functions Remaining Intact
Episodic memory	Semantic memory
Working memory	Reference memory
Declarative functions	Procedural functions
Data base learning	Skill learning
Memory for specific events	Habit
Analysis for meaning	Analysis for structure

[a]Impaired functions, are included under the general rubric of "episodic"; unimpaired functions are known variously as "procedural," "semantic," or "structural." For further descriptions, see Chapter 11.

It is clear that the impaired functions all involve the kinds of activities that are more easily learned by attending while the activities that remain unimpaired are those of a more automatic nature. The first category includes all those activities which are included under the rubric of episodic. The second category includes a variety of automatic activities which according to their functions are labeled procedural, seman- tic, or structural. These will be discussed at length in the next chapter.

As described, Squire (1982) has also distinguished between amnesias due to diencephalic and bitemporal pathology. The differences between these two syndromes seem to be more quantitative than qualitative. Certainly, there appears to be no signifi- cant difference in the kinds of learning abilities that are retained, i.e., procedural* activities; similarly, episodic cognitive memory consolidation and retrieval are im- paired in both syndromes. One gains the impression that both the diencephalon and the bitemporal areas are involved in memory consolidation and retrieval for episodic cognitive material, most probably in a sequentially integrated system. As Squire (1982) summarizes it:

> The importance to memory of the diencephalic and bitemporal structures affected in amnesia is believed to lie in their role in the establishment of memory at the time of learning and in the consolidation or elaboration of memory for a time after learning so as to permit effective retrieval. It also seems clear that this role is narrower than it once appeared to be, in the sense that it applies to particular domains of learning and memory and not to all domains. Thus, motor skills and certain cognitive skills have been proposed to belong to a class of learning that is termed ''procedural.'' This kind of learning is spared in amnesia and therefore is independent of the diencephalic and medial temporal structures that are affected in amnesia. (p. 268)

Even the capacity for episodic cognitive learning is retained to some degree in both of these syndromes, as evidenced by the ability of these amnesics to learn and remember some cognitive material if they are sufficiently cued (Weiskrantz, 1978). This indicates first that the two anatomical regions involved do compensate for one another to a limited extent and second that even episodic cognitive material may be subject to nonconscious processing. That the first premise is true results from the fact that the two key areas are involved in different stages, upstream and downstream, of a single screening process. That the second is equally true is the basis for the thesis that episodic material, like procedural material, can be, and is, effectively processed at the unconscious level (see Chapter 12).

Why it is that episodic types of data are more readily brought to consciousness then procedural or semantic can only be speculated on. Posner's suggestion that the classical sensory tracts appear to have more direct connection to the consciousness- arousal mechanisms than do the parallel routes of processing provides a plausible explanation. Presumably, the serial steps of abstraction through classical sensory routes as described in Chapter 4 provide a more effective method of learning and consolidation than do the short circuitings that occur in parallel processing. In addition,

---

*The term ''procedural'' is used most often in its specific sense to describe mechanical activities such as walking, talking, swimming, and so on. It is also used frequently in its generic sense to include all activities that are automatically processed, i.e., mechanical, semantic, structural, and visceral (see Chapter 11 for further descriptions). In order to avoid confusion between the two meanings, in this book we shall use the term ''procedural'' in its generic sense and the term ''mechanical'' to denote the specific activities.

the normal route of processing for episodic material leads more directly to the ento-rhinal cortex and then onto the amygdaloid–hippocampal complex to involve that unit in the learning, consolidation, recognition, and memory retrieval processes described in Chapter 9. It appears then that episodic data are consciously processed through entirely different channels than are unconscious procedural and visceral materials, channels which because they involve the thalamic–basal gangliar and amygdaloid–hippocampal complexes are directly related to conscious experience.

Anatomy of the Affective Components of Consciousness

The other major category of sensory data that is readily brought to consciousness is that of "feeling," including both those elements associated with sensory stimulation as in somatosensory experience and those associated with the subjective correlates of emotional expression. In Chapters 2 and 3, the physiology of the subjectification of motivational–emotional reactivities was discussed within the parameters of the Papez–MacLean theory. Mentioned there was the importance of the thalamus and basal ganglia in producing the subjective equivalents of the physiological changes associated with emotional expression. In Chapter 7, the sense of feeling was described as inherent in the self-awareness tract (the inferoparietal lobe); it was stated there that the ex-pression of feeling should logically be strongly associated with that part of the brain responsible for the reception of somatosensory stimuli. It appears that both somatosen-sory and emotional processing tracts are closely tied in with the self-awareness con-sciousness system, connections that make eminent biological sense.

Although motivations and emotions, like episodic data, constitute a major ele-ment in conscious experience, it is questionable whether motivational–emotional thoughts and feelings are processed through the same mechanisms as are episodic data. Even though it was pointed out that motivational–emotional sensory stimuli rise through the normal CNS tracts from the periphery to the brain, there appears to be no evidence that such reactivities pass through cognitive cortical centers in anything like the manner postulated for sensory episodic data. At most, affective material stemming from the periphery travels first to thalamic centers, progresses up into the limbic system, and then into the posterior inferior temporal lobe. It is in this area, and possibly also in the posterior sensory association area, that motivational–emotional valence is provided for all of the cognitive engrams anchored there.

Emotional feelings apparently enter the awareness system directly from the limbic system through the contiguous thalamic–basal gangliar complex during upstream pro-cessing. Evidence for this conclusion comes from the study by Kunst-Wilson and Zajonc (1980) previously described in Chapter 8; these authors showed that the emo-tional valence of a percept was recognized significantly earlier than its cognitive meaning. This finding is consistent with our interpretation that affective feelings enter the consciousness system through the thalamic–basal gangliar complex during up-stream processing while cognitive recognition does not occur until the exercise of more specific amygdaloid–hippocampal effects after downstream processing.

Thus all episodic cognitive material in awareness is associated with a specific emotional charge that provides its affective valence. However, the concurrence of episodic data with emotional feelings in consciousness in no way indicates that only here does such an association between cognitive and affective content occur. On the contrary, such an association is invariable be it for unconscious procedural material, unconscious episodic material, unconscious visceral material, and so on. The signal importance of these conclusions will become more apparent in the discussions of later chapters.

Experimental Studies Characterizing Controlled versus Automatic Information Processing in the Brain

The previous theoretical descriptions of conscious episodic data processing are confirmed by experimental psychological studies. On the basis of an extensive experimental program on cognitive behavior, Posner (1978) has listed several characteristics as differentiating between conscious (controlled) and unconscious (automatic) brain processing. He describes conscious brain activity as intentional, aware, limited, and interfering, while automatic brain activity is described as without intention, without conscious awareness, unlimited, and without an interference effect on other ongoing mental activity. These four characteristics of conscious "attentive" brain activity (intentionality, awareness, limited scope, and interference) and the absence of these qualities in unconscious "automatic" activity define in large part the operational differences between the two processes.

The term intentionality implies both self-interest and conscious motivation. Such intention, because it is conscious, must be something more than primitive innate biological drive; it reflects rather the total self-concept of the active individual. In other words, intentionality implies purposive behavior, deliberate and planned and directed toward the fulfillment of long-range goals rather than immediate biological ones. Such behavior is comprehensible only in terms of the involvement of mental constellations representing the entire organism.

In neurophysiological terms, intentionality suggests the integrated involvement of at least several behavioral systems: the motivational system (the limbic system and inferotemporal lobe); the executive planning system (the prefrontal lobe); and the self-awareness system (posterior parietal lobe). As described in Chapter 9 (Fig. 9-3), these structures together with the other cortical centers that constitute the decision-making consortium are considered to act through the hippocampal–amygdaloid complex to activate attention, i.e., conscious cognitive behavior. Consequently, Posner's characterization of conscious mental behavior as "intentional" goes far toward describing the various elements that, acting together, constitute the total phenomenon. Most importantly, intentionality signifies the existence of a strong motivational–emotional mental set directed toward some specific goal compatible with the drives of the total animal, i.e., the self.

Posner's other characterizations of conscious thought as "limited" and as "causing interference with other mental activity" represent important and distinct behavioral and neurophysiological differences from automatic mental behavior. Conscious behavior is limited because it is presumably funneled through the functional bottleneck created by the critical central role of the amygdaloid–hippocampal complex in attention. For the same reason, and because it involves primary sensory tract data, conscious behavior is sequential, so that two coincidental perceptual or cognitive behaviors will interfere with one another.

Utilizing a different set of experimental data from Posner (1978), Schneider and Shiffrin (1977) have investigated the behavioral phenomenology of "automatic information processing," which in the terminology of this volume would be "unconscious" information processing. They compare this with "controlled" information processing, the analogue of what in this volume would be "conscious" information processing. They conclude, on the basis of extensive experimentation and a comprehensive review of the literature, that most information processing is automatic and unconscious but that for certain kinds of learning to take place processing must be controlled and conscious. Their conceptualization of controlled processing is similar but slightly different from that of Posner's.

Conscious activity, or as defined by Schneider and Shiffrin "controlled processing," has certain characteristics. Most conscious activity is limited in the number of units of information that can be handled simultaneously (6–8 chunks); second, all conscious processing is *sequential* (i.e., utilizing one channel at a time) rather than *parallel* (i.e., utilizing multiple channels at a time). In this latter respect, conscious mental activity is like that of the first-line computers that were also essentially limited to sequential processing. However, computers are not limited like conscious thought by the number of variables that can be handled sequentially because computer speed is so great compared with brain speed that sequential processing constitutes no great burden for it (Simon, 1981). Consequently, according to Schneider and Shiffrin (1977), controlled conscious thinking is characterized by slowness, paucity of variables, and sequential processing. As is readily seen, this view is not significantly different from that of Posner's.

Most of the psychological characteristics of controlled information processing are explicable on the basis of the attentional, recognition, memory retrieval, and mental set mechanisms previously described. The sequential and limited quality of conscious thought are ascribed in part to the funneling effect of the amygdaloid–hippocampal complex and in part to the nature of episodic (primary sensory tract) data. The fact that the amygdaloid–hippocampal complex when active generates a θ rhythm at the rate of 6–8/sec is in keeping with a slow rate of processing to account for the limited capacity of conscious thought. The sequential character of controlled data processing is presumably responsible for interference effects. The dominance of left-hemispheric activity in consciousness also contributes to the sequentiality of controlled processing (see Chapter 14). Learning of episodic material is best accomplished with controlled processing because of the active involvement of the amygdaloid–hippocampal complex and the constant recurrence of activation of the same patterns of neurons.

Intermediate Forms of Information Processing

The separation of all thought processing in the brain into two specific categories, controlled and automatic, is itself an oversimplification since experimental evidence indicates that there are other types of processing that are intermediate in nature. For example, the equating above of Schneider and Shiffrin's controlled processing with our conscious processing is only valid in part. In their construct, controlled processing may under certain circumstances remain unconscious even though it is characterized by some of the qualities of controlled processing, i.e., the use of episodic data and the sequential nature of the processing, but not necessarily by all of its constraints. How is one to label such activity? Since the process has most of the characteristics of controlled processing except that it occurs unconsciously, it can be called unconscious controlled processing or alternatively semicontrolled processing. This category of activity is of the greatest importance since by its demonstration, Schneider and Shiffrin offer a justification for the concept of the unconscious processing of episodic material. Since controlled processing is more than merely a descriptive term but indicates also a specific neurophysiological mode of processing, their studies also suggest a putative physiological mechanism for the unconscious processing of episodic data. This concept will be expanded upon in Chapter 12.

A similar contradiction arises in the analyses of the unconscious processing of procedural data. Some of these activities appear completely automatic in nature, while others although predominantly automatic show evidence of some controlled activity. The first category involves procedural activities of a motor nature; their processing is characterized by purely automatic qualities. The second category of activities, although also basically procedural, are more involved with cognitive or semantic types of data processing. Since these are processed through different mechanisms, some of which are automatic and others controlled, their processing may be labeled as semiautomatic (see Chapter 11).

These considerations suggest that the simple division of the modes of information processing in the brain into the two categories, controlled and automatic, is insufficient and that a more complete spectrum running from controlled through semicontrolled to semiautomatic and automatic is necessary. These issues will be discussed in depth in Chapter 11 on the procedural unconscious and in Chapter 12 on the episodic unconscious.

The Various Modes of Conscious Brain Activity

Conscious mental activity may be broken down into three major categories: conscious perception, conscious recognition, and conscious thought. The differences in these three conditions reflect differences in the sources of information being processed and secondly, differences in the neural systems handling those materials. Conscious perception involves perceptual information from the environment that is processed predominantly by the thalamic–basal gangliar complex. Conscious recognition represents the most active interaction between external stimuli and internal memories, with a correspondingly equal involvement of the thalamic–basal gangliar and amygdaloid–hippocampal complexes. Conscious thought involves mainly engrams rising from long-term memory and is implemented through the interaction of the thalamic–basal gangliar and the amygdaloid–hippocampal complexes. Conscious mental activity comprises all of these activities interacting in one form or another.

The question arises: How intact does conscious mental activity remain in those cases where one or the other of these critical neural centers is pathologically destroyed or surgically removed. We have already seen that destruction of the thalamic–basal gangliar complex leads to akinetic mutism with a corresponding absence of conscious mental activity. The damage in diencephalic amnesia is in the thalamic–basal gangliar complex but is anatomically limited so that thought processing in Korsakoff syndrome patients is somewhat impaired but relatively intact. Complete surgical ablation of the amygdaloid–hippocampal complexes was performed in H.M. and if our formulations are correct, there should be markedly impaired capacity for cognitive mental activity remaining.

It is our thesis that in the absence of amygdaloid–hippocampal activity, all that remains is a form of conscious perception. In these cases, such perception is equivalent to the first stage of attention and is limited to those activities that are controlled by the thalamic–basal gangliar complex. It is characterized by a general awareness of the environment, and by retention of the ability to retrieve well-consolidated long-term memories, i.e., of memories more than three years old. In addition, some unconscious episodic recognition may still occur activated directly through the thalamic–basal gangliar complex. This is particularly true for the affective components of perceptions. Attentional mechanisms also remain intact although they are not of the same focused intensity as are those characteristic of amygdaloid–hippocampal activity.

Thus the characteristics of conscious perception are essentially those of the bilaterally hippocampectomized patient H.M., who on the surface has full awareness and full attentional capacities. Actually he is unable to consciously recognize anything he has experienced since the time three years prior to his surgery. H.M.'s attentional and consciousness capacities essentially define the role of the thalamic–basal gangliar complex in these activities since that anatomical complex is all the attentional apparatus that remains to him. It is apparent in H.M. that the activation of the thalamic–basal gangliar complex by the noradrenergic RAS together with the involvement of the neocortex produces most of the qualities of apparently normal attentional awareness. Therefore, the role of the amygdaloid–hippocampus, critical as it is in learning and memory retrieval, is strictly secondary in the implementation of primitive consciousness and attentional activities.

However, in the more specific processes of conscious recognition, the amygdaloid–hippocampal complex does play a critical role in organizing behavior. Since learning and memory retrieval are perhaps the most characteristically human activities, the loss of these abilities essentially destroys the human condition. H.M. remains highly human although largely incapacitated because he had a long history of learning prior to surgery, most of which was available to him after surgery. An infant who at birth had no amygdaloid–hippocampal complex could hardly develop at all because the thalamic–basal gangliar complex could never assume a sufficiently compensatory role.

As to the quality of the inner mental life of an individual who suffered a bilateral resection of the amygdalae and hippocampi even in middle life, Winson (1985) has written concerning H.M.:

> He cannot remember events that had happened only a few moments before. For example, he fails to recognize people he has just met and with whom he has spent many hours. For years H.M. worked at a state rehabilitation center doing simple

manual tasks but during all that period he could never describe his place of work, the nature of his job, or the route along which he was driven every day. Nor can he remember anything about that job today. Having eaten a meal, he will, moments later not recall the experience and will eat another if it is placed before him. His mother has described how H.M. will do the same jigsaw puzzle day after day without any improvement in performance as if the puzzle were new each time, and will read the same magazine over and over again without remembering the content. He has said, "Every day is alone in itself, whatever enjoyment I've had and whatever sorrow I've had." (pp. 11–12)

Conscious thought ordinarily involves the amygdaloid–hippocampal complex because it is based on the continuous activation of memories from the long-term memory store. Nevertheless, even here the thalamic–basal gangliar complex is equally involved since (1) it has major responsibility for the phenomena of consciousness and (2) it retains major capacity for retrieving older (more than three years old) well-consolidated memories. The role of the two major complexes of the attentional system—the thalamic–basal gangliar and the amygdaloid–hippocampal—in the various conditions of amnesia offers interesting insights into their mode of interaction.

The Role of the Unconscious in Conscious Experience

That the phenomena of consciousness consist, at least in part, of the four elements described above, i.e., conscious perception, conscious recognition, conscious thought, and the conscious self, is self-evident. What is less apparent is that conscious awareness is also based on an immense anlage of unconscious experience. For example, as discussed in Chapter 7, the feeling of self, although it seems strongest during alert consciousness, is based predominantly on unconscious sensations that establish the reality and the "sense" of the body. Usually one is not aware of the feeling of his body unless he is in a state of pain or tension, but at such times the sense of identification between the psychic self and the body becomes great indeed. Consequently, the unconscious sense of self is as much a part of conscious experience as are all of the cognitive and emotional sensations of which the individual may be aware.

This paradoxical situation where unconscious input must be considered as part of conscious experience is extended in a multitude of operations other than those which establish the identity of the self. For example, structural and procedural operations (see Chapter 11) prepare sensory stimuli for processing (structural) and integrate motor activities for responding (procedural) in programs without which conscious sensory or motor activities would be impossible. In running, the individual is consciously aware that he is running, but he is not aware of the intricate neural and muscular activities that make running possible. Similarly, in making a decision, we are often not aware of the mental set that determines our decision. Yet these unconscious influences are very real and constitute as large a part of conscious experience as does that limited horizon of which we are aware.

Because the self-awareness system and the entire self-concept system anchored on it are functioning at their most optimal level of activity during the alert conscious state, the subjective sense of self is correspondingly greatest at that time. Equally active is the cortical consortium of behavioral centers which constitutes the decision-making component of the executive self. The interaction of both components of the self-system, the subjective and the executive, at their highest level of activity during the alert conscious state results in actions that are most readily identified by the individual as being his own (intentional). The special character of alert conscious perception and thought is the product of the conditions that characterize that period: the kinematic quality of perceptual images and thought impressions, the nature of controlled information processing, and the high level of activity in both the subjective and executive components of the self-system.

The vividness of conscious thought activity in comparison with the by definition hidden quality of unconscious thought processing has led all too understandably to an exaggeration of the importance of the former and to an equal neglect of the significance of the latter. Even more difficult to encompass is the fact that episodic data can be processed either consciously or unconsciously while procedural operations are almost entirely unconscious. Most important is the recognition that although both episodic and procedural data can be processed unconsciously, the mode of such processing for the two categories is physiologically different. These considerations will be addressed in the next two chapters.

The Procedural Unconscious: Automatic Processing of Mechanical, Structural, and Semantic Data

As opposed to conscious episodic data processing which is governed by a single albeit complicated physiological sequence, unconscious procedural processing involves a variety of types of material each of which is processed through unique and characteristic mechanisms. Consequently the description of unconscious data processing involves not one but many different physiological systems.

The distinctions between episodic and procedural data were described in Chapter 10 (Table 10-1). Episodic data processing defines experience while procedural mechanisms control the processes of gaining experience. Much, perhaps most episodic data, after analysis in the thalamic–basal gangliar complex and possibly the amygdaloid–hippocampal complex, may be evaluated as significant enough to be processed but not significant enough to be admitted to consciousness. Such *unconscious episodic* data processing is of a different order than the *conscious* episodic processing described in the last chapter and the procedual processing to be reviewed here. It will be discussed in Chapter 12.

The three major categories of procedural experience that are processed unconsciously are *mechanical, structural,* and *semantic.* These materials are involved in physical manipulation of motor and sensory activities rather than, as with episodic data, providing for content. As indicated in Table 10-1, procedural data can be learned and retrieved in both the diencephalic and bitemporal amnesic syndromes. However, even though such materials can be learned and retrieved in these syndromes, they can be retrieved only operationally and not to awareness. The inability of procedural material to reach consciousness is not in itself proof positive that such material must be processed through mechanisms other than the thalamic–basal gangliar and the amygdaloid–hippocampal systems. As will be described in Chapter 12, *most* episodic material does not reach consciousness even after having been processed through those very systems. But the difference between the unconscious processing of episodic data and that of procedural data is qualitative. All episodic data can be brought to awareness if the stimulus is strong enough and attention sufficiently directed. Procedural data almost always, and with very few exceptions, cannot be brought to awareness at all.

The term *mechanical* carries the connotation of unconscious activities involving musculoskeletal and equilibrial performance. These are the essential elements that differentiate it from episodic activities. "Fact" (episodic) memory is almost purely cognitive; "skill" (mechanical) memory in most instances involves some form of motor learning. Mechanical problems such as the Tower of Hanoi puzzle, which seems cognitive in character, encompass significant visuomotor and proprioceptive motor activities. Other processes such as walking, running, and swimming are almost entirely dependent on such activities.

Semantic processes include all those involved in speech and communication: (1) the formation of speech by the organs of the mouth and throat, (2) the choice of words for meaning, and (3) the use of the proper syntax. These processes are more accurately labeled, respectively, (1) phonetic, (2) semantic, and (3) syntactic, with the entire operation falling under the rubic of "linguistic." However, since the term semantic has been adopted in this literature to signify all linguistic activities, it will be retained here. Nevertheless, it is clear that of the terms available, semantic, with its connotation of meaning, is probably the least appropriate as a label for the unconscious procedural-like activities associated with oral communication.

The importance of such linguistic mechanisms for communication is obvious; without these unconscious processes, conscious social intercourse between individuals could not take place. In a group conversation, one can readily reconstruct the enormous complexities in conscious programs which must occur if meaningful communication is to be possible: the decision to speak, the shift in attention to a new speaker, the conscious appreciation of communicated meaning both in production and in reception, and many other activities. What is less evident are the immense array of unconscious semantic and motor activities involved in these processes. Certainly those responsible for the production of speech are most obvious. There is evidence to indicate that even silent thinking is associated with the unconscious formation by the lips and tongue of the words encompassing the thoughts; some researchers believe that thinking is an unconscious motor activity of the speech organs of which conscious thought is merely the mental analogue. Without going to this extreme, it is obvious how significant unconscious linguistic processes are in conscious speech and communication.

Purely *structural* functions are also operationally retained in patients with either the mesencephalic or bitemporal forms of amnesia. Structural operations include the mechanisms by which sensory input is organized into specific entities which can be retained and utilized in the brain as episodic data. For example, in the visual sphere, learning to estimate the distance to faraway objects is a structural skill based largely on the innate biological mechanism of binocular vision but involving also the learned elaboration of that inherently endowed ability in the columnar organization of the visual cortex (Mountcastle, 1978a). Other physical qualities of perceived objects such as outlines are identified unconsciously, actually at the retinal level (Kuffler, 1953) in structural operations. Similarly in the auditory realm, melodies are abstracted and translated from one key and rhythm to another without loss of recognition through mechanisms that are completely unconscious. These so-called structural processes are similar to mechanical ones except that they utilize not motor activities, but rather sensory-organizing mechanisms at the unconscious level.

As important as episodic, semantic, structural, and mechanical engrams may be, they constitute only four of the many components of unconscious mental activity; other types of functions (visceral, equilibrial, etc.) provide additional substantive content for the vast activities of the unconscious. Since all of these disparate biological activities are carried out at the unconscious level, it is obvious that conscious mental activity constitutes only a tiny fraction of the whole. Even though we are concerned mainly with those emotionally charged episodic engrams which encompass most human experience, it is necessary to explore the many varieties of unconscious procedural engrams and their modes of processing in order to gain some insight into the mechanisms governing unconscious mental processing in general.

There are an immense number of biological activities that have their control centers in the central nervous system. A partial list is given in Table 11-1 together with a description of the capacity of the different processes for reaching awareness. Psychological studies have established the level of function (conscious or unconscious) of these various processes as well as some of the behavioral characteristics of the mental activities associated with each.

General Characteristics of Automatic Data Processing

Posner (1978) and Shiffrin and Schneider (1977), using unconscious learning of procedural and semantic processes as their experimental paradigm, have described the

Table 11-1 Categories of Conscious and Unconscious Engrams Together with Their Putative Mode of Processing

Type of Engram	Status	Mode of Processing
Episodic cognitive process (idea or thought)	Conscious or unconscious	Controlled Semicontrolled
Mechanical motor process (walking, running)	Conscious or unconscious	Controlled (rarely) Automatic
Semantic cognitive process (reading and talking)	Conscious or unconscious	Controlled (rarely) Automatic or semiautomatic
Structural process (figure–background and stereoscopic visual functions)	Unconscious	Automatic
Emotional motor reaction (body language)	Conscious or unconscious	Controlled (rarely) Visceral or semiautomatic
Voluntary motor movement	Conscious	Controlled
Involuntary motor movement	Unconscious	Automatic
Visceral and equilibrial operations	Conscious or unconscious	Controlled (rarely) Visceral or automatic
Emotionally charged[a] cognitive percept or memory	Conscious or unconscious	Controlled Semicontrolled
Right-hemispheric percept[b] or memory	Unconscious	Semicontrolled
Free-floating emotion	Conscious or unconscious	Visceral Visceral
Orienting response	Semiconscious	Semicontrolled

[a]To be discussed in Chapter 13.
[b]To be discussed in Chapter 14.

behavioral characteristics of such activity. Unconscious "automatic" mental activities are characterized in Posner's (1978) description as the opposite of conscious process and thus lacking in intentionality, lacking the quality of awareness, virtually unlimited in scope, and occurring simultaneously without mutual interference. "Lack of intentionality" implies the absence of the integrating influences of attention and self through the coordinated activities of the several behavioral systems illustrated in Figure 9-3. "Lack of awareness" in our terminology is redundant for "unconscious." "Unlimited" signifies the absence of the functional bottleneck activity of the amygdaloid–hippocampal complex in its attentional capacity, and "lacking an interference effect" speaks for parallel processing as opposed to the sequential processing of conscious attentive mental activity in primary classical sensory tracts.

Shiffrin and Schneider (1977), using a somewhat different experimental design, come to similar but not identical conclusions. According to them, the processing of procedural material (defined by Shiffrin and Schneider as "automatic processing") differs most significantly from that of episodic processing in that the entire reservoir of engrams in the brain is available for simultaneous utilization at any time. Automatic processing of data may be both sequential and parallel, markedly increasing both the speed and the complexity of possible mental manipulations. Consequently, the operations of automatic processing must be considered in many ways superior to those of controlled processing even though not all the data nor the lines of reasoning leading to a given conclusion are available to awareness, as in conscious processing. This accounts for the not infrequent effectiveness of so-called intuitive reactions.

Unconscious processing of procedural data appears to be more diffuse and probably involves more of the brain in an unstructured pattern than does conscious processing. Paradoxically, this is particularly true during periods of alert conscious activity since the entire brain has about twice the activity during active consciousness than it does during periods of mental inactivity (Fig. 11-4). In attended conscious activities, total brain function is more active, more highly structured, and more highly focused, not only because the entire consciousness system is mobilized, but also because at such times the entire unconscious processing system is mobilized. Unconscious mental activities, because they are unlimited and unrestricted both in quantity and mechanisms, and because they are continuous, confer a different type of advantage on the organism. When the consciousness system is relatively or totally inactive, as in sleep or altered states of consciousness, the unconscious continues to function at a moderate level, maintaining not only the visceral integrity of the organism, but a type of behavioral integrity as well. When the consciousness system is actively alerted, then the unconscious operates at its optimal level, even though its effects may be obscured by the effects of consciousness.

Neurophysiological Mechanisms of Procedural Processing

As depicted in Figure 11-1, processing of procedural data is believed to involve entirely different physiological circuits than those controlling the processing of episodic data. The procedural processing circuit comprises both the cerebellum and the putamen and caudate nuclei, centers in the basal ganglia. The putamen and caudate

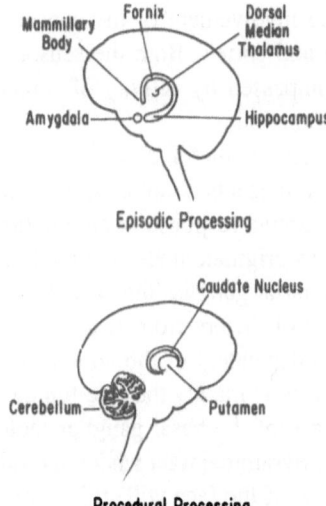

Episodic Processing

Procedural Processing

Figure 11-1 Anatomy of episodic and procedural processing.

nucleus in the basal ganglia are involved predominantly in automatic motor control activity; conversely, different basal gangliar centers of the thalamic–basal gangliar complex are involved mainly in attentional activities. The basal gangliar centers concerned with processing procedural data (i.e., the putamen and caudate nucleus) are separate and distinct from the basal gangliar nuclei concerned with processing episodic data (the globus pallidus, the substantia innominata, and the nucleus basalis of Meynart). The fact that these various basal gangliar centers exist anatomically in contiguous areas does not necessarily mean that they are functionally connected. On the other hand, it is possible that when procedural material is fed into awareness, as it rarely may be, connections to the awareness system may occur from the putamen and caudate nucleus to the contiguous globus pallidus and substantia innominata.

The cerebellum is the organ predominantly responsible for involuntary motor control and coordination, so that it is not surprising to find that it plays a major role in procedural learning. Because of its size and complexity (around 50 billion neurons), cerebellar function is almost as complex as neocortical. Together with the vestibular system and the basal gangliar system of the main brain, it controls most procedural activities. A comparison of the episodic and procedural neural processing systems is given in Figure 11-1.

Specific neurophysiological mechanisms have been described for certain forms of automatic activity. A study by McCormick et al. (1982) provides evidence that conditioned motor learning is accomplished at the unconscious level mainly through cerebellar mechanisms. Animals were taught in a conditioning paradigm to perform a specific motor act to escape punishment. When the skilled motor reaction was well established, a localized area of the cerebellum specific for the musculature involved was excised. With this lesion there was a complete loss of the particular learned motor reaction, although there was no evidence of weakness or of sensory impairment in the extremities involved. This experiment provides evidence that conditioning of skilled motor reactions occurs at an unconscious level through the involvement of cerebellar circuits rather than through the involvement of the conscious voluntary sensory and motor tracts of the brain stem and cortex. Both the sensory and motor elements of a conditioned response are encompassed by activity of cerebellar neurons, half of the cells of which are sensory in function.

A different type of involuntary motor reactivity is associated with emotional expression. "Body language" represents a motor component of emotional expression generated as part of the toal adaptive response to an emotion-evoking experience. Its basic elements are considered to originate under the control of the involuntary motor control system localized in the basal ganglia (the caudate nucleus and putamen). This type of involuntary motor control differs from that of cerebellar involuntary motor control; the former is largely independent of the voluntary motor control system (the pyramidal tract) whereas the latter is mainly the fine-tuning system for motor control. An example of the independence of the basal gangliar motor control system is illustrated in cases of damage to the pyramidal tract where one side of the face is paralyzed. Under these conditions, that side of the face will still move involuntarily if the person smiles or frowns. Here the involuntary motor control, exercised as the basal ganglia component of an emotional response, remains intact. Since emotional motor responses are not generally under conscious control, they comprise another set of unconscious processes which might be called visceral, involuntary, or semiautomatic.

The critical involvement of the cerebellum as described in the implementation of conditioned motor reflexes is fully in keeping with the well-established role of that organ in regulating and coordinating unconscious procedural motor activities. Similarly, the central role of the basal ganglia in controlling motor patterns of involuntary emotional expression is equally well established. Thus these two major brain centers, together with their associated neural tracts, substantially account for most automatic involuntary motor processing. More surprising is the recent evidence from the laboratories of Squire and his co-workers that these two systems, functioning in an integrated although not yet well-understood fashion, also provide the physiological control system for procedural or semantic learning. These activities contain important motor components, especially in so-called procedural learning; they also contain major sensory elements, particularly in semantic learning. As an example of the latter, patients with mesencephalic or bitemporal amnesias can learn to read sentences written backward (from right to left) as readily as can normals, certainly a task more cognitive than motor. In addition to the cerebellum, Squire and his group have identified the caudate nucleus and the putamen, two major components of the basal ganglia, as critical in maintaining procedural and semantic learning, indicating that these areas may have more significant roles in unconscious processing than had been previously postulated.*

The foregoing discussions appear to implicate specific portions of the basal ganglia (the putamen and caudate nucleus) and probably most of the cerebellum in a well-integrated interacting circuit, the nature of which has not yet been well established. Apparently both of these complexes (the putamen–caudate nucleus and the cerebellar)

---

*Note here also the previously described work of Mishkin (1982) on the role of the basal ganglia in establishing "habit" activities (see pp. 121 and 122).

are involved in the control of a vast array of procedural and visceral automatic functions. By definition it would appear that motor efferent activities of these complexes would be as strongly involved as the sensory afferent receptors in procedural activities, whereas this might not apply for visceral operations. These same neural complexes also appear to determine the motor aspects of emotional expression (for example, facial expressions and body language) so that these too may in a larger sense be called semiautomatic.

The specific characteristics of automatic processing appear to derive from the fact that it utilizes mechanisms of processing largely unassociated with hippocampal–amygdaloid attentional activity. It is assumed that in automatic processing, the various major systems (the cognitive, the motivational, the emotional, and the motor) all interreact in a relatively structured fashion, involving each other intimately, but not in the tightly organized and highly structured manner possible under frontal lobe, hippocampal–amygdaloid, self-awareness system control. However, even though unconscious procedural and semantic operations do not appear to have available to them the complex mechanisms involved in routine episodic data processing (for example, abstraction, association, the formation of engrams, verbal symbolization, the logic inherent in language, and so on), it would be a mistake to assume that the mechanisms of procedural and semantic operations are simpler than those involved in conscious episodic information processing. On the contrary, the complexity of certain procedural tasks such as throwing a ball, recognizing a melody in a different key, or recognizing an object in various positions are unquestionably as difficult as are the most purely cognitive tasks.

Functional Programs in Procedural Operations

As observed by Preston (1983) in the introduction to this volume, the interactions among various sensory and motor modalities necessary to perform certain procedural operations are incredibly complicated. The coordination of muscular activity with vestibular, proprioceptive, and visual sensory input necessary to accurately throw a football to a running receiver 30 yards away would involve enormously complex mathematical computations, all completed in a fraction of a second. Although sports and ballet may represent the highest level of procedural complexity, simple motor operations such as walking or lying in bed involve almost equally difficult mechanisms. All of these operations require complex computations far beyond the capacities of our largest, most sophisticated computers.

The processes by which the minds of vertebrates, down to the most primitive sharks, are able to perform these complex sensory calculations and transform them into equally complex muscular activities are at present largely unknown. Researchers in artificial intelligence are particularly anxious to discover these mechanisms because their introduction into computer technology would bring about a major expansion in capabilities. For want of a better explanation, the term "functional programs" has been used as a label for these mechanism; but this essentially replaces one unknown with another.

The central role of the cerebellum in organizing procedural and structural transformations is quite understandable once one recognizes the immense inputs into it from the rest of the central nervous system. This is particularly true for the sensory input that is essential to allow adequate control of motor coordination. The control of voluntary and involuntary motor activities is an extremely sensitive arrangement where minute adjustments in motor stimulation and inhibition are monitored on a split-second-to-split-second schedule on the basis of sensory impulses returning from the involved muscles and joints. This feedforward and feedback arrangement makes smooth motor activity possible.

However, the coordination of motor activity in the entire organism is much more complex than is encompassed in the relationship of the innervation of the skeletal mass to the cerebellum. In the acts of walking and running, not only must the muscles and joints of the body be synchronized in a steady rhythm, but the body as a whole must be kept on balance. This is accomplished through the vestibulospinal reflex which keeps the head position steady regardless of body movements. Here vestibular apparatus input into the cerebellum is coordinated with the total sensory input from the body musculoskeletal mass to keep the organism in steady equilibrium.

Even more complex is the vestibulo-ocular reflex which, despite constant head movements, maintains a steady retinal image; without this, visual objects could not be continually attended. This reflex involves impulses coming from the retina and from the ocular nerves to the superior colliculus where they connect to tracts to and from the vestibular apparatus and the cerebellum. Through these connections many different modalities interact: vision, eye movements, equilibrial mechanisms, and motor coordination. The physiology of the vestibulo-ocular reflex has generally been worked out (Szentagothai and Arbib, 1974) so that already the dynamics of one complex procedural program are known.

Besides the visual input into the cerebellum from the superior colliculus, similar tracts from the auditory and other sensory centers in the brain stem contribute elements of all sensory modalities to the cerebellar pool. Here they are integrated through the vast machinery of the cerebellum (50 billion neurons) to provide for most of the complex procedural and equilibrial operations in the brain. Since none of this is conscious, the cerebellar component of neural coordination, together with the basal gangliar (caudate nucleus and putamen) component of muscular coordination, account for much of the unconscious activity in the brain.

Grillner (1985) has summarized the role of the basal ganglia and cerebellum in organizing and controlling automatic behaviors as follows:

> In mammals as well as lower vertebrates complex patterns of behavior can be performed by animals lacking a cerebral cortex. Neonatally decorticated cats move around in a way that, to the casual observer, does not appear different from that of intact cats. The locomotion appears goal-oriented, for such animals seek and eat food. They even perform exploratory forelimb movements. Decorticated female cats can copulate, give birth, and care for their newborn. A variety of apparently meaningful movements can thus be initiated and performed in cats lacking a cortex. From these results one may of course not conclude that, under normal conditions, the cortex is unimportant for initiation of such movement patterns. On the other hand, it is important that, with only the basal ganglia intact, the central nervous system (CNS) has the capacity to initiate and generate a complex movement repertoire adapted to the needs

of the animal. This is in striking contrast to animals with a lesion at a lower diencephalic level that leaves only the mesencephalon and lower brainstem intact. Such
animals can be made to walk, chew, or swallow, but the movements are stereotyped
and machine-like and are no longer adapted to the needs of the animal or its environment. (p. 147)*

Quantitative Studies of Neuronal Activity in Different States of Consciousness

In the last section, we described the functions of the procedural unconscious and
the physiological mechanisms underlying its operation. But we did not address the
critical question as to whether the procedural unconscious is operational only under the
direction of purposive consciousness, or whether, rather, it is independently active
during all phases of the conscious–unconscious continuum.

Because the experimental investigation of procedural learning requires an alert
subject, the characteristics of unconscious data processing have been derived almost
entirely from the investigation of unconscious activities during the active alert conscious state. Since we wish to know whether the procedural unconscious operates
independently of consciousness, it is important to explore whether such unconscious
activities (both behavioral and neurophysiological) continue during periods of relative
unconsciousness, i.e., during sleep and in altered states of consciousness.

If the concept of consciousness is difficult to describe because of its ephemeral
quality, the unconscious is even more difficult to analyze because of its inaccessibility.
But such an analysis is essential since, as indicated by Jung's analysis, at any given
moment more than 99% of "brain activity" is at the unconscious level. Whether such
brain activity constitutes real activity, especially during the quiescent state, or rather
quiet inactivity remains the critical question. Depending on the answer, the unconscious may be seen as a dynamic level of interaction of activities continually influencing behavior at all times, or alternatively as a reservoir of inert engrams that are
activated only momentarily when brought into consciousness. Our intuitive response,
influenced certainly by our long exposure to Freudian psychology, leans toward the
former description. But this does not preclude the necessity for an objective exploration of this issue. Furthermore, such an inquiry should not only illuminate the nature of
unconscious thought processing, but might also throw some light on its mechanisms.

A first approach to this question is to examine the most basic level of brain
function, namely that of neuronal activity, in different behavioral states. Although
mental functions are ultimately more than can be expressed in terms of the simple
activity of individual brain cells, the statistical study of the latter is closely relevant to
our inquiry.

Experimental data on these issues stem mainly from single cell recordings from
groups of neurons in the ascending reticular activating system and in the cortex of

---

*The fact that decorticate cats can function as well as they do in a total environment also indicates that
significant episodic processing takes place at a subcortical level (see Chapter 12).

animals during various activities in the waking state and during slow-wave and REM sleep. Evarts (1967) has reviewed the subject with particular reference to his own work on pyramidal motor cells (Evarts, 1965a) and on visual cells in the cortex (Evarts, 1965b), and to the work of Huttenlocher (1961) on neurons in the reticular activating system. In each area, 15 to 50 neurons were individually monitored for spontaneous discharge rate under several conditions of waking, deep sleep, and REM sleep, and a distribution spectrum of activity determined. The findings for two areas are illustrated in Figures 11-2 and 11-3.

The findings in the brain stem and in the cortex are somewhat similar in that in both areas there is a greater concentration of activities in the middle section of the spectrum during deep sleep and a greater dispersion toward the extremes during the waking phase. The general overall level of activity during slow-wave sleep seems roughly half of that during the waking period. A similar relationship is seen in an examination of visual sensory neuronal activity in the striate area as illustrated in Figure 11-4. Here the mean discharge frequencies during slow-wave sleep and during waking without vision are generally comparable. The mean frequencies for REM sleep and for waking with vision are also about equal, but about twice that of the previous set. Again the variability is about twice as great in the waking without vision condition as in slow-wave sleep.

Thus in three areas of the brain of markedly disparate function—the reticular activating system, the motor system, and the visual sensory system—overall activity during slow-wave sleep appears to be about equal to that in the relaxed waking state, i.e., without visual or motor activity. The general level of neuronal activity appears to

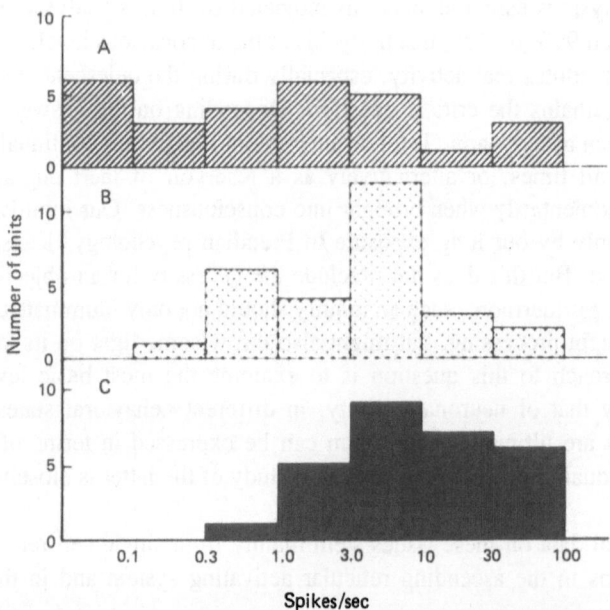

Figure 11-2 Discharge rates in brain stem reticular system during waking, slow-wave sleep, and REM sleep. (From Huttenlocher, 1961. Reproduced with permission.)

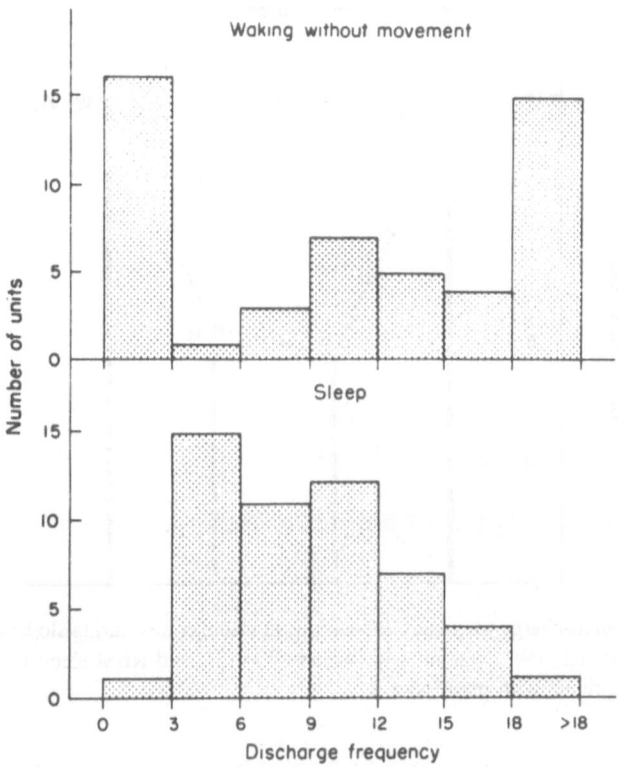

Figure 11-3 Discharge rates in pyramidal neurons during relaxed waking (W) and slow-wave sleep (S). (From Evarts, 1967. Reprinted with permission.)

rise to twice the baseline level in REM sleep and during active sensory or motor performance. It appears that during waking activity there is a shift from the midrange of frequencies of the sleep state to the extremes, both high and low. During REM sleep (and presumably during active sensory or motor processing), there is a marked shift in neuronal activity in the direction of higher frequencies (Fig. 11-2).

These data, although helpful, still do not respond to the question as to the level of frequency discharge at which a given neuron is *functionally* active. Although there are no definitive data on this issue, the work of Morrell (1967) suggests that resting quiescent neurons have a spontaneous discharge rate of about 8–9/sec, at which level the neuron may be considered to be relatively inactive. Using the rate of 9–10/sec as our arbitrary cutoff point, the relationships in Figures 11-2, 11-3, and 11-4 may be reinterpreted to give a more accurate picture of the percentages of very active and of relatively inactive neurons in the different behavioral situations. Within these new considerations, it is probable that the differentials may be somewhat greater than previously calculated. For example, under the REM condition, about half of the neuronal population in the RAS are active (Fig. 11-2), while probably closer to 100% of those in the striate cortex (Fig. 11-4) are functionally involved. For waking without motion or vision (the resting state), only 15% of neurons in the RAS are active, while about 60% of neurons in the pyramidal tract and probably 15–35% in the visual cortex

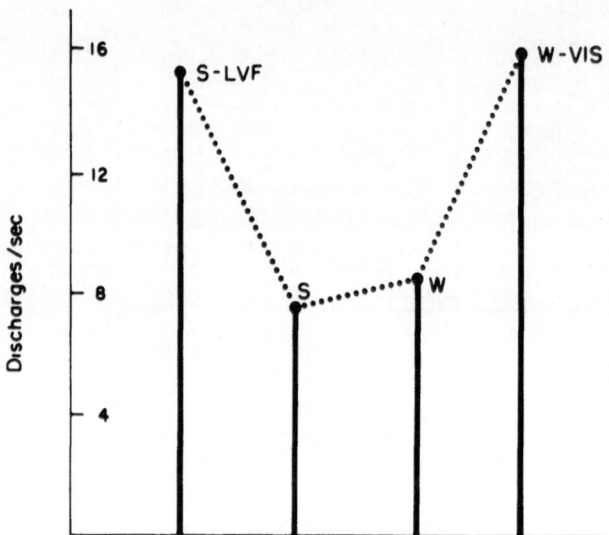

Figure 11-4 Mean discharge frequency for neurons in visual cortex during slow-wave sleep (S), waking in relaxed state (W), waking with vision (W-VIS), and REM sleep (S-LVG). (From Evarts, 1967. Reprinted with permission.)

show activity. For deep sleep, there is presumably still less activity in all areas, although the differences from the quiescent waking state are surprisingly small. The major difference between the relaxed waking and deep sleep stages is in the variability of frequencies, high in relaxed waking and very low in deep sleep.

These physiological data suggest that in high arousal states (waking states associated with vision or motion, and REM sleep) almost the entire brain is functioning actively, though few engrams are being brought into awareness at any given moment. Even in low arousal states it appears that 30–50% of the cortex is still in an active state. By any standards, using either loose criteria of activity (all discharging neurons) or stricter criteria (only those neurons with spontaneous discharge rates of 9/sec or more), a large proportion of the brain appears to be active under all conditions. On the basis of experimental data, the ratios of conscious to unconscious activities described in Jung's analysis appear to have general validity. The physiological evidence not only supports the existence of potentially available unconscious material, but even more of an active unconscious, actively functioning in both high arousal and low arousal behavioral states.

Unconscious Activity in Various Neural Systems

The data just presented offer some insight into activities of three different neural systems of the brain: (1) the reticular activating system, (2) the cognitive system (visual cortex), and (3) the motor system (pyramidal cells). A comparison of the levels of activity of the cells in each of these systems under four different conditions, two of which represent high activation and two low activation, makes it possible to estimate the level of activity at the unconscious level, i.e., the residual at different levels of brain activity, during alert consciousness and during periods of relative inertness. The four conditions represented are (1) waking without vision or motions, i.e., the resting state (2) waking with either vision or motion, (3) deep slow-wave sleep, and (4) REM sleep.

Using 9 to 10 spontaneous discharges per second as our criterion of activity, in the waking state without vision or motion, i.e., the relaxed resting state with eyes closed, only about 15% of neurons in the RAS, about 25–35% of neurons in the visual cortex, and about 60% of neurons in the pyramidal tract are active. The 15% level of activity in the RAS is much higher than Jung's estimate of 1% for the resting state and the levels of activity for the visual cortex and the pyramidal tract are significantly higher. If we assume that visual cortex activity represents cognitive rather than perceptual activity (since the eyes are closed in the resting stage), then it would appear that about one third of the cognitive engrams in the brain anchored in the visual cortex remain active in this condition. A similar extrapolation suggests that during the resting state almost two thirds of motor functions are at least potentially active.

The corresponding figures for deep sleep are surprisingly similar. Again, the number of cells in the RAS with a discharge of 10 or more is about 15%, while the figure for the visual cortex remains about 25–35%. The percentage for pyramidal activity during slow-wave sleep does fall to about 50%, but this is still remarkably high considering that deep sleep is associated with almost complete muscular relaxation.

An exact estimate of the levels of activity in the various systems under fully alert and REM sleep conditions is difficult because of the paucity of data. It seems safe to estimate that in the alert conscious condition, all of the cells in the RAS, visual cortex, and motor cortex are more or less fully activated. In REM sleep, all of the cells in the visual cortex apparently remain activated, but only about 50% of those in the RAS. (No data are available for pyramidal cells.) As described in Chapter 6, in REM sleep the RAS is activated not by the noradrenergic locus coeruleus, but rather by the cholinergic FTG cells of the pons. Consequently this moderately high level of activity in the RAS during REM sleep is obviously of a different quality than that generated by the noradrenergic system during alert consciousness.

The most important conclusions of this analysis derive from the data on the activities of the three neural systems during the resting state (relaxed awake without vision or motion) and during deep sleep. It appears that in both of these states when activity in the RAS is very low (about 15%), cognitive (visual cortex) activity remains moderately high (about 30%), while motor cortical activity remains quite high (about 60%). It makes just as little sense to relate activity in pyramidal cells to voluntary motor activity in deep sleep as it would to speak of moderate visual activity in that condition. What must be hypothesized rather is that in deep sleep, motor engrams anchored in the pyramidal cortex remain potentially active, as do cognitive engrams anchored in the visual cortex.

Having made that assumption, it becomes possible to take the next step and postulate that the levels of motor cortex and visual cortex activities during the resting state and deep sleep represent the levels of unconscious activity in the motor and cognitive systems that persist when the consciousness system is essentially inactive. These calculations again not only indicate that there is an active unconscious, but even suggest that the quantitative composition of that unconscious is mainly motor but partially cognitive. More important, it is unlikely that the visual engrams active in this unconscious are those involved in visuomotor activity since in both the resting state and in deep sleep, the visual system per se is inactive. Therefore, it seems plausible that the visual engrams involved here constitute episodic data that continue to operate in some kind of episodic unconscious.* Conversely, the active motor engrams, representing potential rather than actual motor movements, would presumably constitute the machinery for procedural operations continuing to function in some kind of procedural unconscious.

Experimental Evidence for an Active Procedural Unconscious

It is from the observation of procedural operations during the quiescent resting state and during sleep, when alert conscious activity is suppressed, that we can project our most direct view of automatic processing at work. The fact that one half of the pyramidal cells remain active during deep sleep suggests that this might represent the procedural component of the unconscious as defined by its essentially motor function. Even assuming that the procedural unconscious has control over learned motor activities, one might ask why, during sleep, fully one half of the motor tract has to be kept in a constant state of readiness. During sleep the major functions of the motor tract are to maintain one's body safely in a prone position and to keep the individual from falling out of bed. Both of these functions, although essentially innate, are also learned. An alert newborn infant lying on a high table may easily fall off, but a heavily sleeping man lying on the same table will not fall off. Even in deep sleep, most of the procedural unconscious must remain active to provide for the many exigencies that might occur.

An even more dramatic example of the activity in the procedural unconscious occurs during sleepwalking. Sleepwalking surprisingly occurs during deep slow-wave sleep when the individual is essentially completely out of touch with his environment. The activities of sleepwalking must involve some elements of the episodic unconscious (see Chapter 12), but they must equally involve major elements of the procedural unconscious. The component of voluntary muscle control required during sleepwalking is apparently provided by that portion of the pyramidal cells which is concurrently active; involuntary control presumably continues to be provided by the cerebellum and the caudate nucleus–putamen centers in the basal ganglia.

Thus there is ample physiological evidence (one half of pyramidal cells active) and behavioral evidence (a man in deep sleep does not fall off the bed) to substantiate the concept that the same procedural unconscious that is extremely active in the alert conscious state (walking, running), is also active in the relaxed waking or deep sleep

---

*These data are particularly pertinent to the argument of Chapter 12.

conditions (sleepwalking). But neural systems do not drive themselves; they must be driven by some special energy sources. Both the resting state and sleep are associated with a relative inactivity of the noradrenergic locus coeruleus-driven RAS (only 15% of its neurons active) so that one must look for some additional drive mechanism. As described in Chapter 6, when RAS activity decreases there is a concomitant increase in mildly stimulatory activation from the thalamus in the form of α waves radiating upward over the entire cortex (recruiting waves). This presumably provides the necessary energy component for normal sleep just as the pontine cholinergic system provides the energy for REM sleep activities.

The general situation in REM sleep is even more provocative. In that stage the individual is probably more cut off from external reality than even in slow wave sleep (i.e., more difficult to awaken), yet the neuronal activity in the motor and visual cortices is essentially at its maximum level. If we assume that the portion of neuronal activity directed to procedural control is more or less the same in slow wave and in REM sleep, then there remains in REM sleep a large unaccounted for surplus of neuronal activity. Such activity must be due either to ongoing processing of episodic material or to the action of some unusual physiological process not yet accounted for. If the first were true, then that excess activity would be highly suggestive of the existence of an active episodic unconscious. If the second were true, then one could not reasonably draw such a conclusion.

Crick and Mitchison (1983) have postulated that the widespread neuronal activity in the brain during REM sleep is a physiological activity, the purpose of which is to complete the consolidation of brain engrams experienced during the day. There is much evidence to support, at least in part, this formulation. However, if REM dreams were entirely physiological, they would differ dramatically from nonREM dreams and from the fantasies and day dreams of altered states of consciousness, conditions where there is no evidence for the presence of such physiological activities. But in fact, they do not. Consequently, there is much to suggest that the excess brain activity during REM sleep does indeed derive from the activity of an episodic unconscious. This entire question will be discussed in greater detail in Chapter 12.

The evidence supplied by the demonstrated activity of one half of the neurons in the motor cortex during sleep, by the behavioral evidence of procedural activity both during consciousness and during sleep, and by the existence of additional drive mechanisms during altered states of consciousness and during REM sleep, provides a sufficient basis to postulate and support the concept of an active procedural unconscious at work during consciousness, in the resting state, and in deep sleep states. Can one make a comparable case for an episodic unconscious operating during periods of relative inertness? That is an extremely critical question. The following chapter will explore the issue of whether there is or is not an episodic unconscious similar to the procedural unconscious described here. Establishing the existence of such an entity would be of the greatest heuristic value; only an episodic unconscious would deal with true psychological problems and would be at all comparable with the Freudian ''dynamic unconscious.''

The Episodic Unconscious: Semicontrolled Unconscious Processing of Episodic and Affective Material

In this chapter, we begin to explore in psychobiological terms the Freudian concept of the dynamic unconscious. The question as to whether episodic material is continually processed at some unconscious level during the alert conscious state, during altered states of consciousness, in deep sleep, and during REM sleep is perhaps the most critical issue to be raised in this volume. Granted the importance of unconscious procedural operations, these hardly bear on the kinds of mental activities postulated in Freud's "dynamic unconscious." Procedural and structural operations are merely the processes through which the unstructured stuff of perceptions and behavioral reactivities are organized into manageable entities that can be utilized by the organism to cope efficiently with the demands of the internal and external milieus. In themselves, they do not transmit information; they merely encode that information so as to make it usable. At the opposite end of the stimulus–response spectrum, they organize and implement the motor responses that have been decided on by the conscious–unconscious self.

The sensory input that provides critical information about the internal and external environments is episodic and affective in nature. Episodic data inform the organism as to the state of the external milieu, affective data as to that of the internal milieu. On the basis of the interaction between these two sets of data, decisions are made by the executive self and, with the help of the procedural unconscious and the voluntary motor system, acted on.

That there is a large mass of unconscious episodic engrams in the brain at any given moment cannot be doubted. The immediate question is whether the mass of unconscious episodic engrams constitutes an active or an inert unconscious. There is an immense reservoir of episodic data in the unconscious long-term memory of the Lumsden–Wilson model (Fig. 5-4), but there is no definitive evidence that these engrams do not lie inactive until they are activated as short-term memories (thoughts).

Freud, however, postulated that the engrams in long-term memory are anything but inactive; that they fulminate as in a boiling cauldron; that they interact in a conflictual manner (the dynamic unconscious); that they operate under a set of logical principles peculiar to the setting (primary process); and that the dynamic unconscious is the most important determinant of conscious behavior. His evidence for these conclusions came from his work with parapraxes (slips of the tongue), fantasies, dreams, behavior under hypnosis, and the behavioral distortions deriving from the activities of defense mechanisms. Later in this volume, we will test these assumptions in terms of Freud's own formulations; here it is necessary only to examine them in the light of physiological and biological mechanisms thus far presented.

In order to establish the existence of an active episodic unconscious comparable to the procedural, one must use similar types of evidence. First, there must be clinical and behavioral data indicative of ongoing episodic unconscious activity during all of the various phases of the conscious–unconscious spectrum: the alert conscious state, altered states of consciousness, REM sleep, and deep slow-wave sleep. Second, there must be an adequate source of energy to drive the episodic unconscious during periods of impaired consciousness. Third, there must be reasonable evidence on the physiological mode of information processing, i.e., controlled, semicontrolled, or automatic, that governs the operation of the episodic unconscious during each period of impaired consciousness. If all of these are forthcoming, then and only then would it be plausible to assume the existence of an active episodic unconscious.

Still one other criterion must be met before such an entity could be equated with Freud's dynamic unconscious, namely the demonstration that the episodic unconscious significantly influences activity at other levels of the conscious–unconscious continuum. This is the critical issue that will be considered in depth in Chapter 17. Here we must first attempt to establish the existence of such an active episodic unconscious.

Unconscious Processing of Episodic Engrams during Alert Conscious States

The most common type of unconscious episodic processing is that which occurs concomitantly with conscious controlled attentional activities. As illustrated in Table 10-1, episodic learning and memory recall is seriously impaired in the diencephalic and bitemporal syndromes, giving rise to the often expressed principle that memories of this type cannot be established nor recalled except through an intact attentional processing apparatus. Yet Weiskrantz (1978) has demonstrated that even though there is serious impairment of specific episodic memory consolidation and recall in individuals with diencephalic or bitemporal amnesias, a moderate amount of such learning without conscious retrieval is possible with proper cues and sufficient associations.

In addition to Weiskrantz's demonstration that some episodic cognitive material can be learned and later used in the absence of parts of the memory system, albeit without the individual's awareness, there are other studies that show that even the most purely episodic data are normally subject to some form of unconscious processing. Evidence supporting this conclusion comes from many sources. For example, Forster and Govier (1978) used a dichotic listening paradigm to test this hypothesis. They employed attended and unattended auditory stimuli fed simultaneously into the two ears with the subject's attention directed to one ear. Words presented to the unattended channel were presumed to be operationally "unconscious." Certain words in the attended channel were made emotionally charged through the simultaneous delivery of an electric shock. Repetition of those words in the unattended ear resulted in increased galvanic skin responses (GSR) indicative of an emotional response despite the subject's apparent lack of awareness of the sounding of those words. Similar GSR responses were found with homonyms (sound alikes) of the charged words presented to the unattended ear; the responses were less than were those to stimuli in the attending ear, indicating less efficient processing in the unattended channel. Significant GSR responses to synonyms of the charged words also occurred with presentation in the unattended channel, suggesting processing of emotional valences of unattended stimuli to higher cognitive channels than had previously been hypothesized. These findings supported the interpretation that unattended (and thus presumably unconscious) stimuli could be recognized, at least emotionally, in the same way as subliminal (also presumably unconscious) stimuli.

Other studies indicate that recognition of the emotional valence of a percept may occur in the absence of conscious cognitive recognition of the stimulus itself. Kunst-Wilson and Zajonc (1980), using the paradigm previously described in Chapter 9, tested thresholds for recognition at the cognitive level versus that at the affective level (like–dislike). They found that their subjects were able to express correctly their emotional preference for stimuli at exposures below those necessary for conscious cognitive recognition, even though they did not know why. The authors conclude that affective processing of stimuli is achieved at a lower neural level in the brain than is cognitive processing. They also comment that affective recognition here was unconscious since, because of the experimental design, the subjects were not aware of their own preferences.

An example of simultaneous conscious and unconscious cognitive processing, similar to that of the Forster and Govier study, occurs in the visual sensory modality, the so-called Stroop effect. This occurs when a subject is tested on the interaction between a word color (blue) and an ink color (red) when both are incorporated in a single stimulus (the word *blue* printed in red ink). Posner and Snyder (1975) found relatively few interference effects between these purely episodic tasks and Posner (1978) concludes "these . . . results suggest that color naming and reading go on in parallel and without interference until close to the output" (p. 92). Posner further describes the Warren effect (Warren, 1974) in which auditory and visual input are presented simultaneously, and again gives evidence that parallel processing of differentially activated engrams results in relatively few interference effects. Posner (1978) concludes: "Evidence suggests that pathways can be activated irrespective of the subjects' intentions and without the necessity of their devoting active attention to them. Study of the costs and benefits from priming pathways suggests that it is possible to separate the automatic activation of pathways from attentional processing" (p. 121).

Posner's studies are consistent with the previously described findings of Schneider and Shiffrin (1977) that certain episodic tasks, when performed unconsciously, still appeared to show some of the characteristics of controlled processing but not most of them. This accounts for Posner's designation of such activities as "automatic" in the preceding statement. But I believe that some other mechanisms may be involved. The two simultaneous tasks in the Stroop and Warren effects, although both episodic in nature, represent mechanisms at different levels in the attentional process. In the Stroop effect, the color red represents a primary perceptual quality characteristically perceived during upstream processing while the word "blue" represents a secondary cognitive quality characteristically determined during downstream processing. But if attention were closely fixed on color identification rather than on word identification, then the levels of processing might be reversed. I feel that the absence of interference between two related episodic perceptions is due, in this case, not to the operation of *automatic* processing as postulated by Posner, but to the fact that the two perceptual processes are operating under different *controlled* conditions, one *upstream* and one *downstream*. This interpretation is supported by Posner's own statement quoted above; there is no evidence of interference until "close to the output," i.e., when the primary color perception is raised to awareness by passage through the amygdaloid–hippocampal complex. The perception of the red color in this paradigm is a primary unconscious activity carried out in the lower brain, but transforming that perception into its linguistic form, the word "red" requires the involvement of the cortex and the amygdaloid–hippocampal complex.

It is clear that there is no fundamental disagreement between this position and that of Posner, but merely a difference in emphasis. By labeling the unconscious processing of episodic material "automatic," it seems to me that Posner creates room for confusion in that he does not distinguish between unconscious processing of episodic and procedural material. Since these two processes are physiologically different, even though they share many behavioral characteristics, it seems preferable to separate them and treat them as two distinct entities.

Unattended unconscious processing of episodic data obviously does have all of the qualities characteristic of automatic processing as defined by Posner (1978). It lacks intentionality and the quality of awareness. It is unlimited in scope and can occur simultaneously with other perceptions without causing interference. By these definitions, unattended upstream processing of episodic data is as automatic as is that of any procedural task. But if it were completely automatic then it should not be, unlike procedural processing, markedly impaired in bilateral hippocampal lesions. The fact that it is makes me believe that the unconscious processing of unattended episodic material is fundamentally different in nature from that of procedural material. Hence I prefer the differential usages of the terms "semicontrolled" and "automatic".

The fact that essentially all unattended episodic stimuli that are processed pseudoautomatically can be called into awareness with the slightest effort, further distinguishes them from true automatic mechanical, structural, and semantic operations which cannot be called into awareness at all. Finally, unattended episodic processing takes place exclusively in the early part of the attentional system, i.e., in the thalamic–basal gangliar complex, as opposed to procedural activities which are processed only partially in that complex but more so in the caudate nucleus and cerebellum. To my mind, the sum of all of these differences between the unconscious processing of episodic and procedural materials justifies their being considered as two separate entities.

Attended and unattended perceptual paradigms occur not only in experimental situations, but are part of our everyday experience. The beam of attention described in Chapter 8 is not merely a visual one, although the metaphor employed suggests that interpretation. Actually it applies to every sensory modality, so that there is the attended field of selectivity in vision, hearing, somatosensory activity, and so on. In each case there are areas of greatest attentional intensity, fringe areas of lesser attentional intensity, and large unattended fields. The last are essentially out of the field of consciousness. Another factor in keeping most stimuli from constantly impinging on our attention is habituation as the result of which stimuli of a constant order rapidly fade into the unconscious. The feelings of clothes on the body, which are usually habituated, are readily brought into awareness merely by a concentrated shift of attention. Hence the comparison of attended and unattended perceptual activities is one of the best ways of exploring unconscious episodic activities.

Neurophysiology of Unconscious Episodic Data Processing in the Alert Conscious State

The neurophysiological mechanisms underlying the unconscious processing of episodic data during alert consciousness appear to be those associated with the upstream phase of attentional processing, involving mainly the thalamic–basal gangliar complex. However, operationally speaking, it seems incongruous that unconscious episodic material, often cognitively quite complex, should have its entire processing mechanisms centered in the primitive thalamic–basal gangliar complex. It seems more likely that some unconscious episodic data must traverse the entire cortex in typical downstream processing, up to and including passage through elements of the amygdaloid–hippocampal complex, but not proceeding to the final step of activating the self-awareness system. In that case, unconscious episodic data processing would be almost identical to conscious episodic data processing except for omission of the final step of activating the consciousness system. Such a sequence would certainly deserve the title of "semicontrolled" processing.

An alternative explanation might be that the amygdaloid–hippocampal complex may be involved in unconscious episodic processing, but during the upstream rather than during downstream processing. There is some anatomical and experimental evidence to support this interpretation. The anatomical evidence derives from the previously described close functional association of the dorsal median thalamus with the amygdaloid–hippocampal complex (Swanson and Cowan, 1976). Even closer physiological interactions have been demonstrated between the basal gangliar nucleus basalis of Meynart and the amygdaloid–hippocampal complex (Divac, 1975; Otterson, 1980). Consequently, the anatomical evidence does suggest that parts of the amygdaloid–hippocampal complex may be involved in upstream processing as well as in downstream.

How then to summarize the various modes of processing of episodic material? It appears that in addition to the classical conscious, sequential examination of complex

cognitive abstractions, there are many types of mechanisms necessary for the processing of even very simple physical features. These are described by Sagi and Julesz
(1985) as "detection" and "identification" of simple cognitive elements. Detection
and location in space are accomplished through parallel processing mechanisms, while
even so simple a process as identification of orientation requires serial processing.
Nevertheless, both processes, parallel and sequential, take place at about 80–120
msec, clearly earlier than the time required for classical conscious sequential processing of complex cognitive stimuli (300–400 msec).

As Sagi and Julesz (1985) write:

> Thus, detecting feature (orientation) gradients and locating them can be done in
> parallel, but identifying the features (orientation) and knowing what they are requires
> serial inspection with focal attention. What is surprising is that we find such scrutiny
> to be necessary for as simple a feature as the orientation of a line element that is
> regarded as a basic dimension in vision. This finding is inconsistent with the proposal
> that initial parallel feature processing in nontopographical feature spaces is followed
> by serial processing (with focal attention) to localize different features and to combine
> them according to their location. (p. 1219)

The existence of serial processing at 80–120 msec suggests the involvement of the
hippocampus, even during upstream processing, in the analysis of complex physical or
simple cognitive stimuli. However, it is apparent that this function can be accomplished at the thalamic–basal gangliar level even in the absence of the amygdaloid–
hippocampal complex, as in the case of the patient, H. M. But this does not necessarily
preclude the involvement of the hippocampus in this process normally. In any event,
from these considerations, it seems that there are at least four different methods of
processing episodic data: (1) unconscious parallel processing of simple physical features (semantic processing), (2) unconscious upstream serial processing of complex
physical or simple cognitive stimuli, (3) unconscious downstream sequential processing of complex cognitive stimuli, and (4) conscious downstream sequential processing
of complex cognitive material.

The studies by Posner et al. (1980), Kunst-Wilson (1980), and Sagi and Julesz
(1985) all lead to the conclusion that primary cognitive (episodic) characteristics,
including emotional valence, may be evaluated during the upstream attentional sequence in a manner resembling automatic processing, i.e., in an unconscious, unlimited, unintentional, parallel, and noninterfering mode. All this occurs through the
mechanism of the thalamic–basal gangliar complex with or without direct communication with the amygdaloid–hippocampal complex. Nor is there reason to restrict such
processing to incoming perceptions since old memories (more than three years old)
would have similar access to this unconscious episodic processing system even in the
absence of the hippocampus (Squire and Cohen, 1979). One can also make a plausible
case for such a system based solely on the thalamic–basal gangliar complex without
necessarily invoking the amygdaloid–hippocampal complex as, for example, in the
patient H. M.

The Posner study on the simultaneous processing of color and meaning (Fig. 8-5)
is restricted to two variables only, because of the design of the experiment. There can
be little question that other primary characteristics of the stimulus such as size, shape
of letters (lower case versus capitals), and so on were also being monitored uncon-

sciously together with the designated qualities. Sagi and Julesz (1985) demonstrated experimentally, parallel processing of multiple physical properties of geometric figures, all occurring simultaneously during the preattentive phase. There seems to be almost no limit to such parallel processing of episodic data at the unconscious level of primary upstream perception.

Unconscious Processing of Episodic Data during REM Sleep

The experimental demonstration of semicontrolled unconscious processing of episodic material in the alert conscious state is a necessary preliminary but in itself makes no case for an active episodic unconscious. However, by providing a mechanism through which unattended events may be perceived, incorporated, and acted upon, it lends credibility to such borderline phenomena as subliminal perception and intuitive insights and may even help explain some of the more esoteric claims of so-called extrasensory perception. Probably a better case for the operation of an active episodic unconscious in the alert conscious state could be made by referring to parapraxes, to unconscious defense mechanisms (projection, repression, and denial), and to such activities as body language, automatic writing, and so on. However, all of these phenomena smack heavily of psychoanalytic thinking and as such will be relegated to the last chapter of this volume.

Probably the best evidence for the existence of an active episodic unconscious is that provided by mental productions during periods of REM sleep, non-REM dreams, and of altered states of consciousness. Freud's critical evidence for an active dynamic unconscious was of course dreams, mental productions when the individual was apparently unconscious. Dreams certainly do have at least the surface appearance of an active dynamic unconscious, and one intuitively tends to accept it as such.

Recent work by Crick and Mitchison (1983) has questioned the validity of this assumption. Basing their conclusions on evidence that REM sleep in human fetuses and infants (where it constitutes almost 100% of sleep time) is associated with a neuronal reorganization of the brain, Crick and Mitchison postulate that dreams constitute a physiological rearrangement of engrams rather than an organized reliving of experience. Certainly the occurrence of REM sleep in human fetuses makes it highly unlikely that any associated dreams might constitute in that case an organized dynamic unconscious.

Winson (1985) has presented a modified version of the Crick–Mitchison hypothesis, postulating that REM dreams represent ''off-line'' processing of episodic events that had occurred during the day, for which the brain lacked sufficient prefrontal lobe capacity to process on an ''on-line'' basis. Winson goes further and identifies dreams as the manifestation of critical unconscious concerns analogous in a biological sense to the Freudian unconscious.

Freud (1920) seems to have anticipated this controversy a great many years ago. He wrote:

> Dreams can be divided into three categories in respect of the relation between their latent and their manifest content. In the first place, we may distinguish those dreams which make *sense* and are at the same time *intelligible* which, that is to say, can be inserted without further difficulty into the context of our mental life. . . . There is nothing astonishing or strange about them. Incidentally, their occurrence constitutes a powerful argument against the theory according to which dreams originate from the isolated activity of separate groups of brain cells. They give no indication of reduced or fragmentary psychical activity but nevertheless we never question the fact of their being dreams and do not confuse them . . . with waking life.

> The third group contains those dreams which are without either sense or intelligibility, which seem *disconnected, confused* and *meaningless*. The preponderant majority of the products of our dreaming exhibit these characteristics which are the basis of the low opinion in which dreams are held and of the medical opinion that they are the outcome of a restricted mental activity. (p. 355)

My own feeling is that both viewpoints are probably at least partially correct. They appear to be reconcilable in the light of recent experimental findings that appear to differentiate between the bizarreness and irrationality of early REM-associated dreams and the more rational character of late REM and non-REM–associated dreams (Cohen, 1976). Available evidence suggests that late REM and non-REM–associated dreams probably do represent disinhibited wishes from the unconscious rising to impaired awareness, relatively undistorted and meaning more or less what they appear to mean. Bizarre and totally irrational dreams in this formulation might stem either from bizzare ideation in a borderline psychotic individual or, in the absence of such organic psychopathology, might derive from early REM activity associated with either physiological reorganization or deeper probing of the unconscious.

Freud's judgement that at least some dreams make eminent sense, i.e., are intelligible, is readily supported by personal and general experience. It is further corroborated by the presence of dreams during non-REM sleep. Consequently, there appears to be little basis for the Crick and Mitchison position that all dreams are totally physiological. If dreams do represent a legitimate processing of episodic material during REM sleep, there seems little reason to doubt that such processing can continue during a period of total separation of awareness from the outside world. That would seem to constitute adequate confirmation of the existence of an active, continually functioning episodic unconscious. Further supportive evidence is provided in the next section.

Neurophysiology of Episodic Data Processing during REM Dreams

Winson (1985) describes strong θ-wave activity in the hippocampus of mammals during REM sleep. Activity in the hippocampus during the processing of dreams speaks strongly for the involvement of a more sophisticated level of neurophysiological function in unconscious episodic information processing than merely that of the thalamic–basal gangliar complex. The complexity of dreams suggests that the amygdaloid–hippocampal complex is activated during such operations, not as a component of upstream processing, but rather as the terminal activity of downstream processing after passage through the neocortex. The presence of θ activity in the entorhinal cortex (Mitchell and Ranck, 1980) strongly supports the latter interpretation. Even though the hippocampus may play some role in upstream perceptual processing, most physiological studies suggest that by far the major portion of amygdaloid–hippocampal complex activity occurs during downstream processing (Moscovitch, 1979). The complex nature of the cognitive material that characterizes dreams supports the interpretation that dream processing is completed in the neocortex rather than in the primitive centers of the brain stem. Finally, in dreams the self-awareness system does appear to be at least somewhat stimulated albeit in an atypical manner, as manifest by the peculiar "sense of self" characteristic of dreams. This last fact adds weight to the interpretation that REM dreams more or less activate the entire attentional episodic data processing system, but through the cholinergic FTG system rather than through the noradrenergic RAS system (see Chapter 22).

This formulation suggests that REM sleep, generated from FTG cells in the pons and producing pons–geniculate–occipital (PGO) spikes, activates the cortical part of the consciousness system but not the brain stem segment. The PGO pathway circumvents the general awareness centers in the thalamic–basal gangliar complex even though it appears to utilize other thalamic–basal gangliar centers for cognitive and emotional processing. The fact that the PGO pathway circumvents the dorsal median thalamic nucleus, the critical center of the general awareness system, is consistent with the absence of genuine conscious awareness in dreams. On the other hand, the presence of hippocampal θ activity during REM sleep (Winson, 1985) is consistent with some activation of the self-awareness system, and consequently with the strong feelings of self that do exist in dreams.

The Episodic Unconscious in Altered States of Consciousness

The question remains: Do dream productions represent a unique special state or do they represent an atypical activation of a continuously functioning dynamic unconscious? If REM dreams were the only examples of nonconscious mental activity, one might assume they were unique and atypical. But there are many instances of non-REM dreamlike productions generated during periods of partially impaired consciousness. Such dreamlike productions include fantasies and daydreams during twilight states, hypnosis, transcendental meditation, fugues, and so forth; all periods when the activity of the nonadrenergic RAS is reduced to about 15% (see Fig. 11-2) and when the altered state of consciousness is driven largely by thalamic rhythm.

Such fantasies and daydreams are substantively similar to REM dreams except that they tend to lack the more irrational elements of the latter. Fisher and Greenberg (1977) have made a systematic comparison of the characteristics of REM dreams and daydreams and have concluded that they are essentially similar. They write:

Probably one of the reasons why dream imagery has been regarded as unique is because it takes place in a unique state of consciousness. Other forms of fantasy construction, such as daydreaming and responses to inkblots, occur when the individual is awake. But the dream arises in the sleeping organism. Is this a sufficient basis for assuming that the two classes of fantasy cannot be approached in related ways? Giora (1972) has argued persuasively that although the cognitive processes occurring at various levels of consciousness are different, they still represent a unitary system. It is not clear why one should assume that fantasy production during sleep calls into play an entirely different system than does fantasy production when awake. (p. 64)

But even rational REM dreams differ in quality and content from fantasies and daydreams and each of these differs significantly from the stream of thought characteristic of normal alert conscious mental activity. One can hardly make the case that the types of thought imagery characteristic of irrational REM dreams and of α driven fantasies are at all similar to those of normal conscious thought, even taking into consideration the differences in mental state. In Chapter 22, we shall present a physiological formulation that postulates that the material of REM dreams, ASC fantasies, and normal conscious thinking are only remotely related and derive from different engrammatic reservoirs in the brain. Evidence for this theory will be presented in terms of structural formulations that consider the unconscious to exist as separate, compartmentalized, functional segments of brain activity, differentially activated in different states of consciousness.

There can be little question that the material in altered states of consciousness is both episodic and only somewhat conscious. Its essentially unconscious nature is most obvious in conditions of hypnosis or trancelike states where the individual appears to have turned inwardly and away from the outside world. In these states, mental productions tend to be more rational and less bizarre than those of REM dreams, supporting the idea that they stem from a different reservoir of thoughts. That, together with the difference in state of consciousness from REM states, suggests that, Fisher and Greenberg (1977) notwithstanding, the productions of altered states of consciousness are at least somewhat different from those of REM dreams. In any event, the most important conclusion must be that ASC productions represent an active dynamic episodic unconscious, even though that unconscious may differ significantly from that underlying normal alert conscious brain activity and that underlying REM dreams (see Chapter 22).

If the biological purpose of alert conscious mental activity is to cope most effectively with the demands of the internal and external milieus, and if the biological purpose of REM sleep and dreams is to permit a physiological reorganization of brain engrams, what are the biological purposes of fantasies and daydreams? In humans, at least, fantasies and daydreams seem to provide an opportunity for the individual to come into contact with his own deepest motivations, feelings, and thoughts, elements that are not usually readily available during the *sturm und drang* of alert conscious activity. In fact, fantasies and daydreams may provide the same opportunity for *psychological* reorganization of the brain that REM sleep provides for *physiological* reorganization. The best evidence for this thesis comes from the reputed mentally therapeutic effects of the various altered states of consciousness: hypnosis, transcendental meditation, biofeedback, and so on. Generally such therapeutic effects have been attributed largely to the relaxation associated with these processes but the generation of fantasies and daydreams suggests that some other benefit, possibly exploring one's own unconscious while at relative ease, may be at work as well. These speculations too will be further explored in Chapter 22.

Unconscious Processing of Episodic and Affective Material during Deep Sleep

The foregoing descriptions appear to provide substantial evidence for the concept of a dynamic unconscious that is active in the alert conscious state, in altered states of consciousness, and in REM sleep. In each instance, the three elements necessary to establish the thesis appear to be present, namely, (1) experimental evidence that episodic data can be processed during the three disparate states, (2) physiological evidence of an adequate driving force, respectively, the noradrenergic RAS, the dopaminergic thalamic α system, and the cholinergic FTG system, and (3) clinical evidence of actual ongoing unconscious activity during each state. If these things are true, then there appears to be enough evidence to support the concept of an episodic unconscious, active at all levels of consciousness except perhaps in deep sleep.

Certainly if the dynamic unconscious were at any time inactive in the normal healthy individual, one would expect that period to be during deep sleep. It is at that time that there is no real center for energizing the brain since it appears that the thalamus has shifted from a mildly stimulatory α rhythm to a generally depressing δ rhythm. Furthermore, during deep slow-wave sleep, there is a general relaxation of all bodily activities including body musculature so that the individual is in a more inert state then during any other period of normal existence. Finally, it is difficult even to formulate a theory as to how during deep sleep, episodic memories and thoughts could be activated to permit the functioning of a dynamic unconscious. True, there is sufficient sensory and motor activity to permit us not to roll out of bed during deep sleep, but this reactivity speaks more for a procedural than for an episodic operation.

Nevertheless, two very dramatic episodic behavioral events—one sensory, the other motor—do occur during deep slow-wave sleep. These are, respectively, night terrors and sleepwalking.* Intuitively one would have guessed that these activities would require the powerful stimulatory influence of either the noradrenergic RAS alerting system or the cholinergic FTG REM sleep system. Actual EEG tracings made during such episodes surprisingly reveal slow-wave δ rhythms, entirely at the onset but also partially throughout the duration of the experience. The following excerpt from Mack (1970) provides the basis for these statements:

*In the old nomenclature, night terrors were known as nightmares. Now it is generally recognized that nightmares are anxiety-ridden REM dreams while night terrors occur mainly during deep sleep. Similarly, sleepwalking, which occurs during deep sleep, is sometimes erroneously referred to as "somnambulism"; the latter is more correctly defined as an hysterical dissociative state.

> Although the nightmare has been traditionally regarded as a type of severe anxiety
> dream, Gastaut and Broughton have questioned whether nightmares really are
> dreams . . . This conviction is based on the finding that the majority of nightmares
> they studied in the laboratory in children and adults occurred—as may also be the case
> with enuresis and somnambulism—during arousal from slow-wave (non-REM) sleep
> rather than REM sleep, during which dreaming has more frequently been demon-
> strated. Broughton classes the nightmare, together with enuresis and somnambulism,
> as a confusional sleep disorder because of the poorly coordinated behavior, slurred
> speech, mental confusion, and poor dream recall that regularly accompany abrupt
> arousal or awakening from slow-wave sleep. (pp. 14–15)

The kinds of responsivities displayed both during night terrors and sleepwalking leave little room for doubt that episodic data can be processed at an unconscious level during deep sleep. Night terrors consist of vidid cognitive and affective materials that must reflect an active reservoir of episodic engrams. Sleepwalking is even more dramatic in that the sleepwalker is apparently sufficiently cognizant (one cannot say aware) of his environment to avoid personal harm. Consequently, it seems reasonable to assert that episodic data can be and is adequately processed all during the slow-wave sleep periods associated with night terrors and sleepwalking.

Probably the best evidence for the activity of the dynamic unconscious during slow-wave sleep comes from the not unusual production of typical dreams during such periods. Although it is true that dreams are most often associated with REM sleep when subjects are awakened in the laboratory, it is also true that subjects report fairly typical dreams on about 20% of the occasions when they are awakened during periods of deep slow-wave sleep. This occurrence of fairly rational non-REM dreams during deep slow-wave sleep again supports the concept of the dynamic unconscious continu-ing its activity during such periods. The evidence for episodic data processing in deep sleep during episodes of night terrors and sleepwalking and in non-REM dreams is highly suggestive and appears to establish the idea of a continuous dynamic uncon-scious, active at *all* times.

The Psychobiological Model of an Active Episodic Unconscious

The evidence that the hippocampus is highly active during REM dreams suggests that probably a higher type of cognitive processing must be involved here. This conclusion is reinforced by the nature of such dreams, particularly in their capacity to incorporate presleep material, a reaction that also implicates hippocampal functions. On the other hand, the fantasies of twilight sleep and the non-REM dreams of stage 4 sleep do not appear to be associated with θ activity in the hippocampus (Winson, 1985). This indicates, contrary to the position of Fisher and Greenberg (1977), that there may significant differences between REM and non-REM productions. The ab-sence of θ-wave activity in the hippocampus during light sleep and deep sleep suggests that the hippocampus is not active at those times, as opposed to its activity during REM sleep. If that is indeed the case, then the productions of twilight sleep and non-REM dreams reflect a different kind of unconscious material than would those of REM dreams. It may be that REM dreams appear so much more bizarre than do the productions of twilight states and non-REM dreams because, unlike the latter, they tap a deeper layer of an activated dynamic unconscious.*

All of these considerations lead to a conceptualization of a vast episodic unconscious in the brain that is continually active, mostly so during acute conscious activity and REM dreams, but only moderately less so (perhaps one third as active) during twilight sleep and non-REM dreams. Processing of both external perceptions and internal thoughts is semicontrolled, i.e., unconscious, unlimited, unintentional, parallel rather than sequential, and noninterfering. Processing is largely through the thalamic–basal gangliar complex, but involves the amygdaloid–hippocampal complex as well either during the upstream or more probably after the downstream phase. Early thalamic–basal gangliar processing would characteristically be more diffuse and vague as in twilight fantasies and in non-REM dreams. Late amygdaloid–hippocampal involvement would result in more vivid productions as in REM dreams. Most important is the ubiquitous activity of the episodic unconscious, similar to that of the procedural and visceral unconscious. However, the visibility of the former would wax and wane with the dominant state of consciousness more so than would the latter.

The episodic unconscious is the closest physiological analogue to the Freudian dynamic unconscious and in many respects may be labeled the psychobiological dynamic unconscious. Our view of the episodic unconscious is similar in some respects but quite different in other respects from the Freudian model. In both instances the dynamic unconscious, operating continuously during alert consciousness and during impaired consciousness, determines much of behavior through unconscious influences. But the dynamics of unconscious control are significantly different in the two systems. In the psychobiological model, the episodic unconscious is dominated mainly by rational physiological influences; these are opposed to the predominantly irrational psychological mechanisms of the Freudian model. In the psychobiological model, the episodic unconscious is activated by multiple influences: motivational–emotional, cognitive, and visceral; in the psychoanalytic model, the influences are almost entirely motivational–emotional.

It is worth noting that the physiological and psychological evidence for a psychobiological dynamic unconscious thus far mustered in this volume has been mainly cognitive rather than, as in the Freudian system, almost entirely motivational–emotional. But this is not meant to imply that motivational–emotional influences are not equally important in the psychobiological system. On the contrary, they are every bit as important since the psychobiological system, like the psychoanalytic, is driven almost entirely by motivational–emotional forces. The use of predominantly cognitive evidence has been a deliberate strategy, employed not only to avoid possible pitfalls of the psychoanalytic method, but also because the best available experimental data were mainly in that form. However, it is now essential to address more directly the specific effects of motivational–emotional influences on the operation of the episodic, or in other terms, the dynamic unconscious.

---

*This thesis is expanded upon in Chapter 22.

Hierarchical and Hemispheric Origins of Repression and Other Defense Mechanisms

III

13

The Effects of Emotionality on Conscious and Unconscious Information Processing

Experiential (episodic) data constitute the major components of conscious awareness and in general contribute the most important influences that shape personality. They always carry emotional charge (positive, negative, or neutral), and no discussion of their processing would be complete without a consideration of the influences of such charges. Mechanical and semantic operations are also strongly influenced by motivational–emotional forces (e.g., the effects of stress on stuttering). However, at this time, we shall restrict ourselves to a discussion of the effects of emotionality on episodic material; in Chapter 17 we shall consider the effects of stress on procedural processing.

Given the formulation in the last chapter of the dynamic unconscious as a force that is continually active but particularly so during alert consciousness, it follows that the productions of alert consciousness activity must be considered in terms of unconscious as well as in terms of conscious mechanisms.

More specifically, this chapter deals with the question of the extent to which emotional charge affects the retrievability to consciousness of memories in the unconscious. It is apparent that that question constitutes the most critical issue in any attempt to relate psychobiological explanations to psychodynamic theory. The concept of repression, defined as the inability of highly negatively charged memories to move from the unconscious to consciousness, is probably the central theme of psychoanalysis. From this, Freud's primary assumption, came the natural extrapolation that such highly charged engrams, unable to be expressed consciously, exert an inordinate influence on behavior through their perturbations in the dynamic unconscious.

Because those memories are so subjective and because psychodynamic theory holds that those engrams with which we are most concerned, negatively charged memories, are repressed and must remain unconscious, it becomes difficult to test this basic psychoanalytic thesis in any objective way. Indeed, that is why Freud had to invent dream analysis and free association to provide data for his theory. Since these psychoanalytic techniques are not immediately compatible with our psychobiological approach, it is necessary to utilize some other methodology. Fortunately for our purposes, perception is the external cognitive process of which memory is the internal analogue. As described in the last chapter, perception can readily be broken down into its conscious and unconscious components in a variety of experimental situations, e.g., tachistoscopic presentations and dichotic listening studies. Consequently, even though our main concerns are with memories, the major thrust of our considerations of the effects of emotional charge on the passage of cognitive data from the unconscious to awareness will stress perceptual experiments. Memory studies will also be referred to when available.

Behavioral Studies of Perceptual Threshold and Memory Retrieval

Freud considered all perceptions and memories to have more or less equal cognitive value so that in cognitive processing, motivational–emotional charges exerted the greatest influence. He postulated that all engrams were endowed with positive or negative motivational–emotional charge (cathexis) that either facilitated perception and memory (positive or mildly negative motivational–emotional charge) or inhibited them (highly threatening negative motivational–emotional charge). Moreover, he considered highly threatening negative memories to be so thoroughly repressed as to be incapable of retrieval through ordinary means.

Despite the apparent reasonableness of the repression hypothesis (i.e., the concept that negatively charged engrams may be at least partially inhibited from entering consciousness), only suggestive experimental evidence for this paradigm has been forthcoming. A great deal of work has been done with subliminal stimuli presented on the tachistoscope, an instrument that exposes stimuli, most often neutral or negatively charged words, for fractions of a second. By starting at durations of exposure too brief to allow recognition and by gradually lengthening the time frame, the threshold for recognition (i.e., entry to awareness) can be established. It has been found, by and large, that negatively charged words have higher thresholds, i.e., require longer exposure than do neutral words, and this has been cited as an instance of repression or perceptual defense. About 20% of subjects actually have lower thresholds for negatively charged words, a reaction that has been labeled perceptual vigilance. On the other hand, with positively charged words the great majority of subjects show lower thresholds, i.e., perceptual vigilance.

The applicability of heightened tachistoscopic threshold levels to the concept of repression is not at all clear. For one thing, some reviewers consider that a higher threshold for negatively charged words does not necessarily represent an inability to recognize the word at the lower exposure, but may be the consequence rather of an unwillingness, conscious or unconscious, to report the word. Furthermore, Erdelyi and Appelbaum (1973), themselves proponents of the repression concept, report that some individuals have higher thresholds to emotionally charged words whether the involved emotions are positive or negative. In any event, even if the evidence for some suppression of recognition of negatively charged words were much stronger than it is, that would still not be proof that markedly threatening stimuli could be entirely repressed from awareness, the basic premise of psychoanalysis.

The concept of so-called perceptual defense was introduced by Bruner and Postman (1947) who found that on tachistoscopic presentation, socially taboo words such as bitch, whore, and penis were recognized at significantly higher thresholds than were neutral words of simliar length and complexity. McGinnies (1949) corroborated this result with the additional finding that taboo words were associated with significantly increased GSR responses at just below recognition levels of exposure. Some investigators had objected to Bruner and Postman's conclusion that their study demonstrated perceptual defense on the basis that since the frequency of exposure to taboo words was less than that to neutral words, recognition might be more difficult. However, McGinnies' study indicated that an emotional response to taboo words had occurred either at the conscious or unconscious level at an earlier time, thus negating that particular criticism.

In the field of memory retrieval, similar effects to those for perception apply. The complexity of the interaction between emotionality and cognitive functioning was first demonstrated by the early work of Zeigarnik (1927) on memory retrieval. That investigator discovered that uncompleted tasks tend to be better remembered than completed tasks except where the noncompletion was construed by the subject as a personal failure; in that case completed tasks tended to be better remembered. Subsequent workers found that the attachment of anxiety, guilt, and so forth to the uncompleted tasks consistently resulted in a reversal of the normal tendency to remember uncompleted tasks better. This phenomenon was widely regarded as a laboratory demonstration of repression. These studies indicate that memories, like perceptions, may be subject to some type of impairment in processing when they are associated with anxiety.

In both perception and memory, the question has been raised of conscious reluctance on the part of subjects to accept or admit recognition of socially taboo words in an experimental situation. Many of these experiments are conducted in colleges, not infrequently with female subjects and male investigators, or vice versa. However, other studies by McCleary and Lazarus (1949) and Blum and Barbour (1979), using nonsense syllables made anxiety provoking by electric shock or by hypnosis, have given comparable results to those in the McGinnies experiment. These studies plus a myriad of others reviewed by Erdelyi (1974) and Maddi (1976) strongly suggest that anxiety-associated stimuli may require increased thresholds for cognitive recognition when presented subliminally and that they may be reacted to emotionally (i.e., with increased arousal) prior to cognitive recognition.

That the emotional component of perception is unconsciously identified at a lower neural level than the cognitive component appears well established from the Kunst-Wilson and Zajonc (1980) study described in the last chapter. It seems natural that the presence of an emotional charge during upstream processing should influence the upstream processing of the cognitive component. However, since emotionality is associated with higher levels of arousal, one would expect greater efficiency of cognitive processing (i.e., perceptual vigilance) rather than lesser (i.e., perceptual defense). The fact that there is a differential response to negatively charged stimuli (perceptual defense) than to positively charged stimuli (perceptual vigilance) suggests that the effects of different emotional charges on cognitive processing are qualitatively different—inhibitory for negative charge and facilitatory for positive charge. In that sense, perceptual defense to negatively charged stimuli may be considered a form of repression.

An alternative explanation to repression for these observed perceptual effects, i.e., perceptual defense and perceptual vigilance, has been the concept of interference. This thesis presumes that increased arousal associated with anxiety-provoking experience may actually interfere with normal perceptual processing, reducing efficiency, and producing higher thresholds. This thesis more readily explains the rare perceptual defense responses to positive stimuli described by Erdelyi and Appelbaum (1973) than does classical repression. On the other hand, straight interference theory does not account for any of the responses of perceptual vigilance where both positive and negative emotional charge produce lowered thresholds, i.e., improved perception. A more reasonable explanation for these effects appears to be that perception follows the classical inverted U-curve of the relationship of arousal to performance (Fig. 3-1) where a moderate increase in arousal (positive or negative) produces improvement in performance, while a marked increase in arousal produces a decrement.

The Relationship between Cognitive and Affective Elements in Perception

Where the level of arousal and the level of perceptual efficiency correlate directly, there is no difficulty in conceptualizing emotional charges as being intimately connected with their associated cognitive engrams. However, when, as with very high arousal, there is a reduction in perceptual efficiency, the one-to-one relationship breaks down. Then one must conclude that the association between emotional charge and perceptual efficiency is a loose one depending both on the reactive propensities of the individual and on the special circumstances of a given experience. The demonstration by Kunst-Wilson and Zajonc (1980) that the emotional aspects of a perceptual experience may be recognized at some level (unconsciously) before the cognitive aspects superficially suggests that both components may represent separate and distinct entities. However, this interpretation seems contrary to our previously stated thesis that cognitive and motivational–emotional elements are so intimately involved with one another as to form almost a single unit (Chapter 3).

Actually we are not suggesting that the unconscious recognition of emotional valence prior to the conscious recognition of cognitive significance indicates dissociation between emotions and cognition. Presumably, the early recognition of emotional valence is based on the recognition at an unconscious level of some elemental cognitive characteristics; the latter apparently are sufficiently specific to excite a conscious emotional response, but are too vague and diffuse to allow conscious cognitive perception, i.e., recognition. As Lazarus (1981) has written (quoted in part at the end of Chapter 5):

> . . . it is counterproductive to reify emotion and cognition as independent and merely interactive. In nature they are normally fused (Lazarus, Coyne, & Folkman, in press), as Zajonc himself acknowledges when he writes, "In nearly all cases, however, feeling is not free of thought, nor is thought free of feelings" (p. 154). Even more important, however, such a separation is not required by the fact that emotion occurs at the outset of an encounter rather than later on, after considerable information processing. One need merely recognize that meaning is commonly present at the outset even if it is ill-defined, unconscious, or unverbalizable and the environmental event is barely discernible or ambiguous. (p. 223)

This statement suggests and experimental data appear to support the position that emotional valence may be associated with a cognitive pattern that is too ambiguous to permit conscious cognitive recognition, but is sufficiently structured to excite unconscious arousal of the associated emotion. Apparently, emotional arousal occurs during the upstream phase of information processing, while definitive cognitive identification does not occur until later during the downstream phase. In these terms, every perception may be conceptualized as existing in two forms: an early poorly defined cognitive engram that is sufficiently formed to elicit the emotion associated with the original perception but which is too amorphous to permit conscious recognition, and a later more or less complete engram that may be successfully matched against existing memories and consciously retrieved. For the sake of convenience, we have labeled the first the emotional component of perception and the second the cognitive component, although it is clear that these are merely two aspects of the same complex engram considered at different stages of perceptual processing.

It appears, then, that behaviorally the emotional and cognitive components of perception may have differential thresholds for activating the awareness system (upstream and downstream processing). Negative emotionality is associated with increased arousal which in turn may enhance but apparently more customarily impairs perception (McGinnies, 1949) and memory retrieval (Zeigarnik, 1927). High levels of arousal secondary to positive emotional effects produce enhanced perception and memory retrieval (vigilance), but on occasion may cause impaired perception (Erdelyi and Appelbaum, 1973) and memory retrieval (Holmes, 1972). These behavioral effects are interesting but difficult to interpret, both because of their inconsistency (i.e., a single charge, positive or negative, may cause either perceptual defense or perceptual vigilance) and also because of the unsettled question of voluntary or involuntary reluctance to recognize charged words. Some pertinent psychobiological studies have been performed in this area so that a review of these may help to illuminate these issues.

Psychobiological Studies on the Effects of Emotional Charge on Cognitive Processing

The studies to be described here all illustrate neurophysiological responses to cognitive stimuli before and after positive or negative emotional conditioning of those stimuli. The neurophysiological responses in most of the studies are evoked potentials, but in one they are single neuronal cell responses. The recorded data for the neutral and affective stimuli are designed to provide predominantly cognitive information since the recording electrodes have been located in cognitive pathways. Consequently, any change in the amplitude of the response after emotional conditioning presumably reflects increased or decreased *cognitive* energy. Such energy may vary independently of the presumed increase in *arousal* associated with emotional conditioning. In this paradigm, for example, one might expect a negative emotional charge (high emotional energy) to be associated with either increased or decreased evoked potential amplitude (high or low cognitive energy) as characterizing perceptual vigilance or perceptual defense. Thus, as previously described, the cognitive and emotional components of a cognitive stimulus may appear to be disassociated during processing in the central nervous system.

In a study by Galambos et al. (1956) the electrical response in the cochlear nucleus (brain stem) to a neutral stimulus (a click) became markedly enhanced after that stimulus had achieved motivational–emotional significance through being paired with an electric shock (Fig. 13-1). Engrams such as these are hypercharged, both in electrophysiological and behavioral terms. The high level of emotional charge presumably leads to increased attentional reactivity, and thus to increased accessibility to consciousness.

The response illustrated in Figure 13-1 is apparently the opposite of what one

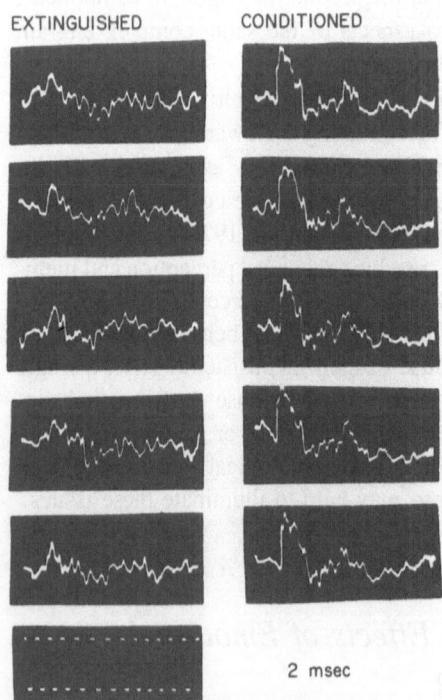

2 msec

Figure 13-1 Effects of conditioning on evoked potentials. (From Galambos et al., 1956. Reprinted with permission).

would expect in perceptual defense and would be characteristic rather of perceptual vigilance. Although Galambos et al. (1956) do not describe the behavioral responses of the animals involved, on the basis of known conditioning procedures one would expect increased arousal, attention, and awareness of the threatening stimulus as well as an increased avoidance response. This experiment then appears to be a psychobiological prototype for the demonstration of perceptual vigilance to negative stimuli at the *conscious* level.

A more complex study measuring neurophysiological responses to *supraliminal* cognitive stimuli with either neutral, positive, or negative emotional charge has been presented by Begleiter and his co-workers (1979) (Fig. 13-2). Using visual evoked potentials as an index of the cognitive energy valence of words with different affective ratings, Begleiter et al. (1979) found the amplitude of the N_1-P_2 wave to be significantly larger for positively charged stimuli than for negatively charged stimuli, and the amplitude of the N_1-P_2 wave for negatively charged stimuli to be significantly greater than that for neutral stimuli. In addition, although this was not reported in the original paper, the P_{300} was also significantly higher for both emotionally charged stimuli than for the neutral (Henri Begleiter, personal communication). Hence those waves of the evoked potential characteristic of increased attention, i.e., the N_1-P_2 and the P_{300}, showed increased amplitude to *supraliminal* stimuli with either positive or negative emotional charge.

An important product of the Begleiter et al. study was the finding that although all emotionally charged stimuli produced larger evoked responses than did neutral stimuli, positively charged stimuli consistently resulted in larger increases than did negatively charged ones. Begleiter et al. discuss the difficulty in equating the strength of negative and positive emotional charges. Nevertheless, it is interesting to note in Figure 13-2 that even mildly positive stimuli (+) produce larger electrical responses than do highly negatively charged stimuli (− −). It must also be emphasized again that the amplitude of the evoked response is a measure of the cognitive energy of the response rather than of the emotional energy; otherwise, the response associated with the highly negative charge (− −) would certainly be greater than that associated with the mildly positive (+).

The greater enhancement of electrical reactivity in the brain by positive affective

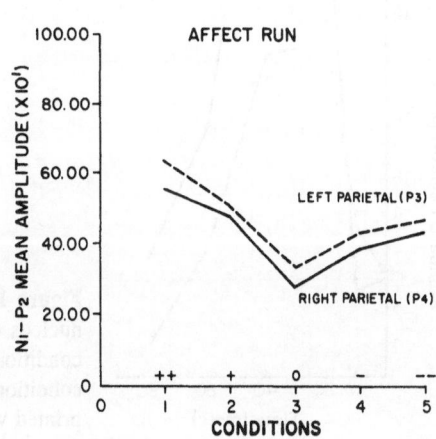

Figure 13-2 N_1-P_2 amplitude from left and right parietal recordings to stimuli of different affect. (From Begleiter et al., 1979. Reprinted with permission.)

charge than by negative, as reflected in the significantly larger N_1-P_2 waves on the positive side of the curve in Figure 13-2, appears to be a general response. This generalization is supported by a study of Olds et al. (1972) on single cell responses to positive and negative conditioning in the medial geniculate nuclei of rabbits. These workers (Fig. 13-3), testing single cell responses in the medial geniculate nucleus, found relative inhibition of responsivity to negative conditioning as compared with positive conditioning (Fig. 13-3). These effects occurred as early as 30 msec after presentation of the stimulus so that they were necessarily *upstream* in nature, suggesting some kind of inhibitory effect in the brain stem (Adey et al., 1957). That negative conditioning should produce no greater activity than the neutral condition is of great interest since it indicates that the quality of responses to negatively charged stimuli may be sufficiently inhibitory to erase the effects of increased arousal. Equally interesting is the fact that the effect of emotional charge on engram reactivity occurs at the subcortical level, an observation that is consistent with our earlier descriptions of upstream information processing. [In an earlier study, Olds (1962) had demonstrated that emotional valence influenced cognitive processing through changes in hypothalamic reactivity.] The absence of any increase in neural activity in the cognitive pathway (the medial geniculate body) in Figure 13-2, despite the presence of strongly negative arousal supports the concept of dissociation between affective and cognitive energy levels.

The Olds et al. (1972) study strongly suggests that some inhibitory effect upon the cognitive response systems occurs with highly negatively charged stimuli during the *upstream* phase of information processing. A similar effect is illustrated in the evoked

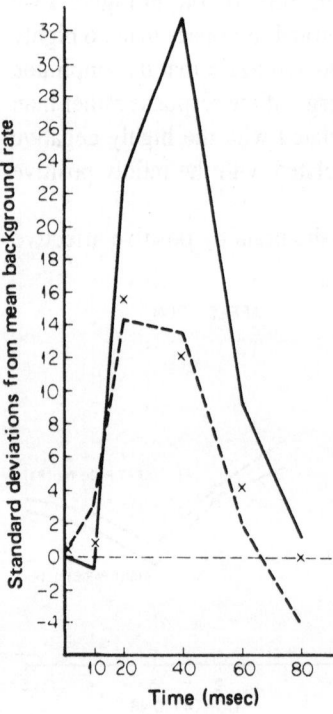

Figure 13-3 Single cell responses in medial geniculate nucleus to positive and negative conditioning. Negative conditioning, X; positive conditioning, solid line; neutral conditioning, dashed line. (From Olds et al., 1972. Reprinted with permission.)

potential phenomena of "augmentation" and "reduction." Certain individuals respond to increasing physical intensity of a flash with diminishing P_1-N_1 waves (so-called reducers), while others (so-called augmenters) respond to all flashes of increasing intensity with increasingly larger P_1-N_1 waves (Fig. 13-4). Presumably, for reducers, increasing physical intensity of stimuli is associated with increasing adaptive responses of an inhibitory nature; these produce protective screening with concomitant attenuation of the brain electrical reaction to the disturbing physical stimulus. Apparently for augmenters no such screening device exists. Not unexpectedly, most normal individuals fall in between (Buchsbaum and Silverman, 1968).

Examples of extreme augmenting and reducing responses are shown in Figure 13-4 (after Buchsbaum and Pfefferbaum, 1971). The earliest wave in the average evoked response (P_1-N_1) is that component which reflects direct access of the impulse to the receiving areas of the lower brain; it becomes progressively larger in the tracings on the left as intensity of flashes increase (augmentation). The same component becomes progressively smaller with increasing stimulus intensity in the tracings on the right (reducing). These latter reactivities apparently reflect the action of an inhibitory "gate" to stimuli of increasing intensity. The mechanisms through which these differential effects are accomplished are presumed to reside in the *upstream* brain stem control centers (P_1-N_1 activity occurs at about 100 msec), similar to those invoked in the early stages of attention (see Chapter 8).

If the augmentation–reduction paradigm is seen as a response to increasing stress where stimuli of increasing intensity constitute a sensory overload, then that phe-

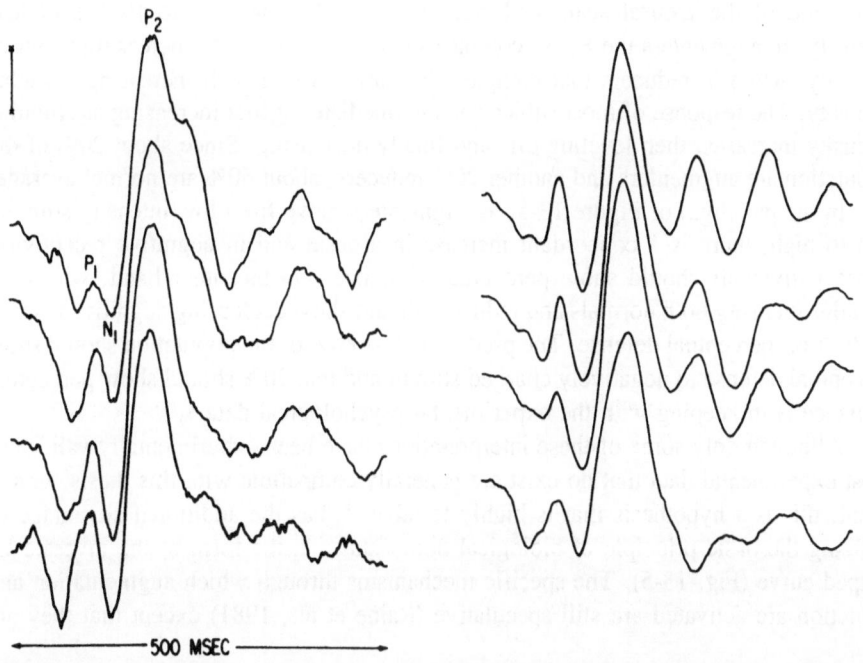

Figure 13-4 Augmenting and reducing. (From Buchsbaum and Pfefferbaum, 1971. Reproduced by permission.)

nomenon can be considered as an organismic response of either increased excitation or inhibition to a condition of stress. This would imply that in certain individuals (reducers) the increasingly loud noise or bright light produces a negative motivational–emotional charge with increased gating in the brain stem and correspondingly reduced evoked potentials recorded over the cortex. For augmenters, on the other hand, bright and loud stimuli apparently lack such a negative motivational–emotional connotation for one of several reasons: (1) augmenters' sensory threshold at low levels may be significantly higher than that for reducers, or (2) their inhibitory mechanisms may be less responsive in reacting to potentially harmful stimuli. Present evidence supports at least in part both of these explanations. Reducers tend to be more sensitive to pain at low levels, but more tolerant to pain at more intense levels (Buchsbaum, 1976). It also appears that reducers are more sensitive to most sensory stimuli, particularly to those of low or moderate intensities. This is evident in the evoked responses of reducers to such stimuli; their early P_1-N_1 complexes are of significantly greater amplitude than are those of augmenters (Fig. 13-4).

The augmentation–reduction paradigm provides the best evidence in humans for an inhibitory effect associated with high arousal. It goes even further. It offers a meaningful paradigm of individual differences in psychological responsivity that would account for the individual differences in psychological responsitivity (namely, different subjects responding with perceptual defense or perceptual vigilance to identical stimuli). A curve representing the different reactivities of different subject populations (augmenters, normal, and reducers), is presented in Figure 13-5. As described by Buchsbaum (1976), augmenters are situated at the lower end of the arousal scale with relatively small P_1-N_1 responses to flashes of low intensity. Reducers are situated at the upper end of the arousal scale with very high P_1-N_1 responses to flashes of low intensity. In augmenters the P_1-N_1 complex increases in size with increasing stimulus intensity, while in reducers that complex decreases in size with increasing stimulus intensity. The response of most subjects is intermediate, at first increasing as stimulus intensity increases, then leveling off, and finally decreasing. Since about 20% of the population are augmenters and another 20% reducers, about 60% are normal average.

In the paradigm of Figure 13-5, as augmenters move from low intensity stimulation to high, there is a concordant increase in arousal and in cognitive receptivity. These individuals should show perceptual vigilance. On the other hand, with high stimulus intensity both normals and reducers should show decreasing cognitive responsivity, i.e., perceptual defense. The prediction that 80% of the population should show perceptual defense to negatively charged stimuli and that 20% should show perceptual vigilance is in keeping with the experimental psychological data.*

Although only some of these interpretations have been experimentally validated, most experimental data that do exist are generally compatible with this thesis. In any event, this is a hypothesis that is highly testable. It has the additional advantage of utilizing the basic principle of biological homeostasis in the form of the inverted U-shaped curve (Fig. 13-5). The specific mechanisms through which augmentation and reduction are activated are still speculative (Raine et al., 1981) except that they are

---

*The relationship of the augmentation-reducing characteristic to personality and the pathogenesis of neurosis is extensively explored in Chapters 19 and 20.

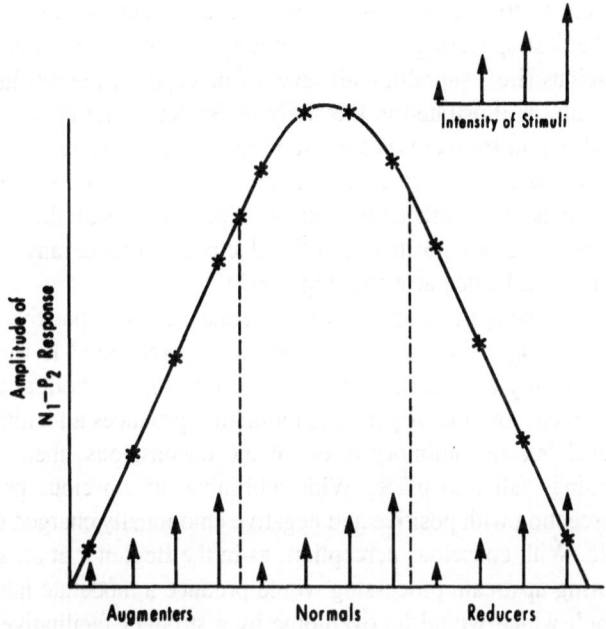

Figure 13-5 The inverted U-shaped curve of augmentation–reduction.

almost certainly subcortical (Lukas and Siegal, 1977). That interpretation is supported both by the finding of Olds et al. (1972) (Fig. 13-3) and by the fact that the major changes take place in the early P_1-N_1 complex of upstream processing.

Differences in Processing Stimuli with Negative and Positive Emotional Valence

All of the quoted tachistoscopic studies on perception as well as the studies on memory retrieval are generally consistent on one point: stimuli with a positive emotional charge tend to be perceived more readily (perceptual vigilance) than stimuli with a negative emotional charge. In itself this is rather surprising since, by and large, negative emotional experiences appear to show evidence of greater physiological arousal than do positively charged stimuli. For example, the increase in associated GSR responsivity is greater for even small increases in negative emotionality than with moderate increases in positive emotionality. If the increase in perceptual efficiency were directly related to an increase in arousal, then negatively charged stimuli should be perceived more readily rather than less readily, than positively charged stimuli.

This is certainly not the case. In most psychological studies of subliminal processing, about 80% of subjects respond to *negative* stimuli with an actual increase in difficulty of perception (perceptual defense). In the same experimental paradigm, with *positively* charged stimuli more than 80% of subjects respond with more rapid perception (perceptual vigilance). At the subliminal (unconscious) level of perception, the difference between reactivities to positive and negative emotionality appears quite dramatic, with the first appearing actively facilitory and the second inhibitory.

At the conscious (i.e., supraliminal) level of perception, the results for positive and negative stimuli, as illustrated in the study of Begleiter and co-workers, (1979), are significantly different from those of the subliminal studies. Here, both positive and negative emotional charge result in increased cerebral activity with the responsivity to the positive charge being consistently greater. Thus, with supraliminally exposed stimuli, neither negative nor positive emotional charge produce any evidence of a significant inhibitory influence at work (Fig. 13-2).

How can we reconcile these apparently disparate effects of positive and negative emotional effects during conscious and unconscious perception? If we assume that positive effects generally exert a facilitory effect on perception both at the conscious and unconscious levels, and that negative emotionality produces a facilitative effect at the conscious level but an inhibitory effect at the unconscious, then most of these experimental findings fall into place. With subliminal unconscious processing, the differences in perception with positive and negative emotionally charged stimuli would be self-explicable. With conscious perception, as in the Begleiter et al. study, unconscious effects during upstream processing would produce a moderate inhibitory effect on negative stimuli which would be overcome by a stronger facilitative effect at the amygdaloid–hippocampal complex level. The final production would be of increased brain excitation, but less than that for positive emotional charge. The exception, of course, would be with intense, negative, *conscious* stimuli in which, as in the Galambos et al. (1956) study, the effect would be markedly facilitative.

This is a very attractive hypothesis which appears to explain most of the psychological and physiological findings; still, it needs direct experimental verification. Thus far, very few reports have addressed this critical question. Kostandov and Arzumov (1980) studied evoked potentials to subliminally displayed words on the tachistoscope where the words previously had had their emotional valence rated by the subject. Stimuli were presented above threshold and subliminally. Negatively emotionally charged stimuli presented at or above threshold produced larger P_{300}'s in the evoked potential than did emotionally neutral stimuli. On the other hand, negatively charged stimuli presented subliminally produced smaller P_{300}'s in the evoked potential than did neutral stimuli. The authors interpret these latter findings to indicate unconscious recognition of the emotional valence of cognitive events at a level at which conscious cognitive recognition had not occurred. Furthermore, they conclude that the same or similarly negatively charged emotional stimuli may evoke perceptual vigilance when recognized consciously and perceptual defense when experienced unconsciously. This report has yet to be validated. It has been questioned on the grounds that, theoretically, subliminal stimuli should not induce P_{300}'s; by definition subliminal stimuli do not reach consciousness and conscious attention is a prerequisite for the production of P_{300}'s. If this objection is not valid and if this study can be replicated, it would be of great theoretical interest, indicating a difference in the way supraliminal and subliminal negative stimuli are processed.

Related experiments by Shevrin and co-workers (Shevrin and Rennich, 1967; Shevrin, 1974; Shervin and Dickman, 1980) help to illuminate this issue. In these studies, Shevrin evaluated the evoked potential responses of repressed individuals (as determined independently on the Rorschach) to threatening and nonthreatening stimuli, comparing them with those of presumed nonrepressors. All stimuli were matched for size, shape, and color. Stimuli were presented both subliminally and supraliminally and evoked potential responses recorded. Shevrin divided the evoked potential responses into two components: early (less than 250 msec) and late (more than 250 msec). With subliminal presentations, repressed subjects showed significantly smaller early component responses to the negatively charged stimuli than to the neutral. With supraliminal exposures, repressed subjects showed significantly larger early component responses to the negatively charged stimuli than to the neutral. Results for late evoked potential components were less clear. The early component responses for nonrepressors also tended to run in the same direction as did those for repressors, but the differences were not significant.

The results of Shevrin and co-workers are not strictly comparable to those of Kostandov and Arzumov, but are sufficiently related to be generally supportive. Effects in the two studies for both subliminal and supraliminal presentations were similar except that Shevrin's effects were in the early evoked response components and Kostandov and Arzumov's in the late. Both components, as previously indicated, are involved in attentional activities so that the difference in findings on the two studies may be reconcilable. In any event, the hypothesis that *subconscious* (subliminal) stimuli with negative charge may be processed subcortically by inhibitory mechanisms while similar *conscious* stimuli are treated cortically with perceptual vigilance is an intriguing one. The fact that negatively charged stimuli produce larger evoked responses in the lower brain stem (cochlear nucleus, Fig. 13-1) and smaller evoked responses in the upper brain stem (thalamic geniculate bodies, Fig. 13-3) again suggests that inhibitory influences are exerted somewhere in the upper brain stem during upstream processing.

There are several plausible mechanisms in the hierarchical control system to account for the distinction between conscious and subconscious processing of negatively charged stimuli. The fact that the emotional component of perception is processed in the early phase of attention (Kunst-Wilson and Zajonc) is anatomically compatible with the location of the thalamic–basal gangliar complex close to the hypothalamus and limbic system. The fact that the response to negative and positive emotional charges is antithetical at this level (respectively, inhibitory or stimulatory) is readily demonstrable (Fig. 13-3) and suggests that the thalamic–basal gangliar complex is actively involved in this process.

Hierarchical Mechanisms for Reducing Excessive Emotional Charge

Theoretically, perceptual defense to overwhelmingly threatening situations makes eminent biological sense. Our presentation suggests that the association of a highly negative emotional charge with a visual or auditory stimulus may, under certain circumstances, inhibit perception of that highly charged stimulus. On first flush this would seem counterproductive since from a biological point of view emotionally charged stimuli, especially those that are negative, should attract greater attention. And indeed, at the supraliminal conscious level both positively and negatively charged stimuli do attract increased attention. However, if negatively charged stimuli were always associated with increased arousal and with increased perceptual efficiency, then a vicious feedback system could develop with a continual build-up of arousal until the biological animal was incapacitated. The introduction of the slowing down of perception would brake the entire process and would prevent the build-up of intolerable arousal. Such a feedback mechanism would assure that whenever there arose a threatening situation in which the emotional charge was too great and behaviorally disruptive, a decrease in cognitive energy and attentional reactivity would occur. That such a mechanism is of more than hypothetical biological significance is evidenced among animals of prey when they are so overwhelmed by fear as to become frozen and immobilized. In such cases the desensitizing of cognitive and emotional valence during upstream processing was apparently inadequate to ward off total and incapacitating fear.*

The putative existence of such a biological feedback mechanism requires an innate neurophysiological system to provide it. On the basis of general physiological considerations, a plausible mechanism. is that described by Skinner and Yingling (1977) in Chapter 8 of this volume and illustrated in Figure 8-1. In their study, Skinner and Yingling demonstrated that somatosensory stimulation of the mesencephalic reticular formation was transmitted to the frontal lobe whence inhibitory influences were transmitted to the reticular thalamic nucleus, and from there further to the medial and lateral geniculate nuclei of the thalamus, the transfer points for auditory and visual stimuli, respectively. In this way the frontal–thalamic system, by inhibiting the auditory and visual systems, served to direct attention to the somatosensory field. Although there is at this time no direct evidence to support the thesis that a highly negatively charged stimulus could provoke the same frontal–thalamic system to inhibit activity in its own sensory modality, the possibility of some such effect or a related one would have to be hypothesized.

The postulated feedback control function of the frontal–thalamic system on subliminal negative stimuli through modulation of perceptual transmission offers a mechanism that seems eminently plausible. Such a function also responds to a frequently posed question: Why is the attentional process divided into two phases and what purpose do those two phases serve? For example, Broadbent (1973) has written of the two-phase structure of attention:

> [It] seems to require a biologically unlikely kind of machinery. . . It seems to mean
> that the part of the brain which analyzes inputs from the environment, and which is
> presumably quite complicated, is preceded by another and duplicate part of the brain
> which carries out the same function, deciding what is there in order to reject or accept
> items for admission to the machinery which decides what is there. (p. 67)

The screening function of the preperceptual upstream phase of attention, which selects on the basis of cognitive criteria those sensory stimuli likely to be most relevant, is obviously an important biological purpose of the two-phase attentional process. This mechanism is apparently implemented through the control activity of the mesencephalic reticular formation–prefrontal lobe–thalamic nuclei system. But the hypothesized negative feedback role for that system in regulating the build-up of arousal secondary to a flood of negatively charged emotional stimuli may serve an equally

---

*Either that or with excessive arousal (terror) the defensive mechanism breaks down. This is presumably what happens in neurotic humans. For discussion of defense mechanisms in neurosis, see Chapter 20.

important biological function, since it would prevent the development of an over-whelming and incapacitating level of arousal. The proven demonstration that the emotional components of perceptive stimuli are processed early during transmission in the brain stem (Kunst-Wilson and Zajonc, 1980; Olds et al., 1972) is at least consistent with this hypothesis. At any rate, this thesis should be readily susceptible to experimental validation or invalidation.

Another system that may be active in these excitatory–inhibitory reactivities is one also previously described (Chapter 8) as involved in attentional activities, namely that consisting of the anterior and posterior hypothalamic nuclei as well as the septum and amygdaloid–hippocampal complex (Isaacson, 1972). There appears to be a feedback circuit between the hypothalamic nuclei and the amygdaloid–hippocampal complex where increased activity in the excitatory elements at either end of the circuit increases similar activity at the other end, whereas increased inhibitory activity at either end increases inhibitory activity at the other. Thus excitatory activity in the posterior hypothalamus is transmitted through the mammillary bodies to the amygdala (see Fig. 2-3) with concomitant stimulatory effects on cognition; conversely, inhibitory influences from the anterior hypothalamus are transmitted through the mammillary bodies to the septum and then to the hippocampus to produce inhibitory effects on cognition.* The fact that these influences are effectuated in the amygdaloid–hippo-campal complex suggests that the latter may be the control mechanism through which supraliminal stimuli are cognitively influenced.

The actions of the two systems, the subliminal prefrontal–thalamic system and the supraliminal hypothalamic–amygdaloid–hippocampal system, are integrated with still another circuit. The prefrontal lobe has a direct connection to the posterior hypoth-alamus which is generally inhibitory in its effects (Nauta, 1964). It seems plausible that with negative emotional stimuli, inhibitory effects at the thalamic level may be trans-mitted to the prefrontal lobe and from there to the posterior hypothalamus to exert inhibitory effects on the amygdaloid–hippocampal complex with consequent cognitive suppression of supraliminal negatively charged stimuli. This mechanism could rein-force the thalamic–prefrontal lobe mechanism, thus accounting for the discrepancy in responses to positive and negative supraliminal stimuli as illustrated in the Begleiter et al. study (Fig. 13-2).

Considering only these very primitive biological reactivities that are implemented through the hierarchical control system, one must conclude that the inhibition of threatening perceptions and memories, i.e., those with strong negative emotional charges, would serve an important biological function. However, the slight delay in perception represented by heightened tachistoscopic thresholds to fairly trivial negative charges seems to represent a relatively insignificant effect. It may be that some other mechanisms designed for monitoring threatening experience also exist, perhaps in the one major control system we have not yet explored, i.e., the interhemispheric. With that in mind, we shall turn in Chapter 14 and 15 to the consideration of the major control system represented by anatomical and functional differences between the two cerebral hemispheres. In Chapter 16, we shall explore the role of the cerebral hemi-spheres in the effectuation of repression and other psychological defense mechanisms.

---

*The role of the amygdaloid–hippocampal complex in the control of excitatory–inhibitory influences is discussed in greater detail in Chapter 19.

14

Differential Cognitive and Emotional Functions of the Cerebral Hemispheres

The major theme in this book thus far has been the description of the structure, function, and operation of the hierarchical control system, both in conscious and unconscious behavior. That control system was defined as the biological organizational structure that determined in its broadest context most mammalian and consequently most human behavior. However, reference has also been made to another control system, the interhemispheric, which apparently contributes an extra dimension, particularly in humans, to the activities of the hierarchical control system. The description of the differences between the activities of the left and right hemispheres presented in Chapter 1 was intended to introduce that dimension, however briefly, at an early point in this volume. Here it is necessary to examine the mechanisms through which the hemispheric system modifies and is modified by the activities of the hierarchical control system.

Cognitive Differences in Hemispheric Function

Biologically, the hemispheric control system represents a rather late development. Although there is evidence of lateralization of brain function in certain of the lower vertebrates, only with the development of significant growth of the cortex in birds (Nottebohm, 1979) and mammals do meaningful interhemispheric differences appear. With the evolution of the speech centers in man on the left side of the brain, the two hemispheres begin to take on significantly different functions. Since language is so important an element in human intercourse and since that activity is largely restricted to the left brain, the two hemispheres have inevitably come to have different specialized roles. As we shall see, there is substantial evidence that hemispheric effects play a much larger role in human behavior than even in that of their closest evolutionary neighbors, the primates.

As an introduction and in order to provide a suitable setting, it is well to start with an historical review of our knowledge of human hemispheric lateralization. Men have known since time immemorial that most humans prefer to act with their right hands to the point where right-handedness is almost universally considered the normal mode of response. As a result of such opinions, in the early 20th century only 2% of the population of the United States were left-handed. In 1972, with decreased social pressure the level had risen to 11%, close to the 12% that is considered to be the natural incidence of this trait. Since motor control, like most other functions of the body, is crossed in the central nervous system, right-handedness is associated with preferential control in the left hemisphere; such lateralization of preferential function is known as left-hemispheric dominance.

Whereas hemispheric dominance for handedness may be changed through training (witness the many natural left-handers who learned to become right-handers) (Michel, 1981; Turkewitz, 1977), the left-hemispheric dominance for speech is innate, biological, and in adults more or less unchangeable. More than a 100 years ago, early investigators such as Broca, Wernicke, and others deduced from their observations in neurological patients during life and on autopsy that lesions in the left hemisphere of the brain, producing paralysis of the right side of the body, were frequently associated with a variety of speech disturbances. Similar lesions in the right hemisphere producing left-sided paralysis appeared to have little effect on either the understanding or production of language. After this major discovery, it was generally assumed that, aside from language control and handedness, other functions of the two sides of the brain were more or less similar. However, the work by Bogen (1969) showing that division of the corpus callosum, i.e., commissurotomy, significantly reduced seizures in temporal lobe epilepsy led to the creation through surgery of a small but significant population of patients with separated cerebral hemispheres. The question was raised by Sperry (1966), then working with Bogen, as to whether these patients might be considered in effect to have two brains. Toward that end, he devised a series of tests in which the two hemispheres could be tested independently. His results, since corroborated by Gazzaniga and others in similar patients, indicate that at least in commissurotomized patients the two hemispheres do have different functions in that (1) they have different ways of processing information, (2) they play different roles in emotional and cognitive activities, and (3) they apparently have different kinds of consciousness.

The fundamental difference between the two hemispheres in their mode of processing cognitive data has been well established both in commissurotomized patients and in normals. In each instance information of various types is fed to one hemisphere or the other through hemifield presentation of visual stimuli or through unilateral presentation of auditory stimuli. The differences in mode of processing are of course most apparent in the commissurotomized patients, where no information can be transferred to the opposite hemisphere, but they are also discernible in intact subjects in terms of rapidity of processing as well as in terms of electrophysiological levels of reactivity.

In general terms, the left hemisphere processes verbal material more quickly and more effectively, and the right hemisphere processes spatial information more efficiently. That the left hemisphere should excel in handling verbal material is hardly surprising; the speech and language centers (Broca's and Wernicke's areas as illustrated in Fig. 5-1) are situated exclusively in that hemisphere in about 95% of humans. Equally significant is the fact that verbal material may be managed, although less efficiently, in the right hemisphere as well. This has been well established in several studies on a series of commissurotomized patients. Communication with the right hemisphere was carried out by flashing words to the left visual field, to which messages the subject responded by arranging Scrabble® letters with the left hand. Although the right hemisphere was able to perform spatial tasks much better than the left, the latter was by no means incapable of such tasks (Gazzaniga and LeDoux, 1978).

At a higher level of intellectual functioning, the left hemisphere has been found generally to employ an analytic method of problem solving and the right hemisphere tends to be more holistic. For example, on a test of facial recognition such as comparing two images for similarity, the left hemisphere might contrast the shape of the nose or the size of the mouth while the right hemisphere would be more likely to make a global judgement based on the general spatial arrangements in the two faces. To a degree, this difference may be a consequence of the verbal–spatial dichotomy, since verbal considerations tend to be analytic and spatial more holistic.

Still a third cognitive difference between the two hemispheres has to do with the management of temporal sequences of events. As Moscovitch (1979) has written:

> Because temporal sequential information is characteristic of language, a number of investigators have suggested that the perception and production of temporal sequences even if they are not linguistic, are mediated primarily by the left hemisphere. Research on a variety of non-verbal tasks strongly supports this view.*

Since time control is one of the highest functions of the brain as indicated by its normal locus in the frontal lobe, it may be this function that accounts most for the general dominance of the left hemisphere in behavior. Various authors have suggested that sequential control of various functions is essential to the development of speech and language and, as described in Chapter 10, of the phenomenology of consciousness. From a biological point of view the specialization between the two hemispheres is of great advantage since it permits a dual approach, analytic and holistic, to all problem solving. On the other hand, the need for a single executive hemisphere capable of imposing unified decision-making control is equally apparent. Under these circumstances, the biological advantage of having such control in the left hemisphere with its special talent for sequential processing and apparently for consciousness, seems logical.

There is, of course, no certainty that the major differences in the functions and roles of the two hemispheres found in commissurotomized patients reflect a similar difference in function and role of the two hemispheres in normal intact individuals. As noted in Chapter 1, the flow of information from one hemisphere to the other throughout the corpus callosum is immense. On the other hand, it is not clear why commissurotomy should consistently result in disparate functions between the two hemispheres and always of the same kind, if those functions were not different prior to surgery. Furthermore, sophisticated techniques for studying each hemisphere indepen-

---

*Linguistic support for this position is evidenced by the fact that in commissurotomized patients, the right hemisphere usually has difficulty in processing verbs but not nouns or adjectives.

dently in normal unoperated individuals have confirmed the existence of differential functions between the two hemispheres even in the presence of an intact functioning corpus callosum. These differences are present in infancy and persist throughout life (Gardiner and Walter, 1977; Harnad and Doty, 1977).

The evidence suggests that in normals, incoming perceptions transverse both hemispheres coequally but are processed differently in each hemisphere. The processed information from each side is freely interchanged with that of the other (Fig. 14-1). The decision-making authority for interpretation and response rests somewhat more in the left brain than in the right, but in the intact individual, the functions of the two hemispheres are entirely integrated. Nevertheless, there is recent evidence to suggest that even under normal conditions, dominance in processing fluctuates constantly between the two hemispheres. Even though both hemispheres are in constant communication, one or the other may operate momentarily at a higher energy level depending on the nature of the cognitive task (Gevins et al., 1983). This subject is addressed in detail at the end of this chapter.

Physiological Mechanisms of Differential Cognitive Hemispheric Processing

Experimental studies demonstrate clearly that there is a tendency for verbal material to be processed differentially in the left hemisphere and spatial material in the

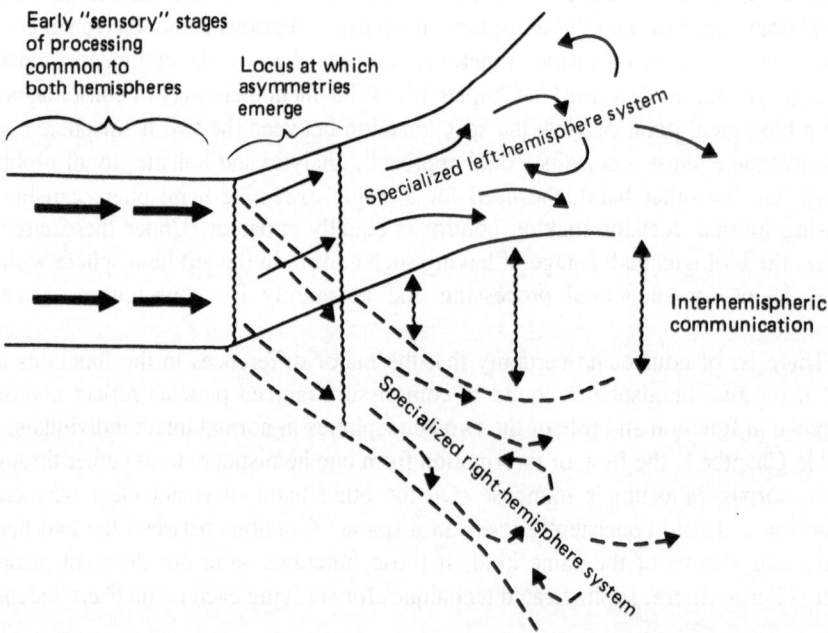

Figure 14-1 Information flow on the two hemispheres. (From Moscovitch, 1979. Reprinted with permission.)

right. However, under certain conditions of mental set or attention, the normal differentiation may be either neutralized or even reversed (Moscovitch, 1979). Under those conditions, processing will take place either equally in both hemispheres or even sometimes predominantly in the inappropriate hemisphere. These findings suggest that there is at least a functional physiological element as well as an anatomical element in the determination of differential cortical processing. Extensive research on the mechanisms involved in "normal" processing as opposed to that in these deliberately manipulated exceptions has not resolved the issue. Two theories have generally been forwarded. The first, the so-called structural direct access model (Kahneman, 1973) presumes that the neural structure of the brain is such that verbal stimuli are automatically directed more to the left brain for processing and spatial nonverbal stimuli more to the right. An alternative theory (Kinsbourne, 1970) presumes that differential processing is the result of differential priming by attentional mechanisms that increase the energy level of one hemisphere or the other to account for the differential efficacy of processing. Most recently, Klein et al. (1976) have suggested that both models are correct so that mechanisms of the direct access model account for "normal" differences in processing stimuli while attentional priming mechanisms may account for the manipulated exceptions. It seems that the Klein model probably has the greatest validity since it explains the fact that differential processing in one hemisphere or the other is associated with greater activation, i.e., electrical activity, in the more involved hemisphere (see Fig. 14-2).

The evidence for structural differences between the two hemispheres derives from the qualitatively different nature of the kinds of cognitive function that the two hemispheres perform. Putative increases or decreases in the energizing force stemming from the brain stem as postulated by Kinsbourne would account more for quantitative differences in the levels of activation. There is no apparent mechanism through which differential priming of one side of the brain rather than the other should result in the qualitatively different modes of cognitive processing in the two hemispheres. These

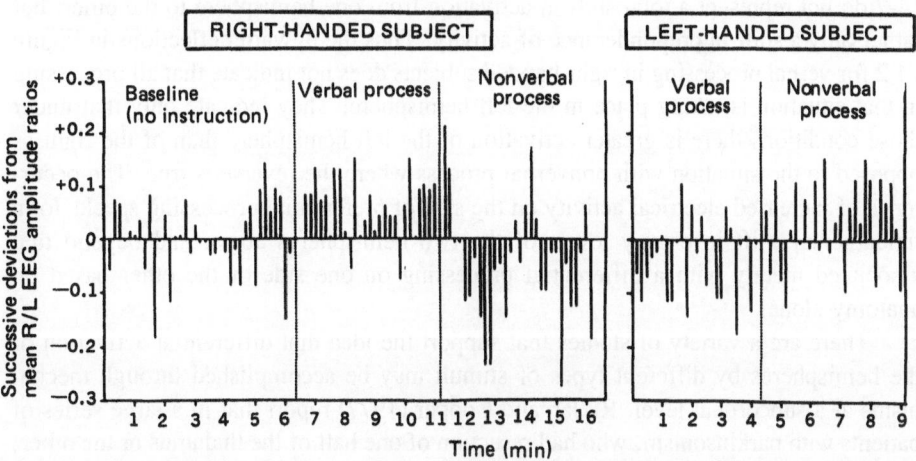

Figure 14-2 Preponderance of hemispheric activity in adults with verbal and nonverbal process thinking. (From Goldstein, 1979. Reprinted with permission.)

differences must be accounted for by structural conditions unique to each hemisphere. As previously noted in the Lumsden–Wilson model of cognitive processing (Fig. 5-4), the two major modes of processing are the associative and the abstractional. Obviously, all mental operations involve both of these sequences. Nevertheless, some operations involve more of one, and some more of the other. In Chapter 5, it was noted that although the derivation of language is highly abstractional, the actual flow of ideas in mentation and speech is even more highly associational. On the other hand, the matching of patterns characteristic of the spatial functions of the right hemisphere is an almost purely abstractional process. From these and other considerations, it follows that the left hemisphere may utilize associational activities more than does the right, whereas the right hemisphere may be more abstractional than the left. Needless to say, both hemispheres utilize both processing modalities so that the associational–abstractional ratio for the left hemisphere may be in the order of 60/40 while that for the right might be 40/60. Such structural differences would account not only for differences in cognitive function between the two hemispheres, but, for differences in other psychological functions as well, as will be described later.

The physiological evidence for Kinsbourne's differential priming hypothesis derives largely from studies measuring electrical activity in the two hemispheres under a variety of behavioral conditions using a technique known as power spectrum analysis. Power spectrum analysis is an electrophysiological technique of ascertaining the average wave length of brain wave activity in one hemisphere versus the other. Since large slow waves (α, θ, and δ, Fig. 6-1) indicate a low level of brain activity, the higher the spectral power, the lower is then the level of brain activity. Figure 14-2 illustrates a study by Goldstein (1979) showing differential electrical activity in the two hemispheres measured in response to verbal and nonverbal stimuli, in one right-handed and one left-handed subject. Major deflections upward indicate increased left-hemispheric electrical activity, those downward right hemispheric. In the right-handed subject, verbal stimuli are associated with increased left-hemispheric activity; in the left-handed subject, the opposite is true.

It should be emphasized that the neurophysiological activities reflected in Figure 14-2 do not represent a total shift in activation from one hemisphere to the other, but rather only a shift in preponderance of activity. Thus the upward deflections in Figure 14-2 for verbal processing in right-handed subjects does not indicate that all processing in that situation is taking place in the left hemisphere. They indicate only that under those conditions there is greater activation of the left hemisphere than of the right as opposed to the situation with nonverbal process where the reverse is true. The occurrence of increased electrical activity on the side of preferential processing speaks for a fundamental shift in energy levels of the two hemispheres above and beyond that associated merely with a differential processing on one side or the other based on anatomy alone.

There are a variety of studies that support the idea that differential activation of the hemispheres by different types of stimuli may be accomplished through mechanisms at a subcortical level. Riklan and Cooper (1977) report that in a large series of patients with parkinsonism, who had resection of one half of the thalamus or the other, left thalamic ablation resulted in significant verbal dysfunctions, whereas right thalamic ablation had only slight effect on spatial processing. They conclude that since representation of language in the left thalamus is less concrete than that in the left hemisphere, the behavioral effects noted were more likely due to difficulties in subcortical activation than to difficulties during the subsequent course of cortical processing. This finding would be compatible with the upstream function of the thalamic–basal gangliar system in perceptual processing, as postulated in Chapter 8.

Ojemann (1977) has described in greater detail the evidence supporting differential "alerting" from the thalamus of the two hemispheres. He writes,

> The suggestion that the right and left human thalamus may not be functionally equivalent is largely the result of observations of language deficits associated with left, and not right, thalamic lesions . . . The nature of this language deficit after left thalamic lesions, when present, does not seem to be identical with any of the described language deficits after cortical lesions of the language-dominant hemisphere . . . Language function may fluctuate widely, from nearly normal, to a silence resembling sleep, depending on the degree of environmental stimulation.
>
> Other functions have also been identified that are altered differentially by lesions of the right or left human thalamus. Deficits in short-term verbal memory appear after left, but not right, thalamic lesions. Deficits in face-matching have been described following right and not left ventrolateral thalamic surgical lesions, and deficits in Porteus-maze performance have occurred following right subthalamic lesions and not left. (p. 380)

At a later point he continues,

> Our model for these effects is that stimulation of left and not right thalamus of man evokes or intensifies a "specific alerting response" that directs attention to verbal information present in the external environment. The more intense this response at the time an item of verbal information is perceived, the more readily that item can be recalled from short-term memory. A low level of specific alerting response accelerates retrieval from short-term memory, while a more intense response blocks the ability to retrieve verbal material already internalized in short-term memory. Thus the thalamus seems to be a site of interaction between alerting mechanisms and short-term memory. At any point in time, the intensity of this alerting response appears to be a gate controlling access to or from short-term memory. (pp. 385–386)

These interpretations are very much in keeping with our previous description of the dorsal median thalamic nucleus as being involved both in upstream perceptual processing and in memory retrieval (see Chapters 8 and 9). They are also compatible with our descriptions in Chapter 6 of the thalamus as one of the subcortical centers for electrically activating cortical function (see also study by Butler in Fig. 14-3 below).

Additional albeit indirect evidence for subcortical (upstream) channeling of control of hemispheric lateralization effects comes from animal studies. Recent work by Glick on laterality in rats has provided evidence to suggest that lateralization in these animals is a function of arousal levels in the basal ganglia with its effects transmitted upward into the cortex. Glick and associates' (1977) work is based on the experimental finding that lesions in the nigrostriatal system of rats (substantia nigra, nigrostriatal bundles, or corpus striatum) result in circling behavior toward the side of the lesion (ipsiversive rotation). These investigators have demonstrated that the administration of amphetamines to normal nonlesioned rats will similarly cause turning behavior with approximately one half of the rats turning characteristically in each direction. They have further demonstrated that the mechanism of this reaction to amphetamine involves differences in levels of dopamine concentrations activating the two sides of the nigrostriatal system. The administration of amphetamine (a dopamine effect enhancer) increases this imbalance, thus precipitating turning behavior. Furthermore, stressful experiences such as electric shocks produce the same effects as amphetamine injections. Thus increased arousal through biochemical or physiological stimulation in the paleocortex produces lateralization, at least in rats.

In humans, a study by Butler (1979) in commissurotomized patients showed that α wave levels in the two separated hemispheres are more or less totally asynchronous. Figure 14-3 shows the EEG recordings from the occipital area in a neurologically intact and in a commissurotomized subject. The EEG rhythms in the two separated hemispheres appear more or less independent of each other. Since alpha is a thalamically generated impulse, discordance of hemispheric activation in split-brain patients appears to stem from subcortically generated differences in levels of electrophysiological activation. (For further discussion, see Chapter 15.)

Perhaps the most compelling evidence for subcortical channeling of hemispheric input is offered in studies by Wood and co-workers (Wood et al., 1971; Wood, 1975). His investigation involved the determination of differences in latency and amplitude of auditory evoked potentials (AEP) as recorded over the two hemispheres in response to auditory stimuli of different characteristics. In his first study, Wood compared AEPs on the two sides with two sounds of different pitch (104 Hz and 140 Hz) and with two sounds preceded by different consonants (bae versus gae). The evoked potential data in this study are shown in Figure 14-4. It may be seen that processing in the left hemisphere for "place" (i.e., bae versus gae) as opposed to "pitch" occurs significantly

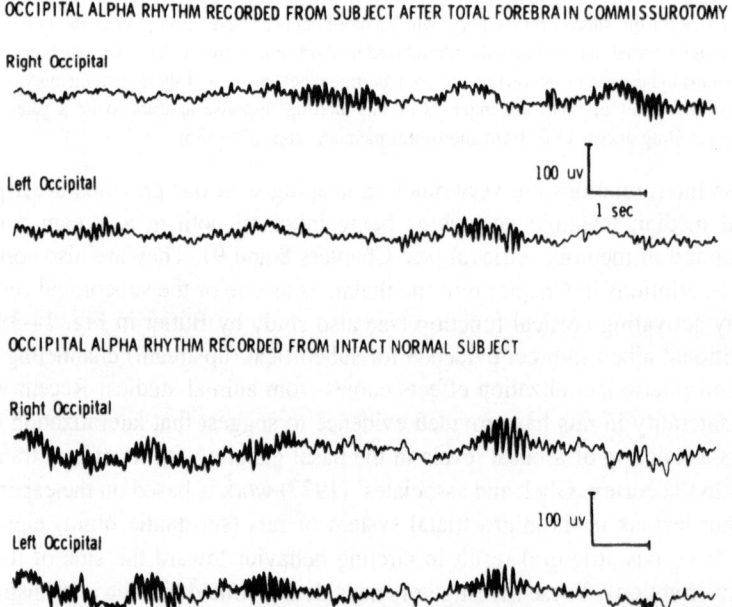

Figure 14-3 EEG recordings from normal and split-brain patients. (From Butler, 1979. Reprinted with permission.)

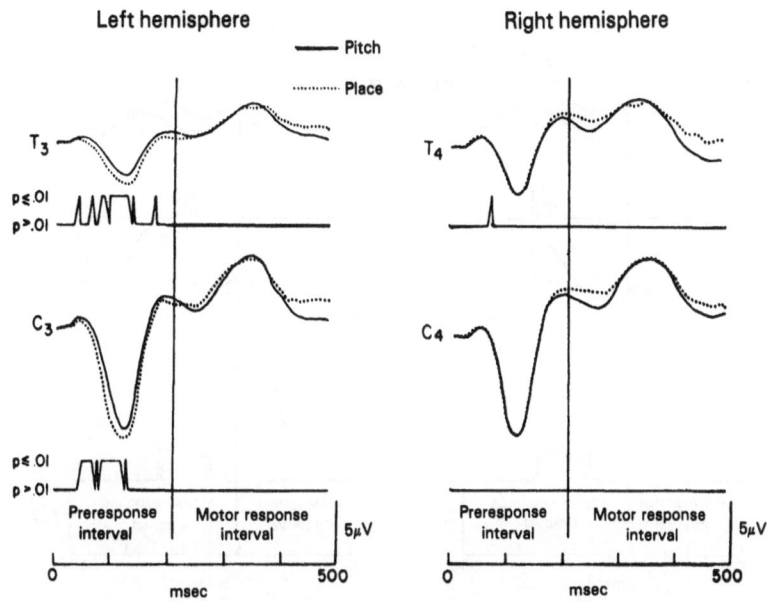

Figure 14-4 Comparison of auditory evoked potential to stimuli of varying "pitch" and "place." (From Wood, 1975. Reproduced with permission.)

earlier and with significantly greater amplitude in the left hemisphere; there are no significant differences in the right hemisphere. More important, the differences in the left hemisphere begin as early as 40–60 msec after stimulation, a latency too short to represent cortical activity. These results are consistent with the interpretation that simple analyses for verbal differentiation are made in the left hemisphere, but begin already at a subcortical level as manifested there by shorter latencies.

In a second experiment (Fig. 14-5), Wood compared the evoked potential response in both hemispheres with sounds of different pitch but also of different pitch contour (i.e., rising or falling inflection). Here, both stimuli were spatial in nature; however, pitch contour was also temporal, requiring greater analysis and processing. Since spatial analysis is a function of the right hemisphere but temporal analysis more a function of the left, both hemispheres showed significant differences in amplitude and latency for the two conditions. However, the differences occurred late in the 250–280 msec range indicating a disparity of late cortical processing rather than of subcortical. Again, the evoked potential data are consistent with the theoretical distinctions previously made between early upstream processing in the first experiment and late downstream processing in the second.

Differences in Hemispheric Processing of Emotional Stimuli

The emphasis here on the subcortical control of activation levels in the two hemispheres with at least some influence on the mode of differential processing is

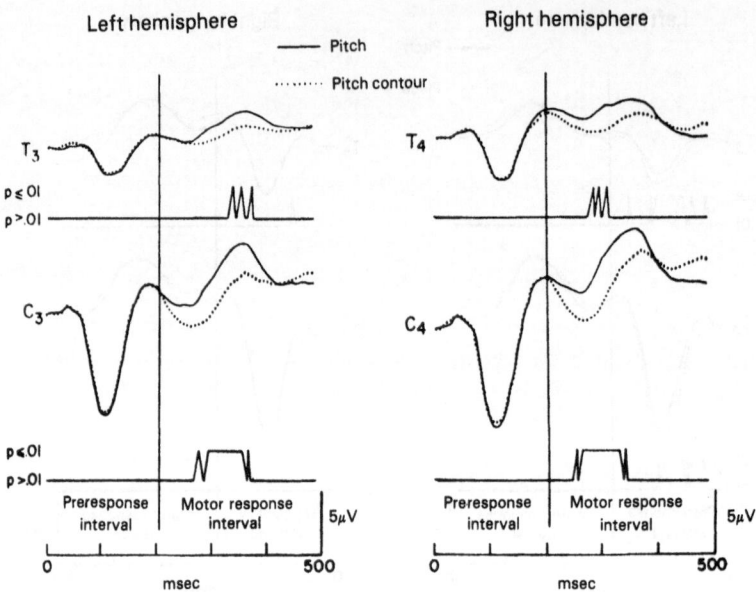

Figure 14-5 Average evoked potentials for identification of pitch contour and pitch. (From Wood, 1975. Reproduced with permission.)

necessary (1) to explain those experimental situations where information processing is preferentially carried out in the inappropriate hemisphere, and (2) to lay the groundwork for the hemispheric differentiation between emotional and cognitive processing. The recent ascendency of cognitive psychology over the dynamic psychologies has tended to raise the level of interest from the subcortex to the cortex; this has probably been overdone. Studies of single neuron responses have shown that learning and recognition can take place in the thalamus and perhaps even the hypothalamus (Olds et al., 1972). As previously described, early subcortical upstream processing may occur in recognizer cells, groups of cells in the basal ganglia that are activated by specific constellations of stimuli (Edelman and Mountcastle, 1978). Even more important, the evidence presented in the last chapter strongly supports the thesis that emotional influences are both evaluated and acted on subcortically at some level in the brain stem, with subsequent determination as to whether the involved stimuli are to be processed consciously or unconsciously.

The differentiation of hemispheric activation illustrated in Figure 14-2 was defined by more or less strictly cognitive criteria. Verbal analytic constellations tend to be processed not exclusively but more effectively in the left hemisphere, and spatial holistic stimuli tend to be processed not exclusively but more effectively in the right hemisphere. A similar situation appears to apply in nonemotional versus emotional thinking. Evidence for the greater shift in activation toward the right hemisphere under conditions of emotional arousal was reported by Goldstein (1979) as illustrated in Figure 14-6. In this study, power spectrum analysis of the two hemispheres was conducted in two schizophrenic patients under either predominantly mental or emotional circumstances. When each of the subjects was doing arithmetical calculations,

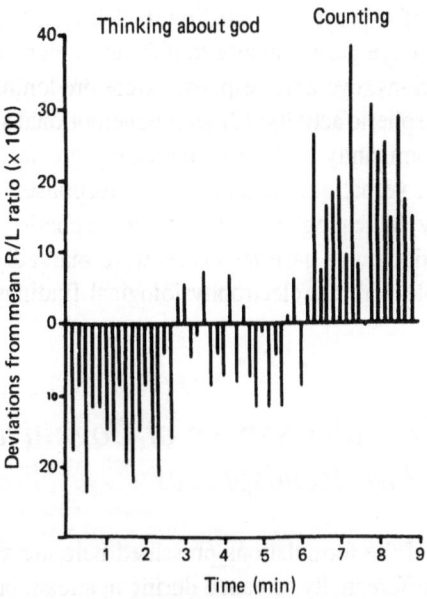

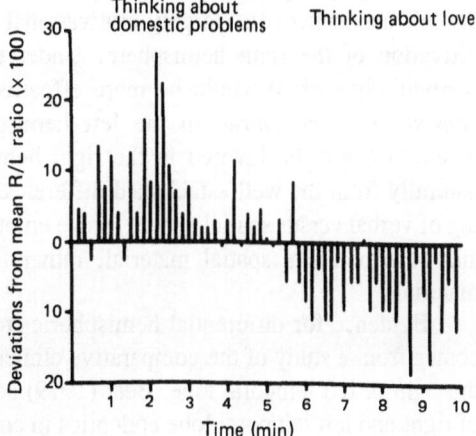

Figure 14-6 Shifts in hemispheric balance of activation with emotional thinking. (From Goldstein, 1979. Reproduced with permission.)

power spectral analysis showed predominance of left-hemispheric activity. On the other hand, when each of the subjects was involved in a highly emotional thought process (thinking about God or thinking about love), there was a marked shift to predominance of activity in the right hemisphere. These data suggest that while the cognitive components of perceptive stimuli are processed differentially by both hemispheres, under the special conditions of increased emotional arousal the right hemisphere may play a larger role in processing all such information. Biologically this would seem reasonable since emotions are vague, generalized phenomena that can be reacted to only holistically and not analytically.

A report by Schwartz et al. (1975) utilizes the techniques of lateral eye gaze to determine hemispheric functional lateralization. Although the validity of this technique as an index of lateralization has been questioned by Ehrlichman and Weinberger (1978), the method appears to have sufficient credibility to warrant the consideration here of experiments based on it. Schwartz and his co-workers found different types of lateral eye gaze response to different kinds of questions: (1) with nonemotional verbal questions, eye gaze responses were predominantly to the right, indicating greater left-hemispheric activity; (2) with nonemotional spatial questions, eye gaze responses were predominantly to the left, indicating greater right-hemispheric activity; (3) with emotional verbal questions, eye gaze responses were predominantly to the left, paradoxically indicating greater right-hemispheric activity; and (4) with emotional spatial questions, eye gaze responses were markedly greater to the left. These data are compatible with the electrophysiological findings of Goldstein.

Differential Storing of Cognitive and Emotional Material in the Two Hemispheres

If the formulations presented here are valid, then it seems to follow that stimuli are differentially screened during upstream processing in the thalamus and basal ganglia with largely cognitive (particularly verbal) stimuli producing increased activation of the left hemisphere and largely motivational–emotional impulses initiating increased activation of the right hemisphere. Under these circumstances, cognitive percepts (particularly verbal) would be more effectively processed but also more effectively *consolidated and stored* in the left hemisphere; motivational–emotional percepts would similarly be favored in the right hemisphere. This differential would follow naturally from the well-established differences in left- and right-hemispheric processing of verbal versus spatial stimuli, since emotional material tends to be vague, diffuse, and patterned like spatial material, rather than specific and sequential like verbal material.

Evidence for differential hemispheric storing of cognitive and emotional stimuli comes from a study of the comparative clinical effects of abnormal hyperirritability in the right or left temporal lobe. Bear (1979) compared the psychological responsivities of right and left temporal lobe epileptics in contrast to those of a group of controls and of nonepileptic neurological patients. The various groups showed entirely different profiles. Both groups of epileptics showed more extreme reactivities than did normal or neurological controls, satisfactorily differentiating between categories. More dramatic, however, were the differences between right and left temporal lobe epileptics; most of the right temporal lobe patients showed severe emotional aberrations while most of the left temporal lobe patients demonstrated severe ideational aberrations. Since in all instances of temporal lobe epilepsy one can postulate increased electrophysiological overactivity (activation or arousal) on the impaired side, Bear's data appear to support the position that the right hemisphere tends preferentially to store emotional material while the left hemisphere tends preferentially to store ideational material.

The reactive constellations that Bear describes as either emotional or ideational are of interest in the light they throw on possible relationship of differential hemispheric activity to different kinds of psychological responsivity. Bear writes:

> An unanticipated feature of the current results was the clarity of the behavioral

distinction between right and left temporal patients. In terms of profile, right temporal epileptics were seen as more overtly or externally emotive: aggressive, depressed, emotionally labile. Patients with left temporal foci developed an introspective, idea-tional pattern of behavioral traits: religiosity, philosophical interests, personality des-tiny, hypergraphia. These findings are qualitatively consistent with the previously reported association of right temporal foci with disorders of mood and left foci with thought disturbance. (p. 88)

Similar results, although not so dramatic, were found in patients studied with unilateral intracarotid injection of sodium amytal, a procedure that causes sedation in one hemisphere while the other remains alert (Perria et al., 1961). Under these condi-tions, sedation of the left hemisphere has been reported to result in catastrophic feel-ings of guilt and depression, whereas sedation of the right hemisphere produced more euphoric states. However, these reactivities were very transitory and less marked than those described by Bear, possibly because they were so short-lived or possibly because there was no state of increased arousal in the alert hemisphere. Finally, Gainotti (1979) has described similar differences in emotional expression in a group of patients who had major segments of one cerebral hemisphere or the other removed because of tumor. In a study on the overall emotional effects of severe damage to one or the other hemisphere, Gainotti (1979) found:

Anxiety reactions, bursts of fears, imprecations, sharp refusals, or depressed abandon-ment of the task were significantly associated with left hemispheric lesions. Whereas indifference reactions, a tendency to joke, anosognosia (unilateral neglect syndrome)* and minimisation of the disability were significantly more frequent in right brain damaged patients.

There is evidence that differentiation of affective and cognitive function between the two hemispheres may be even more specialized and localized, particularly in the language modality. Just as cognitive aspects of language are localized in specific areas of the left hemisphere (Broca's and Wernicke's), so are the affective aspects of lan-guage localized in the corresponding anatomical segments of the right brain. Kandel (1981) has written:

In addition to the propositional aspects of language, represented in Wernicke's area and Broca's area in the *left* hemisphere, there is an affective component to language, consisting of the musical intonation of speech (called *prosody*), emotional gesturing, prosodic comprehension, and comprehension of emotional gesturing. Elliott Ross at the University of Texas and Kenneth Heilman at the University of Florida have recently found that these affective aspects of language are represented in the right hemisphere and that their anatomical organization mirrors that for propositional lan-guage in the left hemisphere. Damage to the right temporal area homologous to Wernicke's in the left hemisphere leads to disturbances in the *comprehension* of the emotional aspect of language, whereas damage to the right frontal area homologous to Broca's area leads to difficulty in *expressing* the emotional aspect of language. Thus, specific affective disorders of language can be localized to particular regions of the brain and these disorders—called *aprosodia*—can be classified as sensory, motor, and conduction, in the same way that the aphasias are classified. (p. 10)

There is also some recent work that suggests that the two hemispheres may differ

*Further support for the thesis that the bodily self-image is more actively represented in the right hemisphere.

in the kinds of emotional material that they process and hence in the kinds of emotional engrams that they contain. Davidson et al. (1974) studied the effects of positively and negatively charged emotional stimuli on electrical activity in the two hemispheres. They found that emotional stimuli with negative charges tend to arouse greater activity in the right hemisphere, whereas those with positive effect tend to differentially stimulate the left hemisphere. These results have been replicated in adults by other investigators in similar studies. Recently, Davidson and co-workers have demonstrated these same effects in infants indicating that the hemispheric differentiation of positive (happy) versus negative (unhappy) stimuli is innate.

One further speculation may be based on general neurophysiological principles. Gazzaniga and LeDoux have hypothesized that in infants, because of the poor development of the corpus callosum, engrams in the two hemispheres might be formed almost independently from one another as opposed to those which developed subsequent to the full maturation of the corpus callosum. Gazzaniga and LeDoux (1978) write:

> In spite of the preponderance of left hemisphere dominance in adults, it appears that linguistic mechanisms emerge bilaterally during early development and only later consolidate in the left hemisphere. During this early period, it is as if the child has split brain. The interhemispheric connections do not fully myelinate, especially those fibers innervating the language areas, until late in development. Until then, each side could be storing engrams, more or less independently, because of certain ignorance each hemisphere has of what is going on in the other. (p. 82)

Since full maturation does not develop for at least six months and may not occur until after one or two years, it would appear that early engrams, devoid of verbal connotation and probably heavily fraught with raw emotional overtones, may be preferentially processed and consolidated in the right hemisphere rather than in the left. If these considerations are correct, then engrams in the right hemisphere might be more primitive, more emotional, less verbal, and of more negative affect than those in the left.

That such conclusions are more than sheer theoretical speculations is supported by the following experimental study reported by Marx in *Science* (1983):

> Victor Denenberg described experiments performed in his laboratory on the effects of environmental stimulation during early life on behavioral and brain asymmetries in rats. The experiments were aimed at testing the hypothesis that early experiences are stored in the right hemisphere.
>
> The Denenberg group compared the performances of adult rats that were not handled during the first 21 days after birth with animals that were. Early handling altered the behavior of the animals in a number of tests. For example, control males did not show an overall preference for turning one way or the other, but handled males had a marked preference for turning left. Handling also reduced the tendency of male rats to kill mice. Experiments in which either hemisphere was destroyed before testing the animals led to the conclusion that the brain changes that produced the altered behaviors in handled rats occurred in the right hemisphere, as predicted. (p. 490)

The studies by Bear (1979) and Denenberg (1981) suggest that the two hemispheres not only process cognitive and emotional materials differentially, but also differ in the kinds of cognitive and emotional material for which they act as repositories. This, in itself, is of enormous consequence in evaluating the significance of hemispheric differential functions on psychological reactivities. Perhaps even more important is the fact that the right hemisphere has a highly unusual kind of consciousness, if indeed it can be called consciousness at all. This is of particular significance in any inquiry of the locus where the postulated dynamic unconscious may be found, and will be the topic for discussion in the next chapter.

15

The Disparate Levels of Consciousness in the Two Hemispheres

With the development of commissurotomy as an acceptable treatment for intractable temporal lobe epilepsy, a significant group of subjects with two essentially separate, functioning cerebral hemispheres became available for study. The differences of hemispheric function in the cognitive and emotional modalities were described in the last chapter. But of all the functional differences that became apparent in commissurotomized patients, certainly the most dramatic was that of the apparent lack of conscious awareness of the right hemisphere to stimuli presented in the contralateral field. However one concludes that there may or may not be a right-hemispheric consciousness, it is certainly true that the kind of consciousness and awareness in the two hemispheres appear to be different. Eccles (1963) summarized the thinking up to that time as follows:

> In conclusion, we can say that the right hemisphere is a very highly developed brain except that it cannot express itself in language, so it is not able to disclose any experience of consciousness that we can recognize. Sperry postulates that there is another consciousness in the right hemisphere, but that its existence is obscured by its lack of expressive language. On the other hand, the left hemisphere has a normal linguistic performance so it can be recognized as being associated with the prior existence of the ego or the self with all the memories of the past before the commissural section. On this view there has been split off from the talking self a nontalking self which can't communicate by language, so it is there but mute, or aphasic. (p. 213)

LeDoux et al. (1979) reported a study in a split-brain patient, a 15-year-old boy, P. S., who demonstrated on right-hemispheric testing similarly rational responses to those on left-hemispheric testing; however, the responses tended to be different. Consciousness in both hemispheres appeared to be separate and distinct and only responses to left-hemispheric testing could be verbalized. The conclusions of LeDoux and coworkers (1979) read:

> These observations suggested to us that the right hemisphere in P. S. possesses qualities that are deserving of conscious status. His right hemisphere has a sense of

223

self, for it knows the name it collectively shares with the left. It has feelings, for it can
describe its mood. It has a sense of whom it likes, and what it likes, for it can name its
favorite hobby. The right hemisphere in P. S. also has a sense of the future, for it
knows what day tomorrow is. Furthermore, it has goals and aspirations for the future,
for it can name its occupational choice. (pp. 545–546)

These conclusions of Sperry (1969) and of LeDoux et al. (1979), based on
numerous experiments and observations in commissurotomized patients, make it unlikely that the locus of the dynamic unconscious, as has been suggested by some
investigators, is confined solely to the right hemisphere. It seems rather that there is a
sort of consciousness in the right hemisphere that in the split-brain patient is less
available to articulation. Particularly interesting is the relative lack of effect of commissurotomy on the self-awareness system. Despite the separation of the right brain
from the aware left brain, there is no evidence in these patients of a unilateral neglect
syndrome. If only the left brain had consciousness and if there were no input from the
right inferoparietal lobe (where clinical considerations suggest that self-awareness is
probably mainly centered), then one would certainly expect some evidence of a unilateral neglect syndrome. The absence of such a syndrome in split-brain patients tends
to support the interpretations (1) that there is awareness in the right brain, although it
may be of a different quality than that in the left, and (2) that the self-awareness system
is represented in both hemispheres, but probably more heavily on the right.

Given the formulations in this book on the structures and mechanisms involved in
the phenomenology of consciousness and the self-awareness system, how does one
account for the fact that in the commissurotomized patient there is a different kind of
awareness in the right hemisphere than the more normal everyday awareness of the left.
Several hypotheses have been presented. One point of view holds that "awareness" in
the two hemispheres may be the same, but that the left is able to make itself known more
readily through speech; in these terms, the right hemisphere in these patients is merely
mute. This may be true at least in part; one has similar difficulties communicating with a
totally aphasic patient. However, in the latter case, when communicatory contact is
made, the level of awareness seems greater than that exhibited by the right hemisphere of
the commissurotomized patient.

A second view attributes the inability of the right hemisphere to carry the normal
quality of consciousness to the special structural organization of the right hemisphere
that permits it to manage spatial material more effectively than verbal. The state of
alert awareness, as defined in Chapter 10, is one of rapidly shifting inputs introduced at
the rate of 20–25/sec with each frame lasting about 0.04 sec. Consciousness exists as a
kinematic experience with 20–25 frames/sec, but with each element in the frame
lasting 0.20 sec to give the entire sequence continuity. It appears that the mechanisms
for maintaining sequentiality are anatomically built into the structure of the left hemisphere; this may possibly be connected in some way with the presence of the verbal
centers. This interpretation is supported by the overall superiority of the left hemisphere in handling sequential tasks of which kinematic consciousness is certainly the
most prototypical.

The right hemisphere is notable in that it has less of the anatomical organization to
provide for sequential functioning and more of the structure associated with abstractional operations. Apparently its organization is such as to lead to single-shot holistic

judgments of data rather than to more gradual time-locked evaluations. In any event, lacking the mechanisms for sequentiality, apparently it similarly lacks the mechanisms for the usual garden variety type of consciousness.

Differences in Activation of the Two Hemispheres

A third viewpoint on the origin of the hemispheric discrepancy in levels of consciousness holds that the right hemisphere may have a different kind of electrical activation than the left, as a consequence of which it may have a different type of awareness. In a group of 14 subjects tested with bilateral power spectra under the conditions of verbal or nonverbal stimulation, Goldstein (1979) reported an interesting difference in the predominance of electrical activity in the two hemispheres. He found the characteristic shift to greater activity of the left hemisphere (higher R/L EEG amplitude ratios) with verbal activities and a characteristic shift to increased right-hemispheric activation with nonverbal activities (Fig. 15-1). However, where for the 14 subjects the R/L EEG amplitude ratio for verbal activity was greater than 1, it was just 1 for nonverbal activity, a significantly different finding. The interpretation of

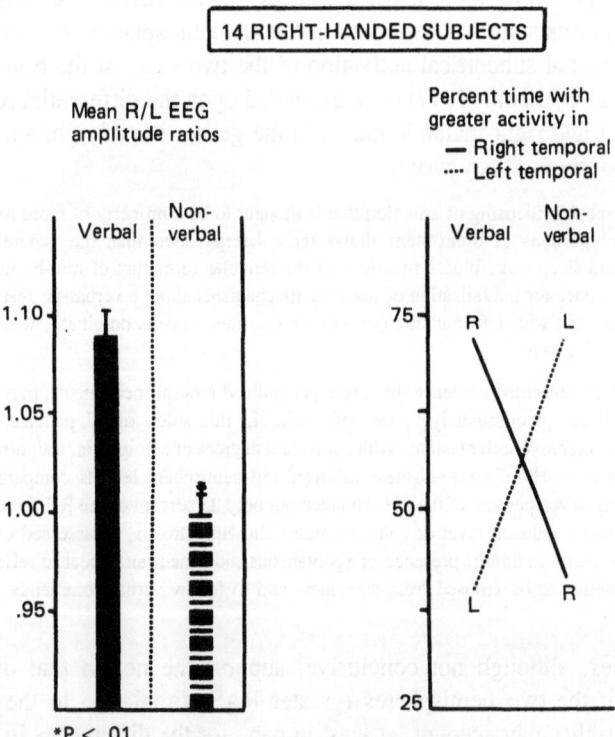

Figure 15-1 Hemispheric electrophysiological balance in verbal and nonverbal activity. (From Goldstein, 1979. Reprinted with permission.)

these data suggests that during verbal activity in these patients, the left brain was more highly activated than the right, but that during nonverbal activity both hemispheres were equally activated. Extrapolating back to an intermediate neutral noncommittal state, i.e., neither verbal nor spatial, one would postulate a somewhat greater activity of the left hemisphere than of the right.

Since power spectra during alert behavior are determined mainly by the ratio of α- and β-wave activity, one could explain this finding on the basis of either greater β activity in the left brain, greater α activity of the right, or most likely both. Cobb (1963) has provided evidence to support this thesis. He writes:

> By the rough estimate of which the eye is capable—there are factors of distribution, time and voltage to take into account—the mean alpha activity in the two hemispheres is different in perhaps 30% of normal individuals and markedly so in 5 or 10%, the difference being mainly in amplitude but sometimes in forward spread. In a high proportion of cases which show asymmetry the greater amplitude is on the right side. (p. 238)

Cobb hypothesizes that the increased α activity in the right hemisphere may actually be due to increased "α blockade" in the left hemisphere, secondary to inadvertent attentive behavior. He bases this conclusion on the established dominance of the left brain rather than on any direct experimental evidence. If his conclusion is valid, it would speak for more direct connections between the activating mechanisms of the brain stem and the left hemisphere as opposed to those of the right. Otto and Kobryn (1969) report even more marked evidence of increased α activity in the right hemispheres of normals and of β activity in the left hemispheres, consistent with the concept of differential subcortical activation of the two sides of the brain.

Whitaker and Ojemann (1977) have expanded upon the differential role of activation from the left and right thalamic nuclei in the generation of right and left cortical levels of consciousness. They write:

> . . . the specific focusing of attention that is thought to be a property of more rostral (thalamic) portions of brain stem shows more lateralization than the generalized arousal and sleep-wakefulness functions of the reticular formation of mid-brain and pons. Evidence for lateralization of thalamic mechanisms along a verbal-visuospatial dichotomy, but with left thalamic (verbal) alerting mechanisms dominant, was presented by Ojemann.
>
> Albert *et al.* presented evidence that more generalized arousal mechanisms may also be lateralized, predominately to the left brain. In this study of 47 patients with unilateral cerebrovascular lesions, with equivalent degrees of hemiplegia, a significant reduction in levels of consciousness followed left-hemisphere lesions compared to right. Fifty-seven percent of the LH-damaged but only 25 percent of the RH-damaged patients had a reduced level of consciousness following strokes, as assessed by response to painful stimuli, presence of spontaneous movement and specific reflexes, and the ability to be aroused from sleepiness and to follow verbal commands. (pp. 455–456)

Such studies, although not conclusive, support the notion that differences in arousal levels of the two hemispheres (greater RAS stimulation to the left, greater thalamic to the right) may account, at least in part, for the differences in the levels of consciousness between the two hemispheres. Lehman (1971) has presented evidence that alpha activity in the cortex is concentrated predominantly in three foci—a small component in the anterior-central portion of the right hemisphere; a larger component in the occipital area of the left hemisphere; and the largest component in the occipital area of the right hemisphere. Lehman (1971) hypothesizes that there are at least two subcortical generating sources for these disparate foci of activity—one for each hemisphere—and possibly three, i.e., two for the right hemisphere. These formulations are consistent with the thesis of Albert et al. quoted in the Whitaker and Ojemann (1977) excerpt in which they postulate that the level of consciousness in the two hemispheres may be differentially determined by differences in the kinds of electrical stimulation emanating from the two thalamic centers. It is also consistent with the presence of significantly greater α activity in the right hemisphere than in the left.

This subject has been reviewed in some depth by Butler (1975). He writes:

> During relaxed wakefulness it is the alpha rhythm which is usually the most prominent feature of the EEG. This waveform is believed to be generated by synchronous activity on the part of large pools of neurons in the cortex, but the mechanism responsible for their synchrony has long been the subject of debate. The observation by Morison and Dempsey (1962) that phasic stimulation of a small region of thalamus could promote widespread cortical synchrony led to the idea of a single central pacemaker for spontaneous rhythms. The concept survived and was perhaps strengthened by Moruzzi and Magoun's description of the brain stem activating system (1949). However, observations that the alpha rhythm could vary in its distribution over different regions of the head led to the proposal that there could be numerous pacemakers each operating on its own area of cortex. Andersen and Andersson (1968) suggested that such pacemakers might rely on local thalamo-cortical circuits, and that there can be at least as many as there are thalamic nuclei. (p. 73)

Butler's (1975) description of the dissociation between the α rhythms of the two hemispheres in split-brain patients (Fig. 14-3) provides supportive evidence that the subcortical driving elements for alpha (probably in the thalamic nuclei) (Andersen and Andersson, 1968) are presumably separate and distinct and may under special circumstances, operate independently. On the other hand, Butler (personal communication, 1985) did not find evidence of increased right-hemispheric α rhythm in split-brain patients, a condition in which one would certainly expect it. Nevertheless, Butler writes (personal communication, 1985):

> In both normal and split-brain subjects it is very much easier to find tasks which cause suppression of the alpha rhythm over the left hemisphere than any which cause suppression of the right. This is true whether one estimates the asymmetry in absolute terms or in relation to the individual's own EEG "at rest." Moreover the alpha asymmetry is not as great during "right hemisphere tasks" as it is during verbal and mathematical ones. Various hypotheses have been put forward to explain this—from distributed processing in the right hemisphere, to a cultural tendency to involve the left hemisphere even when purely spatial strategies of thought would be more appropriate. However, a model which held that the right hemisphere existed at "a lower level of consciousness" would predict just this effect.

Differences in Hemispheric Electrical Activities in Sleep and in Arousal

It is generally difficult to demonstrate differences in α activity during the normal alert state since any kind of mental activity produces α blockade with a consequent diminution bilaterally. The optimal condition for studying α waves is the so-called twilight state, the stage 1 or stage 2 phase of sleep when α productivity is at a maximum. Although the data are somewhat equivocal, a study by Goldstein (1979) on hemispheric electrical activities during sleep is suggestive (Fig. 15-2). Wakefulness and REM sleep, both associated with high levels of arousal, showed increased right-hemispheric activity, whereas stage 2 sleep showed increased left-hemispheric activity (as did stages 3 and 4). Since stages 2–4 are known as low arousal states, it is probable that the apparent shift to left-hemispheric predominance represents a relative increase in right-hemispheric slow-wave activity rather than an increase in left-hemispheric β activity.

These reactivities reflect the inverse relationship between α and β rhythms. In the normal state of alert arousal, the left hemisphere has a high level of β waves and a low level of α waves. Under the same condition, the right hemisphere has a somewhat lower level of β waves and a moderate level of α waves. The overall effect of these activities as measured by power spectrum techniques would be greater activity in the left hemisphere than in the right, i.e., left-hemispheric dominance (Fig. 15-1).

There are relative changes in these relationships and in power spectral balance during periods of high emotional arousal. Under those conditions, both the left hemisphere and right hemisphere would show high levels of β activity and almost no α activity (α blockade). Consequently, in emotional arousal, particularly that associated with negative valence where more energy is directed to the right hemisphere (Davidson et al., 1974), the two hemispheres would either show essentially equal power spectral levels of activity or the right might actually show slightly greater activity. However, even in the first instance of equality, the experimental data would show a shift to the right because of the change from left-hemispheric dominance in the normal alert condition.

There are still other imbalances during states of low arousal (stage 2 sleep, hypnosis, altered states of consciousness). The left hemisphere would be characterized by low levels of β and moderate levels of α activity. The right hemisphere would show low levels of β wave activity and high levels of high-amplitude α activity. The overall power spectral effects would show a relative shift to the left hemisphere even though the actual activity of the left hemisphere was markedly decreased. These interpretations are consistent with the experimental findings of Goldstein (Figs. 14-6 and 15-2).

Right-Hemispheric Consciousness as an Altered State of Consciousness

It appears then that under normal or low arousal conditions, the left hemisphere may tend to be driven more by RAS β activity and the right hemisphere probably more by thalamic α activity. The thesis is suggested here that at low levels of arousal, the right hemisphere has greater activation through thalamic α control and thus experiences a different type of awareness than that of the left hemisphere under RAS β stimulation. On the other hand, with very high arousal levels, the right hemisphere

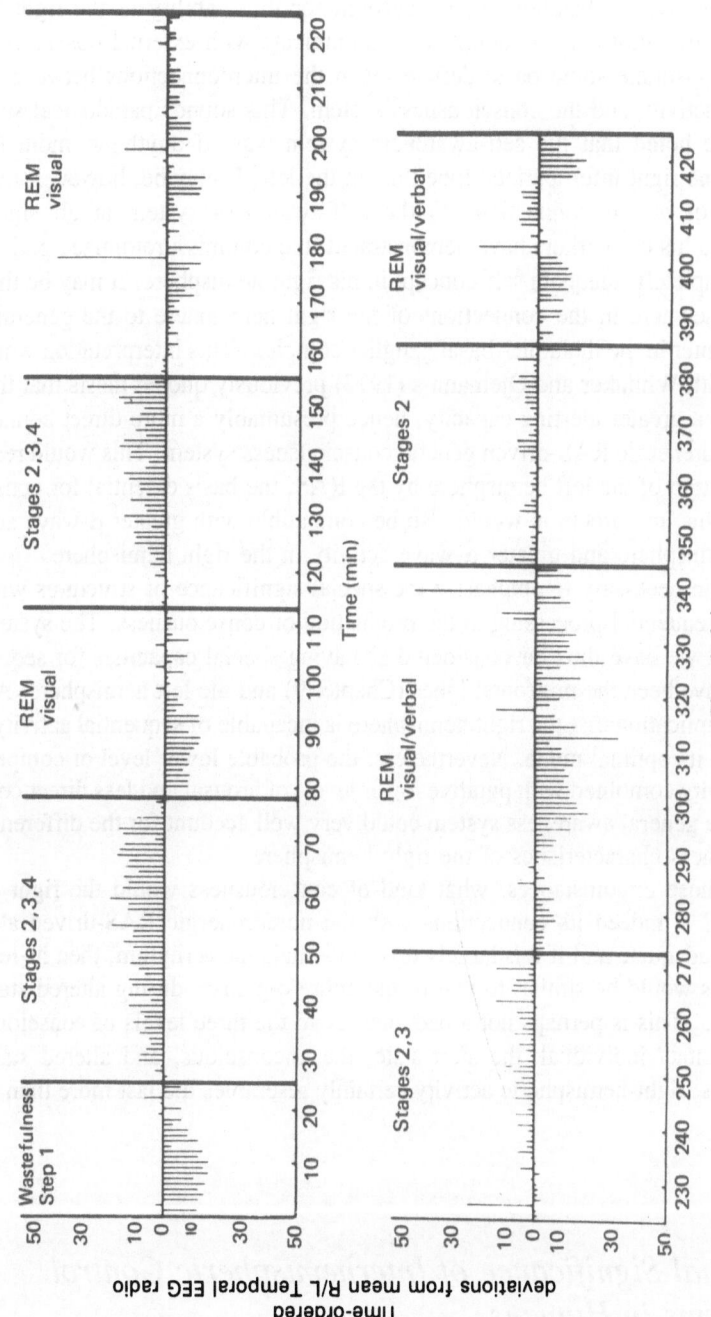

Figure 15-2 Shifts in hemispheric balance of activation during sleep. (From Goldstein, 1979. Reprinted with permission.)

appears to be more directly activated by the RAS β-wave system and assumes an equal or even greater level of excitability than the left hemisphere. However, even here, because of the inherent structural differences between the two hemispheres, the right hemisphere would still lack the normal awareness of the left hemisphere.

These putative explanations might account for the inability of the right hemisphere of commissurotomized patients to communicate with external observers. One must almost postulate some basic deficiency in the interconnections between right-hemispheric activity and the consciousness system. This sounds paradoxical since in Chapter 7 we noted that the self-awareness system was, if anything, more firmly grounded in the right inferoparietal lobe than in the left. It may be, however, that the problem is not in the connections to the self-awareness system at all since, as Gazzaniga and his co-workers have demonstrated, the commissurotomized patient, P. S., had a completely adequate self-concept in his right hemisphere. It may be that the deficit is somewhere in the connections of the right hemisphere to the general consciousness center in the thalamic–basal gangliar complex. This interpretation would be in keeping with Whitaker and Ojemann's (1977) previously quoted thesis that the left thalamus had a greater alerting capacity, hence presumably a more direct connection with the noradrenergic RAS-driven general consciousness system. This would result in greater activation of the left hemisphere by the RAS, the basis essential for conscious awareness. This interpretation would also be compatible with greater β-wave activity in the left hemisphere and greater α-wave activity in the right hemisphere.

It is again necessary to emphasize the special significance of structures with the capacity for sequential processing in the production of consciousness. The systems of the brain that we have thus far considered as having special capacities for sequential processing have been the prefrontal lobes (Chapter 9) and the left hemisphere. Again, there is no implication that the right hemisphere is incapable of sequential activity; that is merely not its optimal mode. Nevertheless, the probable lower level of competence for such activity combined with putative lower levels of arousal and less direct connections with the general awareness system could very well account for the different kind of consciousness characteristics of the right hemisphere.

Under those circumstances, what kind of consciousness would the right hemisphere show? If indeed its connections with the noradrenergic RAS-driven alerting system are inadequate and if it is largely driven by thalamic α rhythm, then its level of consciousness would be similar to that of the entire organism during altered states of consciousness. This is perhaps not a bad analogy to the three levels of consciousness seen in the intact individual: the alert state, the unconscious, and altered states of consciousness; right-hemispheric activity certainly resembles the last more than either of the others.

The Special Significance of Interhemispheric Control Mechanisms in Humans

In view of the tremendous level of transcallosal activity, a serious question has been raised as to whether in the neurologically intact individual the two hemispheres ever operate at different functional levels. If one accepts the thesis that differential activation in the two hemispheres is associated with different levels of function, then the answer seems highly affirmative. A study by Gevins et al. (1983) provides the best available evidence in normal humans for differential activation of the two hemispheres in different types of cognitive processing. In their experiment, numeric calculation (left hemispheric) and visuospatial estimation (right hemispheric) activities were combined in a move–no move target manipulation paradigm, and event-related brain potentials elicited. Through complicated mathematical analyses, the relative dominance of latency and amplitude changes of N_1-P_2 and P_{300} waves were calculated for electrodes placed on different sites over both hemispheres. A high correlation was found between numeric calculations and left-hemispheric electrical activity and between visuospatial estimation and right-hemispheric electrical activity. Most remarkable were the rapid changes in hemispheric dominance with corresponding changes in behavior. As the authors write, the study, "yielded a sequence of clear-cut between-task different patterns involving split-second changes in the localization and lateralization of mass neural activity. Appropriate studies of neurocognitive functions should take into account this rapidly shifting network of localized and lateralized processes" (p. 99).

One must assume that this model of rapidly shifting dominance of hemispheric function holds for general psychological functioning as well as for experimental–cognitive motor tasks. Within this paradigm, emotionally charged engrams of a given type are consolidated in both hemispheres, but more so in one hemisphere or the other. In addition, under different experiential circumstances, engrams from the two hemispheres representing the same episode may be differentially processed and retrieved. In this way, even in the functionally intact individual, engrams of the same event lodged in opposite hemispheres may exercise different effects which are finally integrated in left-hemispheric consciousness. However, in sleep and in altered states of consciousness where left hemispheric dominance has been removed, right hemispheric productions may rise to reduced consciousness. Such postulated mechanisms will be discussed in Chapters 17 and 22.

Finally, mental set has been demonstrated to affect differential processing in the interhemispheric system just as it does in the hierarchical. A study by Phelps and Mazziotta (1985) on hemispheric activity during the task of remembering music revealed that nonmusicians tended to show increased activity of the right hemisphere, whereas musicians tended to show increased activity of the left. (These effects were demonstrated through radioactive metabolic scanning of the brain rather than by electrophysiological monitoring, but the results are equivalent.) On further investigation, the authors found that nonmusicians remembered melodies by humming them and retaining the music in their heads (a spatial operation), whereas musicians remembered tunes by analyzing the notes and visualizing them as musical notations (an analytic function). Apparently the mental set of the observer determined whether the right or left hemisphere would be more utilized in the processing of the same stimuli.

Presumably, the mechanisms producing the Phelps and Mazziotta hemispheric effects are similar to those involved in hierarchical mental set phenomena. In this paradigm, influences from the prefrontal cortex would send differential inhibitory or stimulatory impulses to the thalamic nuclei, as in the Skinner–Yingling paradigm (Fig. 8-1), but here they would be inhibitory to one side and stimulatory to the other. The differential pattern of arousal and inhibition established by impulses from the frontal lobe to the brain stem would be associated with a corresponding dominance of process-ing in one hemisphere or the other with corresponding behavioral effects. Thus differ-ential hemispheric processing of incoming perceptual stimuli may be determined either by the nature of the stimulus itself or in a feedforward paradigm by an established mental set. Most probably, elements of both mechanisms are involved in all cognitive processing in the characteristic feedforward–feedback style of brain function.

This formulation appears to give greater credibility to the concept of a somewhat independent function of the two hemispheres even in the normal alert and intact human—a concept we have generally inveighed against in this volume. But having acknowledged the appropriate caveats against overemphasizing the role of hemi-sphericity in mental activity, we must now ask ourselves whether it may not be just this anatomical and functional specialization that accounts for the variety of psychological mechanisms and other unique qualities of human behavior. It is true that earlier in this chapter we presented evidence of hemisphericity in lower mammals and even in birds, but it is even more true that advanced hemisphericity is largely confined to man. Not even primates show much evidence of it. Hamilton (1977), an investigator in this field, writes:

> It is disappointing to find no evidence for hemispheric specialization in monkeys and therefore to be forced indirectly to support the opinion that cerebral asymmetries appeared during the later evolution of our human ancestors. (p. 58)

But this is really not so surprising if one considers that cerebral lateralization is to a large degree the consequence of the development of the human speech center in the left hemisphere. As Gazzaniga and LeDoux (1978) write:

> Specialization theory assumes that the phylogenetic emergence of the human brain was associated with, and even dependent upon, the radical reorganization of cerebral function, whereby lateral symmetry, which largely typifies the phyla, gave way to bilateral specialization. In short, specialization theory assumes that this type of neural organization underlying the unique mental functions of the left hemisphere is inap-propriate for and even incompatible with the neural organization that sustains the cognitive style of the right hemisphere, and as a consequence, adaptive evolutionary forces provided that these distinct modes be distributed in separate hemispheres. (p. 47)

Thus the development of language in man has given rise to two distinctly unique characteristics of human behavior: hemisphericity (a neurophysiological consequence of language development) and symbolism (the basic character of language). Through-out this volume we have consistently stressed the fact that the hierarchical control system provides the basic functional control for central nervous system activity and that hemispheric specialization merely finely tunes that control. This is undoubtedly biologically correct. But perhaps more important from our perspective are the specific influences of hemisphericity that provide the unique characteristics of human mental activity. Thus in our final deliberations we must consider hemispheric lateralization as a major influence in the total complex pattern of human behavior.

These somewhat philosophic considerations are pertinent only if there is evidence that in the neurologically intact individual, i.e., the normal noncommissurotomized adult, the hemispheres do act differentially to contribute differential influences on behavior. The powerful anatomical connections between the two hemispheres provided by the corpus callosum strongly suggest that in general, both bodies act more or less as one. But the importance of differential priming from subcortical centers described in various studies in this chapter suggest that within the context of integrated action, one hemisphere or the other may exert maximum influence at different times. As illustrated in the study of Gevins et al. (1983), this shift in dominance may occur literally many times a second. These neurophysiological shifts in energy are highly correlated with functional shifts in cognitive behavior (spatial versus arithmetical analysis) but there is no reason to believe that they are not equally associated with changes in emotional state and in the level of consciousness. Consequently, the shifts in hemispheric neurophysiological dominance appear to be associated with shifts in behavioral activities, suggesting that behaviors associated with one hemisphere or the other do predominate at different times.

These conclusions assume particular significance in the area next to be considered, i.e., the effects of emotional factors on conscious and unconscious mental activities in the two hemispheres. However, differences in behavioral responsivities that are attributed to differential involvement of one or the other hemisphere should be seen as resulting from the integrated activities of interacting hemispheres functioning under the overall influence of the hierarchical control system and not from independent activities of the two hemispheres.

Psychological Defense Mechanisms as Interactions between Hierarchical and Hemispheric Functions

In Chapter 13, we described the biological defense against the danger of the organism being overwhelmed by an excessive emotional reaction to threat as a brain stem mechanism that reduced the arousal level of emotionally threatening stimuli by inhibiting the cognitive component. That response was illustrated in animals by the Olds et al. paradigm in which negatively charged stimuli provoked no greater cognitive response than did neutral stimuli in thalamic nuclei (Fig. 13-2). A related effect in humans was demonstrated in the Begleiter et al. study (Fig. 13-3) where negatively charged stimuli, despite being associated with a higher level of arousal than positively charged stimuli, consistently produced evoked cortical responses of lower amplitude. The putative explanation for this latter finding was given as a presumed inhibition of negatively charged stimuli during upstream processing in the brain stem, with subsequent enhancement during processing to consciousness. The case for the differences between unconscious and conscious processing of negatively charged stimuli—inhibition for unconscious stimuli and excitation for conscious stimuli—was supported by the studies of Kostandov and Arzumov (1980) and by Shevrin et al. (1967, 1974, 1980).

Although these effects are unquestionably important in biological survival (witness, for example, the fatal freezing of small mammals when overwhelmed with fear), they do not appear to express the full flavor of psychological defense mechanisms exhibited in humans. For one thing, these subcortical mechanisms do not seem powerful enough to explain the total denial of threatening events that often occurs in humans. For another, psychological defense mechanisms in humans take a variety of forms, some of which are inhibitory, others merely distort cognitive awareness of threatening stimuli. Therefore, it seems that some more complex mechanisms must be involved in human defensive activities than in those of lower animals. The special activity of the interhemispheric system in humans makes it a reasonable candidate for this role; experimental evidence further supports this interpretation.

The thesis to be developed in this chapter holds that in humans, as in all mammals, the primitive brain stem defense mechanism against excessive levels of arousal operates as a first level of defense. However, in humans further modulation of arousal levels is accomplished by differential channeling to the two hemispheres where differential processing in each hemisphere is associated with a diminution in the level of anxiety. Processing in the right hemisphere is characterized as desensitizing (i.e., associated with a reduction in cognitive strength), whereas, processing in the left hemisphere is characterized as sensitizing (i.e., associated with an increase in cognitive valence, but with a decrease in arousal level). The mechanisms through which these effects are accomplished are considered to be a function of the anatomical and physiological nature of the two hemispheres.

Hierarchical and Hemispheric Defense Mechanisms

The previously described McGinnies (1949) and Forster and Govier (1978) experiments represent the prototypes of hierarchical defense mechanisms. In these studies, unconscious stimuli (i.e., subliminal or unattended) with negative emotional charge were responded to with increased GSR, indicating recognition of the emotional component at some unconscious level (unconscious arousal paradigm). The effect was associated with some level of cognitive inhibition. In unconscious arousal, the emotional components of stimuli are recognized before the cognitive component. As in the McCleary and Lazarus (1949) and the Kunst-Wilson and Zajonc (1980) studies, unconscious recognition of the emotional component apparently occurs at a subcortical level, presumably during upstream processing in the thalamic–basal gangliar complex. Cognitive inhibition in this paradigm may occur through the feedback control mechanism involving the thalamic nuclei and prefrontal lobe, or through the amygdaloid–hippocampal complex. Here the increase in arousal provides the signal that an emotionally charged (positive or negative) stimulus is en route, but that it is not sufficiently cognitively defined to permit recognition.

On the other hand, if the negative motivational–emotional charge on a stimulus is at such a level that its suppression might constitute a physical or psychological danger to the organism, then the entire event is raised from the unconscious level to the conscious with a corresponding increase in emotional arousal levels above that associated with neutral stimuli. In that case, the situation has changed from the unconscious paradigm of "perceptual defense" to the conscious paradigm of "perceptual vigilance" (see Fig. 13-1). However, the earlier inhibitory effects of the negative emotional charge during upstream processing persist, and the final conscious cognitive reaction still remains lower than it would be for a comparable positively charged stimulus (Fig. 13-2). In that way the immobilizing effects of excessive negative emotional arousal are also minimized.

But situations may arise that are so psychologically threatening as to make the defenses available through the hierarchical control system insufficient. For example, it would seem that many Jews in Nazi Germany refused to acknowledge their own imminent danger even though every sign pointed to it. Some individuals totally ignored the evidence all around them as though it did not exist while others attempted to rationalize it away. One can only surmise that the unconsciously perceived danger to self and family had become so immense as to have made impossible any attempt to deal with it rationally. The only biological analogy to such total incapacity would seem to be the infrequent "freezing" reaction that occurs among the smaller prey of predatory animals.

Mechanisms capable of dealing with psychological threats of this quality are apparently not available through the hierarchical system. The type of inhibition of cognitive significance provided by the Olds' mechanism (Fig. 13-3) does not seem sufficient either to deal with the complexities of human thought nor to suppress sufficiently the extreme anxiety associated with highly threatening events. For this, the interhemispheric system with its different repertoire of defense mechanisms appears to be necessary.

Desensitizing and Sensitizing Defense Mechanisms

Not all defense reactivities are necessarily excitatory or inhibitory; there could be other more subtle types of psychological defense mechanisms. Theoretically, these might prevent arousal levels from exceeding the optimal midlevels of the inverted U-curve of performance by some form of cognitive distortion other than repression, perhaps by cushioning in a different way the impact of highly threatening stimuli. A number of experimental psychologists, using laboratory tests of perceptual defense and memory retrieval, conclude that some such mechanisms do exist, but in a more complex form than simple repression. Eriksen (1963) writes:

> . . . the critical concept of repression is more sophisticated than to assume that all people or even a majority of people automatically repress any sexual or aggressive ideation, or that all anxiety-arousing thoughts or feelings are repressed. Instead, repression is a defense mechanism used sometimes by some people to handle anxiety-arousing thoughts or feelings whose anxiety-provoking nature is a function of the individual's own unique past experiences. Thus one would not expect a great deal of communality among people in terms of the kind of stimuli that should lead to repression. Furthermore, theories of personality dynamics also recognize that there are other types of defense mechanisms. Repression is not the only way individuals defend against ego-threatening stimulation. (p. 42)

Eriksen describes the alternative defense mechanisms, intellectualization, reaction-formation, and projection, as characteristic of the sensitizing defenses that permit anxiety reduction through an intellectual manipulation of the experience, which in Freudian terms "decathects" it. Eriksen then writes:

> These differences in defensive mechanisms would be expected to have different perceptual concomitants. In the case of repression or denial one might expect a tendency for the subject to manifest avoidance or higher duration thresholds for stimuli related to the sources of conflict. On the other hand, those manifesting defenses of intellectualization, reaction-formation or projection might be expected to show a lower duration threshold for anxiety-related stimuli. (pp. 42–43)

This formulation of defenses against anxiety-producing stimuli as being either desensitizing (denial or repression) or sensitizing (intellectualization, reaction-formation, or projection) expands the range of defense mechanisms beyond that of simple inhibition or excitation and presents psychological reactivities that might explain increased awareness to threatening stimuli (perceptual vigilance) as well as decreased awareness (perceptual defense). Apparently both of these types of psychological defense mechanisms can actually diminish the level of arousal associated with threatening stimuli. A series of experiments by Lazarus and co-workers (Lazarus and Alferth, 1964; Lazarus et al., 1962, 1965) illustrates the effects of these two major defense mechanisms—denial (repression) and intellectualization—on emotional arousal, as measured by skin conductance (GSR) in response to emotionally threatening stimuli (Fig. 16-1). In these studies, different groups of subjects were exposed to movies of extremely cruel and bloody puberty rites among primitive societies and were tested for their emotional reactivity to these viewings. Those individuals who received no prior explanation of the events (controls) reacted with the highest GSR responses throughout the film with particular peaks at the moments of the greatest atrocities. A second group were told before the film showing that the pain evidenced by the victims was not nearly as extreme as their reactions indicated; these individuals (condition of denial) reacted with significantly lower GSR responses than did the controls. A third group were given a different set of pre-film-viewing instructions, namely "we have made numerous studies of puberty rites; this is how primitive people establish the new status of a young person." The subjects in this group (condition of intellectualization) responded with the lowest level of arousal, i.e., anxiety, as manifested in the measures of skin conductance. In addition, there was a significant correlation between level of education and

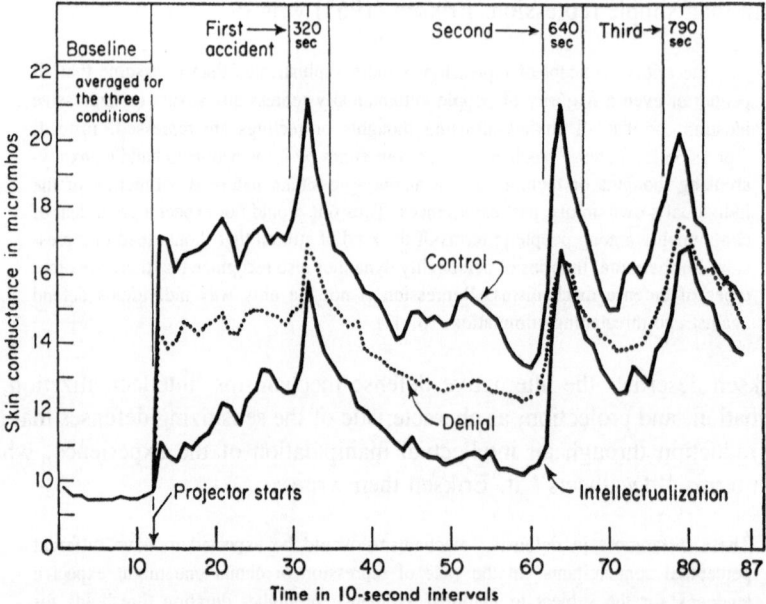

Figure 16-1 Effects of denial and intellectualization on "arousal." (From Lazarus, et al., 1965. Reproduced with permission.)

the effectiveness of intellectualization as a defense so that better-educated subjects scored significantly lower (i.e., showed less anxiety) under this condition than did less well-educated subjects.

The Lazarus et al. (Lazarus and Alferth, 1964; Lazarus et al., 1962, 1965) studies suggest the following tentative conclusions: (1) both sensitizing and desensitizing ego defense mechanisms are designed to reduce arousal (anxiety); (2) sensitizing defense mechanisms (intellectualizing) may be more effective than desensitizing (denial) in this goal; and (3) better-educated individuals will probably find sensitizing defense mechanisms more effective, whereas less well-educated individuals will probably find desensitizing defense mechanisms more effective. This last finding is of interest since it suggests a possible correlation between the mode of intellectual functioning and types of defense mechanisms utilized.

The Lazarus et al. experimental results do not seem at all explicable on the basis of the thalamic–frontal feedback control mechanism. That mechanism might explain how high arousal would interfere with efficient cognitive perception, but it would not explain why a given mental set (defense mechanism) reduces the physiological manifestations of arousal. It seems to me that this study suggests, particularly for intellectualization, that a functional disassociation occurs between the cognitive and emotional components of the stimulus which is different from that caused by plain inhibition of the cognitive element.

Hypothesis on the Neurophysiology of Sensitizing and Desensitizing Defense Mechanisms

Sensitizing and desensitizing defense mechanisms tend to be more complex than the hierarchical unconscious arousal variety, and thus presumably involve more complex neurophysiological mechanisms. Much evidence suggests that these processes may depend on a variety of interhemispheric effects that appear to play a larger role in human mental activity than in that of lower forms. The differences in cognitive and motivational styles and in the levels of consciousness in the two hemispheres could readily contribute mechanisms within the interhemispheric system capable of accomplishing these disparate defense reactivities.

In Chapter 14, evidence was presented that substantive cognitive material in the right hemisphere differs from that in the left in that it tends to be more primitive, less conscious, more emotional, and of more negative affect. Engrams in the left hemisphere would, contrariwise, be more positively charged affectively (Davidson et al., 1974), less emotional generally, and more conscious. The two hemispheres also differ significantly in their cognitive mode of processing so that the left hemisphere tends to utilize sequential associational processing and the right hemisphere preferentially utilizes parallel abstractive processing. These characteristics in themselves suggest that differential hemispheric processing may be involved in sensitizing and desensitizing defense mechanisms.

First, it is necessary to examine the role of "level of consciousness" in hemispheric processing. If we postulate that in the alert conscious state the left hemisphere is more strongly activated and consequently at a higher level of consciousness than the right, then it might follow that supraliminal negatively charged engrams would tend to be shunted toward the left hemisphere and receive increased attentive processing there. On the other hand, subliminal negatively charged stimuli, because they lack the quality of cognitive consciousness, might more likely be shunted to the right hemisphere. There they would be subject to the general unconscious condition of the right hemisphere, and as a result would tend to remain unconscious.

What experimental evidence is there to support the concept that subconscious stimuli (subliminal, unattended, etc.) are differentially channeled to the right hemisphere and conscious attended stimuli to the left? Davidson (1980) reviews the literature on this issue. He describes a number of studies dealing with deficits in motor activity resulting from brain damage to one hemisphere or the other. In most instances, damage to the left brain produced greater impairment of conscious voluntary motor activity, whereas comparable damage to the right hemisphere produced greater deficits in automatic motor functions. In the area of more cognitive function, Davidson (1980) writes:

> Data such as these have led some investigators to propose that the right hemisphere may generally be more involved with nonfocal, incidental and "less conscious" information processing (e.g., Luria and Simernitskaya, 1977). In a recent study on the effects of localized brain lesions on focal (voluntary) versus incidental (involuntary) learning and memory, Luria and Simernitskaya (1977) have found that left temporoparietal lesions resulted in relatively greater impairment in voluntary memory while comparable right hemisphere lesions were associated with greater deficits in incidental memory. In the domain of writing behavior, Luria and his colleagues have shown that left hemisphere lesions result in deficits in consciously executed writing, while right hemisphere lesions impair automatic and nonconscious writing such as signing one's name (Luria, Simernitskaya, and Tubylevich, 1970; Simernitskaya, 1974). On the basis of these related data Simernitskaya (1974) suggests that "a lesion of the cortical areas of the left hemisphere induces a disturbance in the extensive conscious fulfillment of a psychic function, but does not affect the execution of stable automatic operations . . . The structures of the nondominant hemisphere are involved in accomplishing subconscious levels of automatic integration" (p. 343). A similar argument is presented by Luria and Simernitskaya (1977). (p. 27)

Thus it appears that there are three dichotomies of preferential processing in the two hemispheres: verbal–spatial, nonemotional–emotional, and conscious–unconscious. Although the evidence is not conclusive, it is highly suggestive that differential channeling occurs at the subcortical level, possibly in the basal ganglia (the globus pallidus and the nucleus basalis of Meynert) and in the dorsal median thalamus. Such channeling would presumably occur during upstream processing with subsequent differential treatment in the two hemispheres (Chapter 14).

If defense mechanisms are a combined function of increased negative affective charge and of level of consciousness, it is neurophysiologically plausible that repression is a more characteristic condition for prototypical right-hemispheric processing and intellectualization more characteristic for prototypical left-hemispheric processing. In a sense, the interaction of emotional and consciousness influences would determine the route of processing to one hemisphere or the other. Stimuli (perceptions or memories) that were most threatening would have their cognitive components most strongly inhibited through the subcortical mechanisms of the hierarchical control system. As a consequence they would be cognitively less conscious but affectively still negatively charged. Such stimuli would tend to be channeled to the right hemisphere and repressed. Subliminally presented negatively charged stimuli would tend particularly to be channeled to the right hemisphere. Supraliminal stimuli with less negative charge or even with high negative charge might be channeled to the left hemisphere for a different type of more conscious but nevertheless defensive processing.

According to this hypothesis of sensitizing and desensitizing defense mechanisms, impulses directed to the right hemisphere would tend to be less verbal, more emotionally negative, and less conscious (subliminal or unattended), while those shunted to the left hemisphere would tend to be more verbal, less negatively charged, and more conscious (supraliminal or attended). The ultimate determination of whether a percept would reach consciousness would be made at a subcortical level (in the thalamic–basal gangliar complex during upstream processing) where it would be decided how completely or incompletely a percept was to be shunted to one hemisphere or the other. In all instances, shunting in one direction or the other would be only partial with the corresponding defensive treatment predominating.

Experimental Evidence for the Role of the Interhemispheric Control System in Psychological Defense Mechanisms

The previous considerations are of theoretical interest, but the question remains as to the extent to which they are supported by experimental studies. There is fairly convincing evidence to support the concept that the differential character of the engram reservoir in the two hemispheres is associated with differential channeling of different types of material to each. The previous description in Chapter 14 of the work of Denenberg (1981) and his group on the lateralization of early traumatic experiences to the right hemisphere in mice provides specific experimental evidence for this thesis. In addition, Bear's study (1979) indicated that in patients suffering from temporal epilepsy, those with right temporal hyperirritability showed significantly greater emotionality, while those with left temporal hyperirritability showed greater intellectualizing tendencies. But apart from these variations in temperament, there were other differences between the two groups studied by Bear that suggested that differences in mode of psychological defense reactivities might be associated with increased activity of one hemisphere or the other.

In a study of the same patients' self-evaluation of social responsibility, Bear (1979) compared their self-reports with evaluations made by professional raters. He found that on socially approved items, left-sided lesion patients tended to underscore themselves, whereas on socially disapproved items, they tended to overscore themselves. Right-sided lesion patients had the exact opposite tendency. On the basis of these discrepancies, Bear labeled right-sided lesion patients "polishers" and left-sided lesion patients "tarnishers," in terms of their self-image evaluation. On a scale reflecting these tendencies, the two groups of patients were significantly different. Right-sided hyperactive patients reacted like the repressors described by Eriksen (1963); they exaggerated positive effects, but "repressed" negative ones. Left-sided hyperactive patients responded like Eriksen's "intellectualizers" or "sensitizers," i.e., they showed increased sensitivity to negative effects, but decreased sensitivity to positive ones.

These findings were substantially supported in a study by Gur and Gur (1975). They write:

> Using an inventory developed by Gleser and Ihilevich (1969) to measure individual differences in modes of defense, we tested the hypothesis that left-movers differ from right-movers in their characteristic defense clusters. It was predicted that left-movers would score higher on a defense cluster that internalized conflict in a holistic and preverbal fashion, whereas right-movers would score higher on defense clusters that externalized conflict and involved verbal elaborations.
>
> The Defense Mechanism Inventory (DMI) was administered to a group of 28 right-handed males, whose eye-movements' directionality had been previously determined using the battery of 60 questions developed by Gur, Gur and Harris (1975). The DMI classifies people according to the kinds of defense they tend to use more frequently. Five major defenses are identified by this test.
>
> 1. Turning Against Others (TAO), characterized as dealing with conflict "through attacking a real or presumed external frustrating object."
>
> 2. Projection (PRO), characterized as expressing aggression toward an external object "through first attributing to it, without unequivocal evidence, negative intent, or characteristics."
>
> 3. Principalization (PRN), characterized as dealing with conflicts "through invoking a general principle that 'splits off' affecting from content and repressed the former."
>
> 4. Turning Against Self (TAS), characterized as "directing aggressive behavior toward S (subject) himself."
>
> 5. Reversal (REV), characterized as defenses such as repression, denial, negation, and reaction–formation which "deal with conflict by responding in a positive or neutral fashion to a frustrating object." (pp. 270–271)

The results, illustrated in Figure 16-2, show that right-movers (left-hemisphere dominant) used intellectualizing defenses more frequently than did left-movers (significant differences for "turning against object" and for "projection"), while left-movers (right-hemisphere dominant) used repressive defenses more frequently (significant difference for "reversal"). A similar study by Packer (1975) confirmed the findings of Gur and Gur. Even conceding the as yet unproved status of eye movements as an index of lateralization, these studies, combined with the findings by Bear, are highly suggestive.

Finally, Davidson (1985) found that in subjects who were repressors, negative emotional visual stimuli presented to the left visual hemifield (and thus received in the right hemisphere) were transmitted to the left hemisphere for verbalization more slowly (i.e., they had slower reaction times) than did (1) neutral emotional stimuli presented to the right hemispheres of repressors, (2) neutral or negative stimuli presented to the left hemispheres of repressors, or (3) neutral or negative stimuli presented to either hemisphere of nonrepressors. Davidson interprets these findings to indicate delayed transmission of negative emotional stimuli through the commissures in respressors and this interpretation cannot be ruled out. However, the mechanisms postulated in this chapter of inhibition of cognitive valence during upstream processing of negative

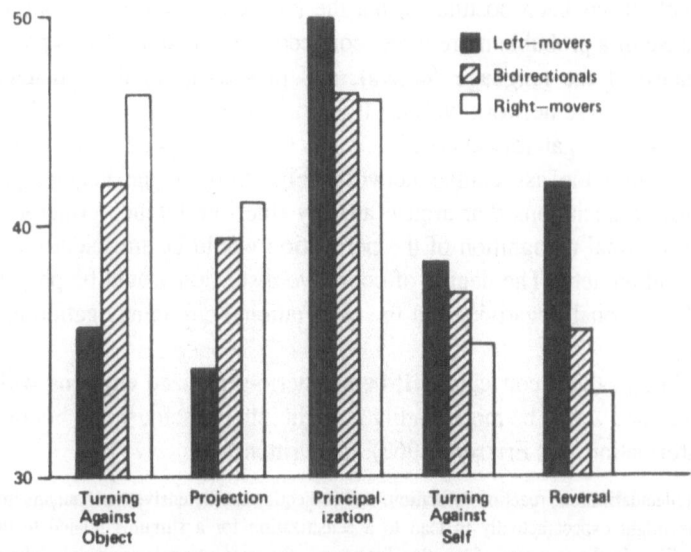

Figure 16-2 Comparison of defense mechanisms of "right-movers" and "left-movers." (From Gur and Gur, 1977. Reproduced with permission.)

emotional stimuli and delayed passage through the right hemisphere provides an equally or perhaps more plausible explanation (for further discussion, see Chapter 17).

Interaction between Hierarchical and Hemispheric Defense Mechanisms

The putative interaction between hierarchical and hemispheric defense mechanisms is also nicely illustrated here. According to this formulation of defense, more threatening percepts would be cognitively decathected in the hierarchical system during upstream processing and would become, because of their lower energy level, less likely to reach the consciousness threshold. As a consequence, they would tend to remain unconscious and by the reasoning outlined above, would probably be shunted to the right hemisphere for processing. This mechanism would explain not only the tendency to suppress negative perceptions, but also the tendency to have difficulty in retrieving unpleasant memories.

Having reached the right hemisphere for processing, such strongly threatening stimuli would tend to remain unconscious because the cognitive valence on the engram had been significantly reduced (with a consequent reduction in associated arousal). Right-hemispheric material would also tend to remain unconscious when the left hemisphere was most active, i.e., in alert consciousness. Thus the defense mechanisms of unconscious denial and repression would have been exercised in the alert conscious state.

The processing of percepts and memories shunted to the left hemisphere would be quite different. It has been postulated that the left hemisphere is predominantly conscious (because of a probable more direct connection with the RAS), is predominantly verbal (because of the language centers), and processes cognitive material mainly through the associative network because it is predominantly verbal (see Figs. 5-4 and 5-5). Accordingly, negatively charged percepts directed to the left hemisphere would be guided through the associative network (Fig. 5-5) by the general principle of avoiding those associations that arouse anxiety (the interference principle).* In this formulation the final recognition of the perception would be sufficiently distant from reality to avoid anxiety. The degree of cognitive distortion would be proportionate to the level of emotional negativity and the associational circumnavigation necessary to avoid anxiety.

According to these concepts, left-hemispheric-sensitized engrams with negative emotional valence would be more readily brought into consciousness, but only through some transformation. As Eriksen (1963) has written:

> Intellectualization, reaction-formation, and projection are defensive mechanisms that one might expect actually to lead to a sensitization for a stimulus related to the conflict. In the instance of reaction-formation, the person manifesting this defense seems to be particularly alert to finding and stamping out the evil that he denies in himself. Similarly, in the case of projection, those manifesting this defense are considered to be hyper-alert to detecting the presence of the defended-against impulse in others. Intellectualization frequently leads to a considerable preoccupation with the subject matter of the unacceptable impulse.

Thus in the case of perceptual vigilance to negatively charged engrams, the process of raising such engrams to consciousness would be accomplished through some distortion, while for perceptual vigilance associated with positively charged engrams entrance into consciousness would be direct without modification.

The Role of Mental Set in Psychological Defense Mechanisms

The paradigm for processing highly threatening perceptions and memories is extremely complex since it involves human personality factors as well as the more primitive brain stem mechanisms. If a stimulus is predicted to be highly threatening, under ordinary circumstances it would qualify even at the brain stem level for entry into consciousness; only under special circumstances would it not do so. Those circumstances, as in the Lazarus et al. study (Fig. 16-1), would presumably involve a specific mental set that through feedforward mechanisms from the prefrontal cortex to the brain stem would establish the conditions for processing such stimuli. The mental set may be established experimentally (as in the Lazarus study), or it may reflect the characteristic

---

*These reactions could be guided by the inhibitory influences of the hierarchical control system characteristic of "upstream" brainstem processing. On the other hand positively charged events could pass through the association network without detours.

reaction style of the individual. The latter in turn might be biologically or psychologically determined by the physiological dominance of either left- or right-hemispheric function. With left-hemispheric dominance, a more excitatory milieu would be established in the brain stem, whereas the overall effect with right-hemispheric dominance would be more inhibitory. In the first case the stimulus would be channeled to the left hemisphere for either direct management as a threatening event or, depending on the individual personality, to be treated with one of the intellectualizing defense mechanisms. In the case of an inhibitory mental set, the impulse would be channeled to the right hemisphere with consequent desensitizing (repressive) reactivities. Consequently, the specific mode of handling threatening impulses either from without or from within becomes the product of hierarchical and interhemispheric physiological mechanisms operating under the influence of mental sets determined by the total individual personality.

Such considerations are obviously of the greatest significance. The mode of processing (i.e., the psychological defense mechanism) employed for a given experience is determined only partially by the qualities of the event itself; it is determined even more by the mental set (personality parameters) of the specific individual involved. Just how important mental set factors may be in determining neurophysiological processing of a given stimulus is illustrated in the Phelps and Mazziotta (1982) and Mazziotta et al. (1982) studies in which music ordinarily processed through the right hemisphere was processed through the left brain in analytically oriented musicians. No single event can mean the same thing to different individuals, nor can their reactions to that experience be the same. Consequently, mental set must be seen as a function of personality which in turn is the product of experience. Only in this paradigm does the entire complex of interactions make sense.*

Summary of the Behavioral and Physiological Characteristics of the Psychological Defense Mechanisms

The overall hypotheses expressed in this chapter may be described as follows:

1. Early upstream processing of perceptual stimuli (early phase of attention) involves screening in the thalamic–basal gangliar complex (Hassler, 1978; Coyle et al., 1983). The affective components of percepts are processed more efficiently at this level than are the cognitive components (Kunst-Wilson and Zajonc, 1980). In this way subliminal (McCleary and Lazarus, 1949) and unattended (Forster and Govier, 1978) percepts may stimulate emotional arousal without cognitive awareness. Under these unconscious conditions perceptual defense (i.e., heightened perceptual thresholds) is presumably a function of some variation of feedback control where positive charge facilitates perceptual processing while negative charge somewhat inhibits it (the "unconscious arousal" paradigm).

*These preliminary ideas are extensively expanded upon in Chapter 19 on Psychobiological Mechanisms in Personality Development.

2. Unconscious suppression of arousal to anxiety-producing stimuli may also involve differential hemispheric processing. In the Lazarus et al. (1965) study, unconscious suppression of arousal was accomplished by producing a defensive mental set of either denial or intellectualization. Mental set operates in part by directing feedforward influences onto the subcortical control centers to establish either a stimulatory (augmenting) or inhibitory (reducing) influence in those centers. Associated with these effects is a differential priming of the thalamic–basal gangliar complexes on the two sides with consequent channeling of impulses to either the left or right hemisphere.

3. Early upstream processing in the thalamic–basal gangliar complex apparently also involves early screening for preferential shunting of stimuli to one hemisphere or the other, depending on stimulus characteristics. Screening parameters include both cognitive (verbal versus spatial) and emotional characteristics (Davidson et al., 1974; Schwartz et al., 1975). More negative emotional and nonverbal stimuli tend to be shunted to the right hemisphere; somewhat less negative emotional and more verbal percepts tend to be shunted to the left hemisphere. Similarly, supraliminal percepts tend to be shunted to the left hemisphere while subliminal ones tend to be shunted to the right. This last interpretation would also help explain the findings of Shevrin (1974) and of Kostandov and Arzumov (1980) that supraliminal negatively charged percepts arouse increased attention, i.e., increased early and late evoked response (ER) components, while subliminal negatively charged percepts are associated with decreased attention, i.e., decreased early and late ER components.

4. Depending on the interaction among the four major variables (cognitive, emotional, level of consciousness, and personality), stimuli are directed either to the right or left hemisphere. Stimuli shunted to the right hemisphere tend to be treated with denial mechanisms; those shunted to the left are processed with intellectualization mechanisms (Gur and Gur, 1975; Bear, 1979). According to this hypothesis, denial mechanisms are the consequence of inherent structural and psychologically imposed characteristics of the right hemisphere; percepts directed there tend to elude awareness. Contrariwise, because of the nature of left-hemispheric organization, stimuli directed to that hemisphere are treated with the mechanisms of intellectualization, the degree of resulting distortion varying with the level of the negative emotional charge.

5. The mechanisms of intellectualizing defenses are considered to be inherent properties of the left hemisphere: because of its postulated closer connections with the RAS and the consciousness systems, because of its analytic potential, and because of its greater use of the associative network. The mechanisms of denial are postulated to be inherent in the right hemisphere: because of its poorer connections with the RAS and the consciousness system, because of its lesser analytic potential, and because of its greater use of the abstractive network (see Fig. 5-4). The major determination of whether a stimulus is treated with denial or intellectualization: is made subcortically during upstream processing, is transmitted through the appropriate channeling apparatus to the cortex, and is implemented through subsequent processing in one hemisphere or the other.

6. Certainly the cognitive, emotional, and consciousness characteristics of a perceptual stimulus or a memory are extremely important factors in determining the mode of processing for a given stimulus. Probably the most important factors are the mental set effects influencing the level of stimulation or inhibition established at the subcortical level through feedforward impulses from the cortical executive decision-making self complex (Fig. 9-3) onto subcortical directional mechanisms. Mental set determines both the hierarchical and interhemispheric mechanisms involved in the psychological management of threatening impulses (perceptions or memories). Mental set may be established experimentally as in the Lazarus et al. study, but customarily is a function of the personality of the individual involved. Since personality is the product of all genetic hereditary influence and all lived experience, ultimately psychological defense mechanisms can be understood only in terms of the entire organism (see Chapter 19).

The considerations in this and the previous chapters have prepared the groundwork upon which a more comprehensive model of conscious and unconscious mental function may be based. The psychobiological system to be presented in the next section derives completely from the conclusions of earlier chapters. Yet it bears a remarkable resemblance to the Freudian psychoanalytic model. Whether this effect is a natural consequence of the argument of this volume or whether it only reflects an unconscious prejudice on the part of the author should become more apparent in the presentation itself.

IV

Psychobiology and the Pathogenesis of Neurosis

VI

A Psychobiological Model of Conscious and Unconscious Brain Activity

The descriptions of the physiological processes underlying mental activity presented thus far in this volume provide only the skeleton for a comprehensive psychobiological theory of mental behavior. Any system that is designed to provide a full explanation of human behavior must consist of more than a series of neurophysiological mechanisms. The attractiveness of Freudian psychoanalytic theory lies as much in its comprehensiveness as it does in any one of its specific explanations. Freud attempted to integrate the known biological principles of his day with the growing awareness of the importance of development and experience into a unitary concept that would still be compatible with clinical phenomena. As a consequence, psychoanalytic theory has a universal approach to human behavior that has probably contributed more to its general appeal than has any specific effort at scientific validation. It follows then that a broad comparison with the Freudian system might provide an excellent context in which to expand the implications of the psychobiological model of mental activity. Indeed, such an evaluation is only fitting and proper since it is mainly from psychoanalysis that the general interest in unconscious mental activity derives.

At the time Freud began his explorations into abnormal psychology, the dominant psychological schools were those of Wundt and Titchener, who restricted their research of the mind to the analysis of purely conscious experience. The later development of behaviorist psychology, with its emphasis on the observation of behavior as opposed to investigation of introspective experience, led even further away from any concern with unconscious mental activity. As a medical practitioner, Freud was interested in psychopathology and its dynamics. His clinical exposure to hypnosis introduced him to the concept of a functional unconscious as the major dynamic mechanism involved in that process. The partial success of hypnosis in treating some forms of psychopathology convinced him that unconscious mechanisms were central to such mental dysfunction. The theoretical formulation of the "dynamic unconscious" followed naturally.

On the basis of this level of reasoning, Freud established the topographical organization of consciousness and the unconscious, as illustrated in Figure 17-1A. Consciousness or awareness constitutes the "tip of the iceberg." All unconscious material that can readily be brought into awareness is conceived as lying in the contiguous area of the preconscious; the ease of transfer from preconscious to conscious would presumably be governed by mechanisms similar to the attentional processes described earlier in this volume. To the bottom area of Figure 17-1A, the unconscious, Freud relegated those highly charged negative engrams that threaten the psychological homeostatis of the individual. In order to explain the ability of the mind to keep those engrams from entry into conscious awareness, Freud constructed the "repressive barrier" to actively repress those engrams back into the unconscious. There such engrams, fomenting with pent-up energy, create disturbances that are translated into normal behavior or into one or another neurotic symptoms.

This theory, which in itself is not unattractive, is extremely difficult to prove or disprove. Within the psychobiological structure, many of the mechanisms postulated by Freud have been more or less demonstrated: the influence of motivational–emotional charge on attentional valence, the presence of both excitatory and inhibitory influences in attentional mechanisms, and the semicontrolled processing (primary processing) of unconscious engrams. Nevertheless, it is not clear that these individual mechanisms are organized in the specific structure postulated by psychoanalysis, particularly in respect to the putative existence of the repressive barrier. The concept of an active repressive barrier is especially difficult to fit into a psychobiological mold since it introduces the idea of a homunculus in the brain: the "ego," which decides what should and what should not be admitted to consciousness. However, if we equate the ego with the psychobiological self-system, even that reconciliation may not be impossible.

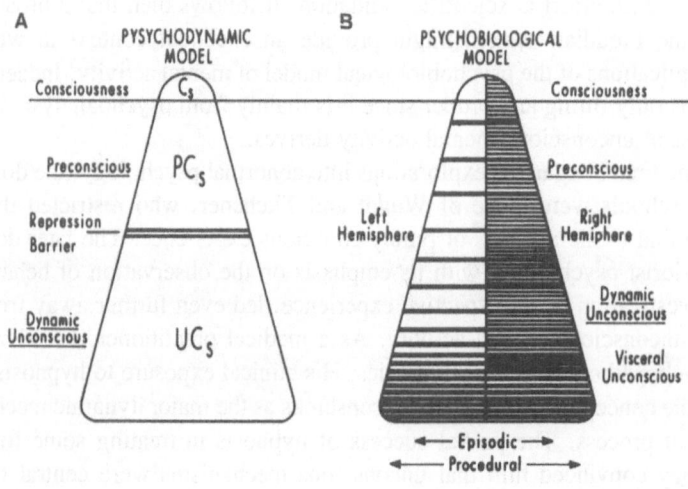

Figure 17-1 Freudian and psychobiologic structure of the conscious–unconscious continuum.

Hierarchical Control Mechanisms in the Psychobiological Model of the Unconscious

In the psychobiological model of mental function as here conceptualized, all activity is sustained in the consciousness–unconscious continuum, operating at different levels according to the shifting needs of the human organism. The entire continuum acts as a single entity so that the passage of activity from one level to another is controlled by a set of fixed principles. The order of the components of the consciousness–unconscious continuum runs from the most conscious to the least conscious as follows: the alert conscious state, the preconscious, the dynamic unconscious (with its two components, the cathected and decathected unconscious), and at the lowest level, independently, the procedural and the visceral unconscious. Since the regular route of passage of influence is directly from a given level to the next, the dynamic unconscious plays the critical role in the control of both consciousness and the preconscious, and of both procedural and visceral function. In terms of function, the six compartments may be divided operationally into three layers: the first consisting of the alert conscious state and the preconscious, the second of both sections of the dynamic unconscious, and the third of the procedural and visceral unconscious. These relationships are illustrated in Figure 17-1B.

The Alert Conscious–Preconscious Level

The alert conscious state and the preconscious obviously differ in level of consciousness, but they are similar in that they both utilize episodic data almost exclusively; they are governed by controlled and semicontrolled processing respectively, and both interchange information with one another readily and smoothly. The constant interaction of the material in both compartments is governed as much by cognitive as by affective influences. Thus with the presentation of emotionally neutral stimuli, perception leads readily to recognition through identification with engrams in the preconscious long-term memory. On the other hand, engrams with strong positive or negative emotional charge would tend to be stored in the dynamic unconscious, from where they could be recaptured more or less readily into the preconscious.

It may seem strange to place the alert conscious state and the preconscious into the same operational level when one is conscious and the other unconscious. However, in this instance the level of consciousness is merely a function of the immediate relevancy of a generally *emotionally uncharged* perception or memory in a particular situation. Since that relevancy is essentially cognitive, the two compartments may be considered operationally to function more or less as one.

The kind of episodic material processed in the preconscious is by definition unconscious but also by definition so close to consciousness as to be essentially inseparable from it. It represents those perceptions, thoughts, and memories which in the stream of consciousness have just returned from short-term memory to long-term memory, or those which are about to be summoned up from long-term memory to awareness. In addition, it comprises all the perceptions, thoughts, and memories which, because they are not defended against, offer no barrier to immediate entry into consciousness. In a word, they constitute the sum total of those engrams on which the emotional charge, if any, is facilitative rather than inhibitory.

An important quality of conscious–preconscious thought processing and behavior that derives from the essentially "controlled" nature of its physiology is that most experienced entities are conceptualized as individual events rather than as complex patterns of automatic procedural reactivities. The distinction between these two categories of phenomena lies in the fact that the first is a series of different associated "episodic" events that all together constitute an episode, whereas the latter is a sequence of more or less stereotyped activities encumbered under the rubric of an automatic procedure. It is necessary to emphasize this distinction because it illustrates the truism that the contents of the episodic conscious and preconscious are of a different order of structure and function than are the contents of the procedural and visceral levels of the unconscious.

The episodic conscious–preconscious is the seat of verbal, episodic, controlled process material, whereas the procedural and visceral unconscious is the seat of nonverbal, procedural, and visceral automatically processed material. The first is sequential and differentiated and is activated through the thalamic–basal gangliar and amygdaloid–hippocampal complexes. The second, as described in Chapter 11, is organized into complex reactive patterns through programs in the putamen and caudate nucleus and cerebellum. How these two sets of disparate material intermesh in the dynamic unconscious is one of the more important issues in this volume.

The Dynamic Unconscious

Both psychobiology and psychoanalysis agree that the dynamic unconscious is the major control area for all behavior. Their conceptualizations, however, are quite different. Freudian theory views the dynamic unconscious as consisting largely of repressed material. Psychobiology conceives of the same entity as containing the memories of all experience, positive and negative, and as influencing behavior on the basis of the sum total of that experience. Nevertheless, there is some congruence between the two systems.

The fact that repressive and intellectualizing defense mechanisms are readily demonstrable in clinical situations and can be shown to have dramatic anxiety-relieving effects (Lazarus et al., 1965), to my mind constitutes convincing evidence that emotional influences affect mental activity at the unconscious level in a different way than do cognitive processes, namely by introducing inhibitory influences. Without accepting the Freudian concept of a "repressive barrier," we can substitute the idea of an "interference effect" in which an excessive negative (highly threatening) charge on an engram would result in atypical processing of that engram in both the hierarchical and hemispheric systems. A collection of such threatening engrams would constitute a separate subsection of the psychobiological dynamic unconscious. Furthermore, the treatment of these engrams would be determined by mechanisms somewhat different from those controlling less negatively or positively charged engrams. The sum total of all strongly negative hypercharged engrams in the brain, exercising their effects in some as yet undisclosed fashion, would resemble most closely the Freudian concept of a dynamic unconscious.

As a result of such considerations, the compartment previously designated as "the psychobiological dynamic unconscious" may now more accurately be subdivided into two subcompartments, depending on the subset of the material contained: (1) that for normal affective and cognitive experience (the "cathected" subset) where cathected indicates that there has been no de-emotionalizing of the cognitive events, and (2) that for highly negatively emotionally charged material (the "decathected" subset) where de-emotionalizing has occurred. The psychobiological dynamic unconscious (cathected subset) is governed by "normal" physiological mechanisms and as such is not suitable for comparison with the Freudian dynamic unconscious. But a brief reconsideration of some of the experimental data presented in Chapters 13 and 16 on the influence of emotions on the *decathected* subset makes it evident that these engrams are processed through mechanisms that are different from those in the *cathected* unconscious and more similar to those postulated in the psychoanalytic system.

Although this *decathected* segment of the psychobiological dynamic unconscious is in many respects comparable to the Freudian dynamic unconscious, there are still significant differences. For one thing, this segment constitutes a relatively small portion of the psychobiological dynamic unconscious, probably somewhat larger in individuals with psychopathology, but even there significantly smaller than the cathected component. Second, there is still no repressive barrier in the Freudian sense, only an interference effect implicit in each threatening engram. Finally, even though the decathected unconscious plays a role similar to that of the Freudian unconscious in producing psychopathological behavior, the mechanisms involved, as will shortly become evident, are qualitatively different.

General Characteristics of the Dynamic Unconscious

The two compartments of the dynamic unconscious, the cathected and the decathected, are basically similar in their operation and function except for the differences in the underlying operations implicit in their titles. Their similarities consist of the facts that in both instances, they deal not only with episodic but also with procedural and visceral activities; that both are governed by semicontrolled mechanisms of information processing, intermediate between those of controlled and automatic; that their contents are more difficult to bring to awareness, particularly those in the decathected unconscious; that passage from the top conscious level down to the deep unconscious procedural and visceral levels and back again is always through the dynamic unconscious; and that consequently between them, they are probably the major determining influences in behavior.

The differences between the cathected and decathected compartments of the dynamic unconscious stem from the differences in the previous treatment of the engrams within them and from the differences in the consequent characteristics of their activities. The term cathected, as applied to engrams in the cathected unconscious, signifies that the original emotional charge on that engram, positive or negative, was sufficiently tolerable to the organism so that no special treatment of its cognitive component was necessary to reduce the associated level of arousal. Hence, engrams in the *cathected* unconscious, unlike those in the preconscious, may have quite substantial positive or negative emotional valence. In general, engrams with positive valence will have greater input in the cathected unconscious since negative valence is almost always at least partially reduced during upstream processing at the thalamic–basal gangliar level (see Chapter 13 and Fig. 13-2). Nevertheless, such partial decathecting may be minimal so that the residual engram will still function as relatively undefended in the sense of not having been exposed to hemispheric sensitizing and desensitizing defense mechanisms.

The operation of the *decathected* unconscious is of course of an entirely different nature. Here, probably all engrams are of such quality as to constitute a serious threat to the biological or psychological integrity of the individual. Consequently, the original process of decathecting at the brain stem level would have been significantly substantial to assure the submission of the perceived event or memory to defensive treatment in one hemisphere or the other (Chapter 16). In many instances, the engrams in the decathected unconscious will have been sufficiently decathected to permit normal behavioral adaptation to a threatening unconscious conflict. In such cases, only when external perceptions or internal associative thoughts would inadvertently reactivate the cognitive component of the decathected engram, would abnormal arousal (anxiety) occur. On the other hand, where the process of decathecting is insufficient to contain the associated level of anxiety, a variety of other defensive treatments, most often neurotic in nature, are utilized. These sequences are discussed in detail at the end of this chapter and again in Chapter 20 in the discussion on the neuroses.

The unique function of the *dynamic unconscious,* which applies equally to both of its elements albeit in different ways, derives from its central position in the consciousness–unconscious continuum. Because it is highly dynamic, influences from it are directed upward onto the alert conscious–preconscious level of operation and downward onto the procedural and visceral unconscious levels. The vital quality of the dynamic unconscious stems not only from the episodic and affective material draining into it from the alert conscious–preconscious, but equally from important procedural and visceral material rising upward into it from the deeper procedural and visceral levels. Consequently, because of the dynamic quality of its operation (in the sense of its engrams being highly cathected, i.e., highly emotionally charged, or highly decathected, i.e., complexly defended) and because it receives material from both the most conscious and least conscious compartments (episodic and affective from above, procedural and visceral from below), the dynamic unconscious becomes the dominant intergrating influence in all psychological and behavioral functions.

The physiological basis for these complex integrating activities of the dynamic unconscious lies in its semicontrolled mode of data processing that permits it to send and receive messages both to and from the conscious–preconscious level above it and to and from the procedural and visceral levels below it. The ability to both receive and respond, i.e., to communicate in the language of episodic data with the conscious–preconscious compartment, allows the dynamic unconscious to influence, or more probably to determine to a large extent, conscious behavior. Its comparable ability to communicate with the deeper procedural and visceral layers in their own language provides the mechanisms through which psychological activity can affect basic physio-logical functions or conversely be affected by them. Because only the dynamic uncon-scious has the "language" to speak to both the controlled and to the automatic levels of processing, all integrated activities must be consummated through it.

Upward and Downward Influences of the Dynamic Unconscious

The evidence for the foregoing conclusion lies in both clinical and experimental circumstances. Evidence of unconscious influence on conscious behavior is so substan-tial as hardly to need validation. The most obvious example, the one used by Freud, is that of parapraxes, slips of the tongue that are unconsciously motivated. Although the psychobiological model does not view all parapraxes as dynamically motivated (many are considered merely cognitively derived errors), others certainly are. In a similar fashion, unconscious motivations may inspire particular actions, the origins of which are frequently unknown to the individual himself until after the act is consummated. The tendency to drive in an accustomed direction when one means to drive in an entirely different direction is a good example of such an effect. Finally, the meaning of defensive behavior, particularly as in the sensitizing defenses of projection, reaction-formation, and intellectualization, is often patent and transparent to all observers, but hidden from the individual himself.

The upward influence of the dynamic unconscious in neurotic behavior is again too apparent to require much substantiation. In these cases, the individual exhibits a variety of behaviors, for example hand-washing in obsessive–compulsive neuroses, that make sense to no one, including the individual himself. Whether one does or does not accept the Freudian explanation of compulsive hand-washing, it would appear that within any psychological system, a dynamic unconscious would be a necessary ele-ment to explain, however inadequately, such behavior.

Evidence for the downward influence of the dynamic unconscious on procedural and visceral functions is even more convincing. A concrete example of the manner in which directives fed directly into the dynamic unconscious can affect procedural func-tions in a way not possible with conscious control is provided by musculoskeletal control under hypnosis. Hypnosis is a technique that, by circumventing the conscious–preconscious level, is able to introduce information directly into the dynamic uncon-scious. Under hypnosis, individuals are able to achieve and maintain postures of extreme rigidity (catatonic stances and opisthotonos, i.e., a back rigid enough to form a bridge between two chairs) that they could never accomplish in the conscious state. This is probably the best experimental example of how the dynamic unconscious can control procedural responsivities in a manner not available to the conscious–pre-conscious component.

An even more dramatic example of the potency of the dynamic unconscious in the control of deeper unconscious activities is evidenced in the effects of hypnosis on a variety of visceral activities. Writing on the subject of the true nature of the unconscious, Lewis Thomas (1979) the well-known biologist, has described in an essay on warts his wonder at the fact that these excrescences could be removed efficiently and effectively by hypnosis. He reviews the literature and concludes that there can be no question about the phenomenon. Individuals with warts on both sides of the body, when told under hypnosis that they will lose the warts on only one side of the body, do so completely and thoroughly in a few weeks. Thomas is amazed at the wisdom and skill of an unconscious that, with little instruction from the hypnotist, is able to initiate complex physiological mechanisms, both localized and generalized, to bring about the specified cure. He writes:

> There ought to be a better word than "Unconscious," even capitalized, for what I have, so to speak, in mind. I was brought up to regard this aspect of thinking as a sort of private sanitarium, walled off somewhere in a suburb of my brain, capable only of producing such garbled information as to keep my mind, my proper Mind, always a little off balance.
>
> But any mental apparatus that can reject a wart is something else again. This is not the sort of confused, disordered process you'd expect at the hands of the kind of Unconscious you read about in books, out at the edge of things making up dreams or getting mixed up on words or having hysterics. Whatever, or whoever, is responsible for this has the accuracy and precision of a surgeon. There almost has to be a Person in charge, running matters of meticulous detail beyond anyone's comprehension, a skilled engineer and manager, a chief executive officer, the head of the whole place. I never thought before that I possessed such a tenant. Or perhaps more accurately, such a landlord, since I would be, if this is in fact the situation, nothing more than a lodger. (pp. 79–80)

The viewpoint implied in his half-humorous but very serious statement holds that there is indeed an unconscious that manages and controls much of our behavior, but that, as a level of activity, it is one which is governed by the same basic principles of biological homeostasis as are the functional mechanisms of physiological activity. In these terms, the unconscious is the arena in which the biological forces of heredity, development, and experience interact to determine behavior. Because of the severe limitations that exist for "controlled" thought processing, the amount of information that can be efficiently managed consciously at any given moment is highly limited, so that the mechanisms regulating attention must be carefully attuned to the needs of the moment. On the other hand, the mass of automatic processing of material not immediately accessible to consciousness must be ongoing if the organism is to have continuity and coherence. The integrity of the individual depends not so much on his conscious activity (for this can be interrupted as in sleep or coma without disrupting that integrity) as upon the continuity of the unconscious. To accomplish these ends, as Lewis Thomas writes, the unconscious must be well structured, logical, and efficient.

Although the unconscious mechanisms described by Thomas are not at all known, by their very nature they would seem to be ongoing and continuous rather than occasional and intermittent. Together with the evidence previously described, the picture of a dynamic unconscious begins to evolve as an active arena for interaction among the competing motivational–emotional, cognitive, and visceral drives, an arena that, except in true pathological unconsciousness, is never completely inactive.

Even more importantly, the picture presented by Thomas of unconscious mechanisms as not strange and bizarre, but rather as complex programs integrated into everyday existence, offers a paradigm that fits readily into the general theoretical position of this volume. In this view, the psychobiological dynamic unconscious is not a separate area of the mind dedicated only to working out childhood conflicts. It represents rather the level of interaction for all of the engrams in the brain not being utilized at the conscious level at a given time. As described above, consciousness is the state par excellence for dealing with immediate problems; the dynamic unconscious is the essential psychological mechanism for dealing with continuous ongoing behavior.

The Procedural and Visceral Levels of the Unconscious

The operation of the procedural unconscious was described in detail in Chapter 11 so that it is only necessary here to review those mechanisms that characterize it. The procedural unconscious is involved of course with procedural processes, such as automatic behaviors (walking, talking, singing, etc.), and with particular skills (driving, tennis playing, or piano playing). These processes have in common a large element of motor function and also a complex pattern of interactions among sensorimotor functions that allow a high degree of precision, all accomplished at the unconscious level. In Chapter 11, the complex arrangements in the brain through which these remarkably complicated maneuvers can be made effortlessly were labeled as "programs," a euphemism for unknown mechanisms.

But something must be added about these behavioral programs which was not stressed in Chapter 11. These complex algorithms for behavioral functions are organized not around specific nerve arrangements nor muscle structures, but rather about specific activities. Consequently, there is a program in the brain for walking, talking, washing one's hands, piano playing, and so on. Although the arrangements of procedural mechanisms are strictly physiological, the total function can be defined only behaviorally. But since behavior can also be described episodically (cognitively), then a bridge between the two languages—the episodic and the procedural—begins to become apparent.

A similar situation applies for many visceral functions. Eating, sleeping, urinating, defecating, and sexual activity are all visceral functions that are readily defined in cognitive (episodic) terms. Many of these activities contain major motor (procedural) elements as well. Although the visceral components of these functions presumably are controlled by visceral mechanisms in the brain stem and the motor components are controlled by procedural mechanisms in the putamen, caudate nucleus, and cerebellum, there is obvious coordinated interaction between the two systems in each of the visceral functions listed above.

Processing in both the procedural unconscious and the visceral unconscious is automatic, i.e., unconscious, parallel, simultaneous and noninterfering, and generally unlimited. As previously described, these are the processes that maintain organismic function at all times and in all places. But these processes, which are also influenced directly through environmental conditioning, are not independent of the entire reservoir of episodic experience encompassed both at the conscious–preconscious level and in the dynamic unconscious. Consequently, the modes of interaction among these systems and the physiological mechanisms underlying them are issues of the greatest significance and will be discussed later.

The Operational Sequence of Interactions among the Three Levels of the Consciousness–Unconscious Continuum

If the conceptualization of the dynamic unconscious as the intermediary agent in operations among the three levels of the consciousness–unconscious continuum is correct, then all or at least most interchange between the top and bottom levels should almost obligatorily be through the middle. To a large degree this seems to be true. For example, if one deliberately attempts to consciously control a well-established procedural mechanism such as walking or piano playing, the efficiency of the particular skill involved is usually decreased. Conscious intrusion on an established procedural skill is actually disruptive. On the other hand, if one consciously determines to do better at a given skill without concentrating on the procedural process itself, that skill will often be improved. It seems as though a conscious episodic goal (to improve a skill) is somehow transmitted as a positive potentiating mental set which is translated at some level into a language that improves procedural function. It may be that mental set itself, by establishing a positive emotional milieu, affects procedural skills directly, but it would seem that there must be some more concrete method by which the translation of episodic material (the wish to do better) into procedural process can be achieved. This is presumably accomplished in the dynamic unconscious through the direct translation of cognitive language into procedural language as a result of which the transaction is completed.

A somewhat different example occurs in stuttering. Individuals who have a tendency to stutter or stammer are often almost free of their condition when relaxed, but lapse into a severe state when they consciously try to stop stuttering. This might be attributed to a more direct disruptive effect of anxiety upon procedural process (the characteristic effect of anxiety upon procedural process), the opposite of the direct positive effect of positive motivation upon performance as in the previous example. Here, a better case can be made for the direct effect of a negative affect in consciousness upon operations in the procedural unconscious. But, as in the previous instance, it is still difficult to see how a positive cognitive intention can be translated into greater procedural performance without the intervention of some intermediary step.

The purpose of these descriptions is to suggest the presence of a functional gap between the cognitively structured conscious–preconscious, operating through more or less controlled processing, and the behaviorally patterned procedural and visceral levels of the unconscious, operating through more or less automatic processing. Ordinarily the translation of one into the other would appear to require the intercession of the dynamic unconscious with access to both types of material and both types of processing. The introduction of negative affective influences, as illustrated in the example of stuttering, does appear to circumvent the necessity for the intervention of the dynamic unconscious, but this would seem to apply only when there is no requirement for translation from one operational language to the other.

The need for mutual translation of episodic and procedural paradigms goes even deeper. Flow among the various compartments is of course not merely downward from the conscious–preconscious levels and the dynamic unconscious onto the procedural and visceral levels of the unconscious, but is also upward from the latter to the former. For example, in the case of inadvertently driving along an accustomed route when one means to go elsewhere, it is likely that it is the procedural unconscious, controlling the automatic motor responses, that is misdirecting the dynamic unconscious which is controlling the choice of route. Similarly at the visceral level, unconscious pangs of hunger will influence one's choices in a free-association test. More dramatically, a full urinary bladder will be vividly represented in dreams despite the subject's lack of awareness of it.

Again, in each of these instances where there is a procedural or visceral process of a *conceptual nature* (into which most procedural and visceral processes can be translated), that process may be identified with a comparable cognitive (episodic) engram in a manner similar to that in which two comparable cognitive engrams may be so identified. Furthermore, interactions of this type are most likely to occur in the dynamic unconscious where the physiological mechanisms relateing to both kinds of activities exist.

The Neurophysiology for Mutual Translation of Episodic and Procedural Paradigms

Although the neurophysiology of semicontrolled information processing was discussed in some detail in the chapter on the episodic unconscious (Chapter 12), it is necessary here, because of the differences in the nature of semicontrolled processing in the preconscious from that in the dynamic unconscious, to examine the issue again. From our previous descriptions of semicontrolled processing in the preconscious as opposed to that in the dynamic unconscious, it appears that the first is quite close to controlled processing while the latter has within it many more of the qualities of automatic and visceral processing. These assumptions are necessary to account for the fact that preconscious cognitive directives to procedural and visceral mechanisms are fairly ineffective, whereas similar dynamic unconscious directives are highly effective. One must postulate for the dynamic unconscious, but not for the preconscious, a mode of processing that is capable of communicating both with controlled episodic and with automatic procedural and visceral material.

Unfortunately, the evidence for these conclusions is all circumstantial. There are at present no direct experimental studies to demonstrate that information processing in the dynamic unconscious is of a different nature from the semicontrolled processing in the preconscious (the effects described by Posner) or the automatic processing in the procedural unconscious (the effects described by Shiffrin and Schneider). Nevertheless, the circumstantial evidence is such as to make plausible a neurophysiological hypothesis on the nature of semicontrolled processing in the dynamic unconscious.

If the dynamic unconscious is to have the capacity to translate cognitive episodic directives (as in hypnosis) onto procedural and visceral processes, then it must also possess mechanisms that can communicate (receive and send messages) in both of these operational languages. Episodic (cognitive) engrams were described in Chapter 4 as functional networks of neuronal activity anchored in specifically involved neurons that constitute both the pattern and the locus in the brain that define each abstract conception. Association among cognitive engrams was described as resulting from simultaneous excitation of two different engrams related, however, through the sharing of some neurons or circuits. Reactivation of associated engrams was again ascribed to be effectuated through the excitation of such shared neurons or circuits.

The previously described procedural programs must somehow be structurally similar in nature to those of cognitive (episodic) engrams. Although many procedural programs are wired into the brain genetically (swimming, walking, speaking, etc.), almost all of them require experience for their adequate development. The processing of experience associated with procedural learning, although of a different nature than that associated with cognitive learning, must still depend on the same mechanisms of abstraction (including mechanisms of both convergence and divergence), of consolidation of the sensory components, and of association. Procedural programs may be viewed as similar to cognitive (episodic) engrams in development except that they exist more in the cerebellum than in the cortex.

The cerebellum is so often considered as an essentially motor organ that the fact that the majority of its cells are sensory in function is often overlooked. The development of procedural functions through experience is associated with the development of procedural engrams in the cerebellum superimposed upon genetically wired-in programs. These procedural engrams are associated with the simultaneously developed cognitive episodic engrams and inevitably share some neurons, most likely in the brain stem, but also probably in both the cortex and the cerebellum. Consequently, the interaction of episodic and procedural engrams is not only not surprising, but seems rather inevitable.*

The case for the interaction of visceral and episodic material is of course similar. Visceral processes are, if anything, more genetically hard-wired into the brain stem mechanisms that activate them, but the procedural processes that are associated with them, such as eating, urinating, defecating, etc., are like most other procedural processes, modified by learning through experience. These processes, too, are associated with cognitive episodic learning. Here the three domains, the cognitive episodic, the procedural, and the visceral, are all involved in individually unique, highly motivated, highly emotional activities and become irrevocably chained to one another in physiologically established neuronal associations.

The putative association of the cognitive episodic abstraction for a visceral pro-

---

*It is the fact that a specific procedural program exists for an activity like hand washing and that that program has episodic equivalents; that accounts for the interaction of episodic (mental) and procedural (behavioral) activities in obsessive–compulsive neuroses. See Chapter 20 for further explication.

cess, as for example eating, with the visceral (hunger and satisfaction of hunger) and procedural (breast-feeding, eating) elements of the process is by no means difficult to conceptualize, particularly since there are centers in the thalamic–basal gangliar and limbic system complexes that feed directly into all three modalities. The question may be asked: Why do we assign the area of interaction of the three modalities to the dynamic unconscious rather than to the conscious–preconscious level? The answer of course is that both procedural and visceral activities are almost entirely unconscious whereas the conscious–preconscious level is essentially conscious. Since the activities of consciousness involve an entirely different aspect of brain function—that of consciousness, self-awareness and attention—they are concentrated in different pathways than are those involved in unconscious procedural and visceral functions. That is not true for activities in the dynamic unconscious, which can and do relate to activities in both the procedural and visceral unconscious.

Does this suggest that the dynamic unconscious is located in a different part of the brain than, let us say, the preconscious? The answer is obviously "no," since in the alert conscious state probably all of the brain is involved in both of these activities. What is implied, however, is a difference in functional organization. Elements in the preconscious long-term memory are so cognitively and affectively valenced as to be more susceptible to introduction into awareness. Elements in the dynamic unconscious are so cognitively and affectively valenced, especially those in the decathected unconscious, as to be less susceptible to introduction into awareness. Consequently, the dynamic unconscious, because of the nature of its individual elements, is more prone to remain unconscious and is consequently more prone to interact with the material in the procedural and visceral levels of the unconscious.

Hemispheric Control System Effects in Unconscious Brain Function

Hierarchical control mechanisms as described above appear to present a partial context within which a meaningful model of human behavior may be conceptualized. But these descriptions do not seem to offer adequate explanations for some of the more complex, presumably unconscious, behavioral effects such as sensitizing and desensitizing defense mechanisms, the productions of altered states of consciousness, and so on. For possible answers to these questions, we must look to the interhemispheric system.

The psychobiological model of the unconscious holds as one of its basic tenets that the nature and function of the dynamic unconscious as it is represented in the two hemispheres is basically different. The evidence for differential processing and for differential content and reactivities in the two hemispheres is strongly suggestive. As described in Chapters 14 and 15, support for the putative mechanisms through which the differences in hemispheric content and function are established comprise the following: (1) the evidence that predominantly cognitive stimuli would tend to be more actively processed and hence better consolidated in the left hemisphere while predominantly emotional stimuli would tend to be more actively processed and hence better consolidated in the right hemisphere; (2) the evidence from Davidson et al. that negatively charged emotional stimuli tend to activate the right hemisphere more than the left while the reverse appears to be true for positively charged emotional stimuli; (3) the probability that in infancy, before the development of the higher cognitive functions including language, most perception is holistic rather than analytic so that infantile memories might be better stored in the right hemisphere; (4) similarly, because of the mode of differential hemispheric processing in early infancy and childhood, veridical and abstract engrams may predominate in the right brain while abstract and symbolic (verbal) engrams, may predominate in the left brain (the key word is "predominate" excluding any "either–or" dichotomy); (5) the late development of the corpus callosum in childhood, maintaining a relative separation in the development of early memories that might or might not be modified by future experience (Denenberg, 1981); (6) the lower level of consciousness in the right hemisphere as manifested in commissurotomized patients; (7) the evidence that unconscious activities (subliminal and unattended stimuli and involuntary motor activity) tend to be shifted more to the right than to the left hemisphere (see excerpt by Davison, 1980, in Chapter 15); and (8) the clinical evidence by Bear (1979) and Gur and Gur (1975) that the two hemispheres differ both in the nature of their content (left, intellectual; right, emotional) and in their modes of defense (left, sensitizing; right, desensitizing).

Considerations such as these have made it tempting to lodge the psychobiological dynamic unconscious in the right hemisphere. Various psychobiologists, basing their formulations on psychoanalytic concepts of the unconscious, have attempted to reconcile Freudian thinking with more recent experimental findings by using the differential functions of the two hemispheres as a major mechanism for differentiating conscious and unconscious processes. Arguing by analogy from the situation in commissurotomized patients, Ornstein (1972) and Galin (1974) have hypothesized that unconsciousness is a proven characteristic of engrams in the right hemisphere so that material that is lodged on that side is, under certain circumstances, not available to left-hemispheric awareness. Since ordinarily in the intact individual right-hemispheric material has ready access to left-hemispheric awareness through the corpus callosum, they postulated that repression is implemented through a functional commissurotomy secondary to strong inhibitory influences upon the corpus callosum, either upon specific emotionally charged engrams, or in certain conditions as a more generalized effect on anatomical elements in the commissures.

As Galin (1974) puts it:

> All of the above considerations lead us to examine the hypothesis that in normal, intact people, mental events in the right hemisphere can become disconnected functionally from the left hemisphere (by inhibition of neuronal transmission across the corpus callosum and other cerebral commissures) and can continue a life of their own. This hypothesis suggests a neurophysiological mechanism for at least some instances of repression and an anatomical locus for some of the unconscious mental contents. (p. 582)

Galin goes on to discuss various situations under which such a functional commissurotomy may occur, but does not offer any experimental physiological evidence to support the validity of the concept. In similar explorations in the field of psychosomatic mechanisms, Hoppe (1977) felt that the presence of clinical patterns of alexithymia,* paucity of dreams, and operational thinking in commissurotomized and in psychosomatic patients as reported by Sifneos (1973), and Nemiah (1970) spoke for the existence of a functional commissurotomy in the latter group of patients. Hoppe and Bogen (1977) found evidence of more severe alexithymia in their commissurotomized patients than Sifneos had found in psychosomatic subjects using the same test parameters, and they concluded that in the latter group the functional commissurotomy was relative rather than absolute. They felt that this difference supported the functional nature of the syndrome.

The argument for the existence of a functional commissurotomy is based on analogy rather than on firm experimental evidence. The only suggestive evidence at this time is that by Richard Davidson (1985) on delayed reaction times described in the last chapter. But one can explain the phenomenology of repression on the basis of less unlikely mechanisms and without invoking the unproven functional commissurotomy. The previously described subcortical mechanism of channeling perceptual stimuli for differential hemispheric processing characterized by either distorted processing in the left hemisphere or delayed passage through the right appears to offer a better paradigm. Within this model, differential hemispheric channeling would occur through some form of screening at the subcortical level on the basis of mechanisms described earlier in this volume. Under such circumstances, a kind of functional separation between the hemispheres might be accomplished, not on the basis of a physiological zone of inhibition, but rather on the basis of such differential channeling of different kinds of material to one hemisphere or the other with subsequent differential treatment.

Galin speculates that the right hemisphere may be an important repository for repressed negatively charged engrams and hence, given even a relative functional separation between the hemispheres, one part of the dynamic unconscious. This could be at best only a partial explanation. For example, Hoppe (1977) studied the dream patterns of a woman who had had a total right hemispherectomy for a malignancy. It proved that she, too, reported dreams, even though they were infrequent and characterized by operational thinking. It would be difficult to postulate that part of this woman's dynamic unconscious had been resected even though the nature of her unconscious brain activity may certainly have been modified. At most one can speculate that under certain circumstances, e.g., REM dreaming, engrams in the right hemisphere (those more primitive, more veridical and symbolic, more holistic and less verbal, more emotionally negative, and generally less accessible to conscious awareness) might be more readily activated than those in the left hemisphere and might thus play a larger role in certain types of unconscious brain activity. This interpretation is more or less in line with Galin's thesis.

However, it is important to emphasize that there may also be found in the left hemisphere large reservoirs of negatively charged unconscious engrams, probably equal in number to those postulated to exist in the right. Furthermore, despite the general differences in content and function between the two hemispheres, it is most probable that both repressive and intellectualizing functions would occur in each of them. It would still be true that repression would be more characteristic of right-

---

*A separation of emotional reaction from cognitive awareness.

hemispheric activity, both because of the nature of its engram content (more negatively emotionally charged) and because of the nature of right-hemispheric function (less conscious). Conversely, even though repression could occur in the left hemisphere, its characteristics there would probably be somewhat different from those of the right hemisphere, namely, less complete, possibly involved as much with distortion as with repression, and much more involved with verbal manipulations. In this way, the two hemispheres would operate somewhat independently, but on the whole, concurrently. Then the unconscious, defined as the sum total of all information contained in the brain but not in awareness at any given moment, would have its locus not in any one part of the brain, right hemisphere or otherwise, but in the entire brain.

In this modified form, the speculation of Ornstein (1972) and Galin (1974) that some important elements of the dynamic unconscious may lie *predominantly* in the right hemisphere seems somewhat less implausible than might at first have appeared. Our present formulation has to my mind, however, certain advantages over that of Ornstein and Galin. For one thing, it does not emphasize the right hemisphere to the exclusion of the left, but rather suggests an integrated interactional relationship. For another, it does not require hypothesizing the existence of a "functional commissurotomy," an unproved entity, but substitutes for that differential priming of the two hemispheres, a mechanism for which there is substantial evidence. This present formulation then offers a psychobiological paradigm of a dynamic unconscious where the allocation of engrams to the dynamic unconscious as opposed to the preconscious is the product of three effects: (1) hierarchical mechanisms at the brain stem level producing either cognitive inhibition or stimulation, (2) differential channeling, again at the brain stem level, to the two hemispheres for differential processing, and (3) differential processing in the two hemispheres.

Activities in the Decathected Dynamic Unconscious

In Chapter 13 we presented evidence that highly negatively charged episodic engrams are processed in the upstream phase by de-energizing the cognitive component. There would then be a consequent suppression of the excessive arousal associated with the original highly negative emotional charge. As a consequence of their lower cognitive valence, their lower arousal levels, and their more negative emotional charge, these engrams would tend to be shunted to the right hemisphere where, both because of their hierarchical treatment and because of the nature of right hemispheric function, they would tend to remain unconscious and relatively irretrievable to conscious memory (see Chapter 6). Such engrams would be said to have been "repressed" or "denied," and would constitute the major elements in that special compartment of the dynamic unconscious known as the "decathected unconscious."

Psychoanalysis and psychobiology diverge significantly in their theoretical positions on the level of cognitive arousal associated with "repressed" engrams in the dynamic unconscious. Freudian theory holds that repressed engrams in the unconscious, because they are highly charged emotionally and because they are unable to achieve conscious expression, foment in a constantly agitated manner. (It is this conception of ungratified primitive needs that led Freud to the formulation of the id operating in a dynamic unconscious in which conflicts between opposing forces are only somewhat reconciled.) The present psychobiological interpretation of the activity of repressed engrams in the unconscious is qualitatively different. It holds that desensitization of engrams by denial or repression occurs through an inhibition of the energy level of its cognitive component with an associated decrease in arousal. From this it follows that such engrams exist in the unconscious at a *lower* cognitive energy level and at a *lower* than the original level of arousal. Even if the disassociation process is not completely effective so that the level of arousal remains somewhat high, the inhibition of the cognitive component should still reduce the activity of that particular engram both at the cognitive and affective levels.

Although this formulation postulates a different functional mechanism from that posited by Freud as underlying the development of neurosis, the overall conceptualization presented here is still consistent within the psychoanalytic concept of "free-floating anxiety" associated with reactivation of decathected engrams. If, for example, in a claustrophic individual particular episodic engrams representing an earlier experience have been decathected by some repressive mechanism, the individual's anxiety remains controlled as long as no external or internal event cognitively reactivates those engrams. If a related event does occur, the cognitive engram would be reactivated sufficiently to permit the build-up of unsupportable anxiety (the arousal element), but not sufficiently to permit the engram to rise cognitively to awareness. Under these circumstances, free-floating anxiety could occur without awareness of the underlying cause. This construct is not so very different from the psychoanalytic except that it construes repressed engrams as lying dormant in the unconscious until they are reactivated rather than as existing in a state of constant agitation.

Under these conditions, what effect if any would such repressed engrams have upon conscious behavior? Obviously, a great deal. If external experience associated with the original repressed engrams would lead to exacerbation of severe latent anxiety, then such experience would be assiduously avoided. Because perception of the emotional component occurs during unconscious upstream processing, the individual would be unaware of the causes of his sometimes bizarre behavior. In the psychobiological formulation of the decathected unconscious, repressed engrams exert their influence not as in the psychoanalytic model through the direct effect of hyperactive engrams on behavior, but rather indirectly through the negative effect of hypoactive engrams in a feedback circuit designed to avoid reactivation.

On the other hand, in the psychobiological model where threatening engrams have been decathected in the left hemisphere through sensitizing defense mechanisms, they are considered to exist in the dynamic unconscious at an increased cognitive energy level (perceptual vigilance), but at a decreased level of emotional arousal (see Lazarus et al. study, Fig. 16-1). Such engrams could also exercise a greater than normal influence on unconscious mental activity. Under these circumstances, conscious behavior would be directed not necessarily toward avoiding those experiences that might reinforce the original conflict-producing engram, but would rather be governed by activities, mental or physical, that would reinforce the intellectualistic rationalizing defense mechanism. Here the hypercharged engrams would exert a more direct influence on behavior, similar to that hypothesized in psychoanalytic formulations.

Despite the general emphasis on right-hemispheric unconscious activity, the exercise of sensitizing defense mechanisms in the left hemisphere may represent in some ways a more important normal component of total dynamic unconscious activity. For one thing, in left-hemispheric defensive activity, decathected reactivities would have a more direct, albeit distorted, influence on overt behavior than would the avoidance behavior characteristic of right-hemispheric activity. For another, left-hemispheric behavior would be evident in everyday conscious activity, where such distorted reactions as projection, intellectualization, and reaction-formation are readily observed. This is in opposition to the right-hemispheric behaviors of denial and repression, where the critical conflict is hidden and becomes overt only during periods of suppression of left-hemispheric activity, as for example, in dreams, in altered states of consciousness, and in neurotic behavior when the repressed material can surface.

Finally, while it is true that most normal activity is controlled through the activities of the cathected component of the dynamic unconscious, it is also true that much normal behavior and almost all neurotic behavior stems from the more complex workings of the decathected dynamic unconscious. Nor do we mean to imply that only in neurotics does the decathected unconscious play the major role, although the latter is certainly true. But all humans are exposed to conflictual struggles, if only because of the conflicts associated with being a biological organism living in a highly structured social environment. Hence an understanding of the workings of the decathected unconscious is necessary for the understanding of normal behavior and essential for the understanding of neurotic behavior. The following chapters will deal with the normal human experiences, particularly those of childhood, that through their effects in the decathected unconscious influence personality development and produce neuroses.

18

The Role of Childhood and Adult Stress in the Genesis of the Decathected Unconscious

Much time and space have been given in this volume to a description of the dynamics, the mechanisms, and especially the neurophysiology of the "decathected unconscious," but paradoxically very little experimental data have been presented to describe in any detail the substantive content of that entity. The reason for this omission has been the direction of our interest, which until now has been concerned mainly with the definition of physiological mechanisms. Theoretically, the activities of the decathected unconscious, because of the influences of powerful defensive mechanisms, should be most likely to produce some variety of neurotic behavior. But this is only partially true since defensive measures often successfully decathect threatening material. In order to provide more substantial experimental and clinical data on the operation of the decathected unconscious in normals, we will emphasize in this chapter the normal use of defense mechanisms in the decathected unconscious. Only in the later chapters of the book will we extrapolate to more neurotic behavior.

Normal Behavior and the Cathected Unconscious

First a word about normal behavior and the role of the "cathected unconscious" in its control. It seems clear that because of the nature of cognitive processing, normal conscious episodic cognition is heavily influenced by ongoing processes at the unconscious level. The most behavioristic psychologies would not contradict this position; indeed, by denying the existence of consciousness, behaviorists tend to make all behavior unconscious. The more clinically oriented branch of behaviorist psychology, i.e., learning theory, deals with the question of conscious versus unconscious behavior chiefly by avoiding it. In that system, the reactions of individuals to a variety of

stresses are considered to be established through one or another conditioning paradigms in mechanisms that underlie all future behavior. But the question remains as to
where and how memories of the initial experiences are maintained so that they may be
identified with a new related experience to reactivate the old established behavior.
Certainly such engrams must exist at some procedural or episodic unconscious level in
the brain. Behaviorists acknowledge this, but claim that this unconscious is merely an
inert reservoir in no way similar to the Freudian cauldron of dynamic interaction.
Hence they attach little significance to it.

The psychobiological point of view is intermediate between that of learning
theory and psychoanalysis. Its position is that a dynamic unconscious does exist and is
active but in a different sense than that postulated in psychoanalysis. As in Freudian
theory, the psychobiological model holds that the dynamic unconscious is active at all
times and in all states of consciousness, and that it continually exerts its influences on
conscious, preconscious, procedural unconscious, and visceral behavior. However, it
conceives of the dynamic unconscious not so much as an independent entity, but as one
level of activity in a continuous spectrum of interactions that control both the internal
workings and the external behavior of the organism. One might define these interactions as the result of neurophysiological feedback and feedforward influences, more in
keeping in quality with the conditioned reflexes of learning theory than with the more
anthropomorphic constellations of the conflicts between id, ego, and superego. Despite
this, the overall thrust of the interactions between conscious and unconscious motivations in the psychobiological model prove paradoxically to be more similar to the
sturm und drang of Freudian theory than to the mechanistic views of learning theory.

The shortcomings of learning theory have been excellently summarized by Janis
(1969). He writes:

> The "leakage" of the repressed anxiety-provoking cues into other mental activities
> involves many complications that are difficult to explain by learning theory. This is
> one of the main reasons many psychologists and psychiatrists have severly criticized
> learning theorists and have accused them of oversimplifying complex personality
> functions. They also criticize learning theories as being too narrowly based on a
> simple model constructed from animal experiments on reactions to painful stimula-
> tion. Although few doubts are expressed about the applicability of these experiments
> as a model for human traumatic learning, many serious questions are raised about
> extending the model to include other types of human anguish that often arise in
> stressful life circumstances—grief over the loss of a loved one, shame about failing on
> an important task, guilt about violating one's ethical standards, and those vague
> feelings of self-discontent described so expressively by existentialist writers. These
> emotions have powerful motivating effects, which presumably can become even
> stronger than fear of external harm, since they can compel a person to commit suicide.
> But they seem to be based on cognitive processes that have a uniquely human quality,
> involving conceptions of the self and anticipations of future interaction with fellow
> human beings. Much of the strong opposition to learning theory approaches centers
> upon doubts that these human cognitive processes can ever be translated validly into
> the simple laws of conditioning derived from animal research. (p. 61)

Janis' statement emphasizes both the weaknesses and strengths of learning theory
psychology. Among the major deficits are the lack of reference to the subjective and
executive "selfs," the entities that represent the organism as a whole and which are
ultimately the final arbiters of behavior. Because learning theory is a reductionist rather

than a holistic psychology, it reduces behavior to mechanistic interactions among relatively rigid mental entities rather than seeing them dynamically as fluid interchanges among interacting elements. Psychoanalysis has the latter virtue, but because of its particular theoretical structure, finds it difficult to set up experimental situations to test its theses.

Recent learning theorists have attempted to overcome the deficits in their psychology by borrowing those concepts from psychoanalysis that make learning theory more applicable to human experience. For example, George F. Mahl (1969) has presented a diagrammatic model of a conditioning paradigm of an emotional overreaction. Mahl introduces the concept of the unconscious and even a repressive barrier, but considers the unconscious mainly as the place where memory sets rest before they are brought to awareness. In his concept there is only a moderate influence of such memory sets on behavior and these are through mechanisms that are only implied and not well described.

Both the strengths and weaknesses of learning theory become evident in an analysis of normal behavioral mechanisms as postulated in learning theory as compared with those theoretically determined by the activities of the psychobiological cathected unconscious. In the latter operation, as in learning theory, positive emotional charge is associated with perceptual vigilance and approach behavior; conversely, negative emotional charge is associated with perceptual vigilance, but with avoidance behavior. But against this similarity, the two systems differ, mainly in the emphasis of psychobiology on the derivation of all human behavior from operations at the mental level. Psychobiology insists upon the overall dominance of the two selves—the subjective and the executive—in determining all behavior just as psychoanalysis invokes the ego. Learning theory is much more reductionist in its analyses of behavioral reactivities. But unless one appeals to some higher order of organization, how is one to understand the willingness of a child to insist on learning to ride a bicycle despite repeated painful falls. Except in terms of mental sets established by the self-system, such behavior would be almost inexplicable.

Classical psychoanalytic theory, on the other hand, seems to err in the opposite direction by assuming that most so-called normal behavior is activated by neurotic motivations that must be suppressed. In the orthodox Freudian system, for example, sexual-type reactions are universally dominant and must be reacted against; consequently, there are few uncomplicated direct responses to relatively uncomplicated stimuli. The Freudian unconscious is most comparable to the psychobiological decathected unconscious in that both consist of potentially stressful thought processes. But there is little or no provision made in psychoanalysis for relatively normal behaviors, comparable to those generated in the psychobiological cathected unconscious where reactions are simply and directly related to the emotional charge and significance of the stimulus.

The traditional psychoanalytic position emphasized neurotic behavior at the expense of normal behavior and it may be that this prejudice, deriving from clinical experience, has spilled over into psychoanalytic theory. Indeed, a more recent post-Freudian psychoanalytic theory elaborated by Heinz Hartmann and known as "ego psychology," makes a similar point. Lasch (1984) describes this position as follows:

> In order to become a general psychology, Hartmann (1958) argues in his *Ego Psychology and the Problem of Adaptation,* psychoanalysis has to deal with aspects of

"adaptive development" that are allegedly free of conflict—that is, with those "functions" of the ego that cannot be reduced to defensive mechanisms against the conflicting demands of the id and the superego. These include a remarkably broad range of activities: perception, thought, language, motor development, and even memory. To those who might argue that such matters lie outside the scope of psychoanalysis, Hartmann replies that "if we take seriously the claim of psychoanalysis to be a general theory of mental development, we must study this area of psychology too." (pp. 219–220)

Lasch objects to Hartmann's contention that there is a "conflict-free ego sphere," but psychobiological considerations would tend to support it. Indeed, in our construct, the domain of the conscious (the preconscious and the cathected unconscious) spends its major activities not only on the "conflict-free ego sphere," but even on some conscious conflictual events that are too immediate and too urgent to be treated by decathexis. For example, if one steps out of the way of a speeding car, it is very doubtful how much, if at all, the decathected unconscious is involved. Lasch (1984) fears that eliminating so much of the dynamics of the classical Freudian unconscious will only emasculate the theory. My own feeling, with Hartmann, is that it enlarges and enriches it.

Normal Behavior and the Decathected Unconscious

Where learning theory is probably as effective as is psychoanalysis in explaining most normal behavior, the situation is completely reversed in cases of neurotic behavior. Such patients engage in a variety of activities that clearly do not follow the basic dicta of learning theory nor of the cathected unconscious, i.e., positive emotional charge should produce perceptual vigilance and approach behavior, and negative emotional charge should produce perceptual vigilance and avoidance behavior. In fact, neurotic behavior so often violates these basic learning theory principles as to seem often to operate under an entirely different set of influences. Learning theory does attempt to explain such discrepancies through the invocation of generalizing effects of noxious stimuli, but those explanations are too vague and nonspecific to be satisfying.

Psychoanalytic explanations, on the other hand, are often more specific than the evidence can support. Moreover, patients described in the psychoanalytic literature not infrequently demonstrate symptomatology such as hallucinations and bizarre ideation that appears to extend beyond the limits of simple neurosis into the realm of the "borderline disorders." Since the latter may be considered to represent at least a psychotic tendency and since the dynamics of psychoses are entirely different from those of the neuroses, one should hesitate to utilize psychoticlike material in the interpretation of neurotic behavior.

But within these limits, many psychoanalytic formulations appear to be fully compatible with the psychobiological model of neurosis. Formulations dealing with the nature and content of the Freudian dynamic unconscious and of the psychobiological decathected unconscious are basically similar, despite certain significant differences. Among the latter are the nature of the repressive mechanisms that decathect negatively charged perceptions and thoughts (physiological mechanisms as opposed to the repressive barrier); the degree of irrationality and symbolism in unconscious thought processes (left- and right-hemispheric unconscious processing versus primary process logic); and the nature of the biological motivations in conflict with psychosocial demands (biological drives as opposed to the id). However, the psychobiological dynamic unconscious, both cathected and decathected, is regulated by precise and specific physiological mechanisms, more or less like those of learning theory and unlike those of the irrational churning of the Freudian unconscious. On the other hand, the psychobiological unconscious is, like the Freudian unconscious, a dynamic one where actions and interactions among complementary and opposing drives are continuous, always operating within the rubric of the subjective and executive selves (or the Freudian ego) to determine all conscious and unconscious behavior.

As a consequence of the sharing of these basic principles, psychobiology and psychoanalysis find the construct of a dynamic unconscious critical to the understanding of human behavior. Since clinical access to that dynamic unconscious is mainly through dreams, free association, and altered states of consciousness (Chapter 22), these become important elements in the theory and practice of both of these disciplines. This is less true for learning theory where the unconscious is seen as a relatively inert domain in which memories lie passively until summoned to awareness. Nevertheless, all three systems agree that is is through the effects of some stressful situations, residual either in an active or a passive unconscious, that major changes in personality occur.

The Effects of Stress on Psychological Behavior

Even though psychoanalysis and learning theory agree that the origins of much normal behavior and of almost all neurotic behavior stem from the negative effects of emotional stress, psychoanalysis conceptualizes such stress as mainly an internal mental affair, generated by the conflict of drives in the id against the opposing forces of ego and superego, whereas learning theory perceives stress as coming essentially from the environment. In each case, primary external events are ultimately internalized but in different forms. In psychoanalysis the main battlefield becomes that of the "mind"; in learning theory it remains that of experience reflected neurologically in various conditioning paradigms.

For the purposes of psychobiology, this aspect of learning theory philosophy is fortunate. Responses to external stress are relatively easy to examine experimentally, whereas the Freudian dynamics of internal stress can be explored probably only through psychoanalytic methodology. For example, the understanding of the origin of anxiety neuroses, deduced from couch analysis to stem from memories of childhood separation, can be enhanced by studies of separation experiences in young children (Mahler, 1972) and in a more extreme form, in young primates (Harlow and Zimmerman, 1959). Similarly, isolation and social deprivation studies in infant primates such as those performed by Harlow and Zimmerman (1959) are elaborated by similar clinical observations in human children (Spitz, 1945). Certainly such experimental studies and observations are not contrary to psychoanalytic principles; on the contrary, some of the most important observations in these areas have been made by orthodox Freudians (Mahler, 1972; Spitz, 1945). Consequently, the studies to be quoted should be seen as compatible with psychoanalytic, learning theory, and psychobiological thinking.

The major environmental stresses are considered by Janis (1969) to fall under three main emotional rubrics: (1) anxiety, manifested as fear, shame, or guilt; (2) anger deriving from frustration and resulting in aggression; and (3) grief, deriving from separation, isolation, or some personal loss, and resulting in depression. By no means do these three paradigms exhaust all of the possible patterns of emotional reactivity. However, Janis (1969) considers that among them they explain many of the processes that influence personality development and that may be instrumental in the genesis of the neuroses.

The Normal Role of the Defense Mechanisms in Allaying Anxiety

Anxiety is the biological reactivity to an overwhelming emotionally threatening event in the environment. In certain pathological states, the so-called anxiety neuroses, anxiety may occur in the absence of any apparent overt external cause. Such anxiety is called free-floating and is presumed psychobiologically to derive from unresolved conflict, possibly aggravated by some underlying genetic diathesis.

Freud (1926) differentiated between normal and neurotic anxiety on the basis of how reality oriented the emotional reaction was. He described normal anxiety as evoked by "real danger which threatens from some external object" (p. 151). Janis (1969) defines neurotic anxiety as involving "intense emotional reactions and defensive efforts which are out of all proportion to the relatively mild or non-existent threat to which the person attributes his distress" (p. 113). Janis further refines the concept of "normal anxiety" by redefining it as "reflective anxiety," or anxiety as it exists in the mind of the individual in response to real threats whether such threats be in the immediate environment or whether they exist only among his mental reflections as possibilities of certain eventualities. He classifies such threats as being envisioned as (1) weak, (2) moderate, or (3) strong, and describes the behavioral reaction to each, respectively, as (1) a tendency to deny the threat and to seek reassurance as to its nonexistence, (2) a tendency to become more vigilant and to take planning and precautionary measures, and (3) a tendency to become jittery and upset, to be indiscriminately vigilant, and to lose mental efficiency.

The response curve for effective performance under such increasing levels of anxiety is essentially that described as characteristic of the inverted U-shaped curve relating performance and level of arousal (Fig. 3-1) and is reflected in Janis' three levels of reaction. Janis illustrates this with a study from Zemach (1966) in which college men were exhorted to volunteer for civil rights activities. Three pamphlets were distributed, one generating a mild sense of guilt, the second a moderate sense of guilt, and the third intended to generate an overwhelming sense of guilt. The relative effectiveness of the three pamphlets followed the inverted U-shaped curve, where the pamphlet provoking least guilt produced only moderate results (about 28%), the pamphlet provoking a moderate sense of guilt was most effective in recruiting volunteers (over 50%) and that provoking intense guilt was least effective (about 10%).

The demonstrated impairment of performance is indicative of "reflective guilt," described by Janis as one manifestation of reflective anxiety. Consequently, the low volunteer rate at the highest level of guilt arousal is assumed to be not neurotic, but rather a normal reaction to the generation of excessive anxiety. But in this maximal guilt-evoking situation, no instructions were given to provide a defensive mental set of either rationalization or denial similar to that provided by Lazarus et al. (1965) in the primitive rites study described in Chapter 16 (Fig. 16-1). One would surmise that if psychological defense mechanisms had been experimentally induced by Zemach (1966) as by Lazarus et al. (1965) that the recruitment rate in the high-guilt group might have been significantly higher. The presumed effect of introducing defense mechanisms, sensitizing or desensitizing, is ostensibly to reduce the level of anxiety (guilt) by moving the point of operational effect from the extreme right of the curve further to the left and thus improving the overall performance rate (in this case the level of recruitment).

All of these processes are within the range of normal psychological activity and need by no means be considered neurotic. On the contrary, in this last example of the use of defense mechanisms against a high level of guilt and also in the previously described Lazarus et al. (1965) study (Fig. 16-1), defense mechanisms are effective against normally derived anxiety reactions. High levels of anxiety must be dealt with even in normal behavior. In the psychobiological model, only that highly threatening material is channeled to the decathected unconscious where the disruptive effects of excessive emotionality can be permanently attenuated through cognitive and emotional modulation. The specific management of threatening material is of course dependent on the nature of the material, the defensive style of the individual, and the emotional and social setting of the particular event.

Consequently, it is apparent that the activities of the decathected unconscious are responsible for much normal as well as for most neurotic behavior. Generally, it is as a result of the breakdown of homeostatic mechanisms in the decathected dynamic unconscious that neuroses occur. As with other psychobiological parameters, this may happen when defense mechanisms are either too weak or become overloaded (see Chapter 20). These considerations require an analyses of individual personality and of the different kinds of reactivities that may produce such instabilities. The entire question of the pathogenesis of the neuroses will be addressed in a more detailed fashion in the final chapters of this volume.

Anxiety, Fear, Shame, and Guilt in the Decathected Unconscious

In the previous section, we differentiated between normal or reflective anxiety and neurotic anxiety with the stipulation that both types of anxiety could be divided into subtypes depending on the nature of their derivation. These subtypes of anxiety are fear, shame, and guilt. Fear is the anxiety aroused by some specific threat, real or unreal, to the individual; shame, the anxiety generated by the threat of loss of social status; and guilt, the anxiety stemming from within from some sense of personal neglect or irresponsibility (Janis, 1969).

The anxiety associated with fear is the most typical and is that usually referred to when the term is used. It is accompanied by a more overwhelming sense of disaster and of physiological and psychological disruption than generally occurs with shame or guilt. It has been suggested that the anxiety associated with guilt is separate and distinct from the guilt itself and arises from its association with a fear of personal retribution. In that sense, fear and anxiety may be identical in their patterns of physiological and psychological manifestations, whereas shame and guilt may incur anxiety only as a secondary effect.

Kagan (1969) has differentiated between guilt and shame as follows:

> At a superficial level, guilt and shame seem similar, for both are characterized by an unpleasant feeling that results from violating a standard. At a somewhat deeper level, however, one finds that there are means of differentiating between the two. The behavioral manifestations of shame and guilt are one means of differentiation. Shame is commonly, although not always, accompanied by blushing or lowering of the head and eyes. Guilt does not typically lead to any characteristic set of behaviors that are quite so public.
>
> The conditions that elicit guilt and shame provide another basis for differentiation. The unpleasant feelings called shame are elicited by an expectation that other people will be disappointed in the fact that a standard has been violated. The unpleasant feelings called guilt are caused by expectations that the self will disapprove. The child is likely to feel shame when he believes he has violated a standard that someone has held for him. Shame is therefore tied to anticipation of disapproval from others for violation of a standard that the child accepts. Guilt, on the other hand, is more independent of the expectation of disapproval from another person. The child experiences guilt when he anticipates reprisal from his own conscience for violation of a standard he has set for himself, rather than of one he believes other people have set for him. (p. 471)

These distinctions are enormously important in the dynamics of human behavior. Effects vary greatly depending on whether these emotional reactivities arise from real outside events (reflective anxiety, fear, shame, or guilt), or rather from imagined internal cogitations, particularly those at the unconscious level (neurotic anxiety, fear, shame, or guilt). Each of these emotional reactivities appears to be differently susceptible to personal exorcism. Real fear seems to be most readily accommodated to, real shame somewhat less so, and real guilt least. In the hierarchy of anxiety-producing emotions, the sense of guilt is more commonly incorporated into the deep unconscious in an unsatisfactorily decathected form than are shame or fear and is hence more difficult to eradicate.

According to Horney (1936), most anxiety neuroses stem from an unworked-through sense of guilt. This is probably so because of the fact that of the three anxiety-related emotions—fear, shame, and guilt—the latter is the most internalized and the one least dependent on external reinforcement. Accordingly, it is not surprising that in the psychoanalytic system, where most significant conflict is considered to be between the id and the ego and superego, i.e., completely internalized, some form of guilt is the almost universal progenitor of neurotic anxiety.

The Psychobiological View of the Oedipal Complex

The dominant source of internalized guilt in psychoanalytic theory is the Oedipal complex, the result of a constellation of instinctual reactivities and of personal experiences in early childhood (3–5 years) in which the child's love for the parent of the opposite sex evolves together with an equal hatred of the parent of the same sex. Freud postulated that the depth of the guilt generated derived from the duality of the criminal intent fantasized, first in the desire of the child to have intercourse with the parent of the opposite sex and second in the desire to murder the parent of the same sex. These childhood fantasies were only partially sublimated during development so that deep-seated Oedipal conflicts remain, universally, in a more or less sublimated form in normals and in a decompensated form in neurotics.

The general observation that children tend to prefer the parent of the opposite sex and frequently to reject the parent of the same sex is so common as to leave little question of its validity. But one can reach this same conclusion through the observations of learning theory and psychobiology without invoking fantasies of incest and murder in the minds of 3- and 4-year-olds. There are many reasons why such a reaction should exist. For one thing, the reverse relationship is probably also true; parents tend to prefer their children of the opposite sex and are usually kinder, more gentle, and less demanding with them. For another, during the period of the original infantile attachment of children to their mothers, especially in boys, the father becomes a serious competitor for the mother's affection. However, this is equally true for girls, yet they do not learn to dislike their fathers. Some other factor must be operating.

Ultimately one is almost compelled to accept the existence of some biological instinctive force that determines heterosexual preference, certainly in the parents, but equally in young children. Is this force infantile sexuality as defined by Freud? Yes and no. Certainly some such biological attraction can account for preference of children for the parent of the opposite sex, for the pleasures of masturbation, and for a variety of psychological conflicts that may derive from these impulses. But it still seems psychobiologically improbable that a 3- or 4-year-old can cognitively conceive of either sexual intercourse or murder to create the Freudian constellation of the Oedipal conflict. Nor does it appear necessary to invoke such murderous and incestuous fantasies to justify the existence of the Oedipal conflict. The latter would be just as real if it were based on somewhat less extreme feelings of love for the parent of the opposite sex and of hatred for the other.

Psychoanalysts may smile at my willingness to go halfway with them in the implicit acceptance of infantile sexuality by postulating an instinctual biological preference for the opposite sex, even in children, but resisting the larger concept of fantasies of incestuous intercourse and murder. But my resistance is based not on any illusions about child innocence, but rather on the sense that children are just not sufficiently developed cognitively to entertain such fantasies.

Most importantly, the foregoing considerations appear to lend considerable support to the Freudian position that the Oedipal complex does play a significant role in generating internalized conflict in the decathected unconscious. There, if it is not adequately sublimated or otherwise defended against, it will generate strong feelings of guilt. Similar mechanisms can be hypothesized for feelings of guilt deriving from the earlier stages of psychosexual development—the oral and the anal—where ambivalent feelings of love and hatred are simultaneously generated as some desires are fulfilled and others frustrated.

Frustration, Anger, and Aggression

Hostility and hatred are invoked not only in psychoanalysis, but in learning theory as well. On the relationship of frustration, anger, and aggression, Janis (1969) writes:

> Normal anger . . . is characterized by at least a rough proportionality between the severity of the provocative frustration perceived by the frustrated person and the intensity of his aggressive reaction. The point was first made by Freud, who postulated that aggression would always occur as a basic reaction to frustrating circumstances—whenever pleasure-seeking or pain-avoiding behavior was blocked (1917). This postulate is widely accepted today by most psychologists; moreover it is firmly established by both clinical and experimental evidence. (p. 149)

Frustration has been identified clinically and experimentally as the chief cause of aggressivity; the association has been concretized in the so-called frustration–aggression hypothesis of Dollard et al. (1939). In experimental situations where frustration is a short-term and transitory experience, the first reactions are aggressive and hyperexcitatory, as described by Rosenzweig (1938). When frustration is continued for extensive periods, when aggressive action has proved futile, or when aggressive action is itself punished, then the excitatory phase subsides and a phase of excessive inhibition tends to ensue.

The usual definition of frustration is a situational one where the individual who has a strong drive toward a goal, which is readily observable and apparently achievable, is thwarted in his attempt to achieve that goal by some, to his way of thinking, unreasonable barrier. Under the frustration–aggression hypothesis, such a situation normally leads to either aggressive behavior or, if that is prohibited, at least to aggressive feelings. These in themselves lead to a state of increased excitation, unless there are counteracting influences to prohibit aggressive behavior or to inhibit the conscious awareness of aggressive feelings.

The interesting element in frustration–aggression experiments is the sharp difference between the behavior of the first excitatory stage and that of the second inhibitory stage. In the first stage there is an outburst of irrational activity and inefficient mental responsivity even in adults, activities that resemble the infantile banging of enraged frustrated children. When this reactivity has proven to be unavailing, the second inhibitory phase ensues. Here the individual will react with many forms of repressed anger including sarcasm, irritability, and other poorly camouflaged hostile responses.

Janis continues:

> In many real-life frustrating situations similar indirect or symbolic ways of expressing aggression are likely to be observed, especially in circumstances where people realize that they can get into serious trouble by expressing hostility openly. The subtle manifestations of hostility, however, may be missed entirely by an outsider who is unfamiliar with the subculture of a particular community, social class, or occupational

group whose traditions may prescribe certain types of humor, playful needling, or cool indifference as the preferred means for expressing hostile feelings to one another. (p. 154)

Rosenzweig (1938, 1943) has elaborated an extensive hypothesis of normal and abnormal types of behavior based on the characteristic mode of handling frustration. He postulates that frustration is the most ubiquitous emotionally charged situation that confronts the individual, since it involves a large variety of conflictual situations. These may include the conflict between individual desires and environmental demands, between individual expectations and reality (the kind of cognitive dissonance that occurs in nonreinforced conditioning), and in ambiguous situations where reward or punishment also do not follow along natural lines of expectation. Reasoning from studies in which some subjects tend to remember failures while others tend to remember success, Rosenzweig (1938) attributed these differences in behavior to differences in personal style of handling frustration. He writes:

> When an individual experiences frustration, insofar as he does not allocate responsibility for the unhappy occurrence in an objective way, he may respond in one of the three following typical subjective ways or some combination of them: (1) he may manifest the emotion of anger and condemn the outer world (other persons, objects and circumstance) for his frustration, adopting an attitude of hostility toward his environment. This type of reaction may be termed "extrapunitive"; (2) he may react with emotions of guilt and remorse and tend to condemn himself as the blame-worthy object. This type of reaction may be termed "intrapunitive"; (3) he may experience emotions of embarrassment and shame, making little of blame and emphasizing instead the conciliation of others and himself to the disagreeable situation. In this case he will be more interested in condoning than in condemning and will pass off the frustration as lightly as possible by making references, even at the price of self-deception, to unavoidable circumstances. This type of reaction may be termed "impunitive."

Thus, in handling highly charged emotional situations, the "extrapunitive" response would be in psychobiological terms the most overt and the "intrapunitive" would reflect a turning inwardly resulting in guilt and depression. On the other hand, the "impunitive" response would presumably involve defensiveness that could be either of the "desensitizing" or "sensitizing" variety, characterized, respectively, by either denial or repression of the entire episode or conversely by some form of intellectualization. These reactivities provide a broad spectrum of responses, each of which would lead, in different personalities, to different kinds of neurotic distortions. For example, the extrapunitive style of responsivity may be incorporated in certain sociopathic and sadomasochistic reactivities. The intrapunitive is more characteristic of mechanisms that lead to certain types of reactive depressions. Finally, the impunitive response associated with a general denial of anger and hostility has been identified as involved in the pathogenesis of various psychosomatic illnesses, particularly ulcerative colitis and bronchial asthma.

The Grief Syndrome

A different reactivity, separate and distinct from that either of anxiety or frustration, occurs in very young children and primates when they are separated from their mother for any significant period (Janis, 1964). The experimental prototype of the "separation syndrome" or "bereavement response" was produced by Harlow and Zimmerman (1959) in monkeys. Infant monkeys separated from their mothers at the age of 3–4 months react for the first day with screaming, kicking, and grimacing. This reaction is considered a built-in biological reaction pattern that, because it attracts the mother's attention and usually brings her scampering back to attend the infant, serves a preservatory function in the evolutionary process. The more variable part of the syndrome begins usually on the second day when the infant withdraws into a "defeated" reaction mode which is highly comparable to the anaclitic depressions of unmothered children in orphanages described by Spitz (1945). Characteristically, these infant monkeys sit huddled and withdrawn at the rear of their cages, unmoving, unresponsive to outside stimulation, very inactive, appearing fearful and totally subdued, and manifesting poor appetite and little social interaction. These responsivities remain for as long as the animal remains isolated, and if not corrected are prolonged into adult life.

Ethologists have attempted to explain at least some of the behavioral manifestations as a reaction to the deprivation of biological experiences necessary for maturation. Monkey infants isolated at birth, when they enter the "depression phase," not only huddle over and curl up into a typical defensive position of emotional retreat, but also clutch themselves by crossing their arms and holding their upper arms with their hands, as though to provide the tactile stimulation of their bodies which apparently is so necessary for their normal development. This huddling and self-clutching behavior may be seen as a fixation at the earliest phase of development where continual holding and fondling are so essential to the infant's well-being. Rosenblum and Plimpton (1981) have described these developments as follows:

> The separated infant is faced with the problem of how to reestablish, either within itself and/or through its interactions with others, the range of regulation which the mother has provided. Isolation-rearing studies have provided one example of how an infant will attempt to establish an equilibrium within itself. Stereotyped motor acts are frequently observed in both human and nonhuman primates, raised under various levels of deprivation. Berkson has suggested that stereotyped behaviors are infantile patterns which have been redirected as a consequence of deprivation rearing. When infants are placed into social isolation at birth, at a point when sucking and clasping reflexes are strong, high levels of self-sucking and self-clasping almost always develop (Berkson, 1968). (p. 238)

Further support for this interpretation is provided by the classic experiment of Harlow and Zimmerman (1959) who compared object attachment to two "surrogate mothers" (one made of wire, the other covered with terry cloth) by infant monkeys who were exposed to no other "maternal" objects. The infants were fed milk from bottles suspended from either surrogate mother's chest. Bottles were alternately attached to one "mother" or the other, but regardless of which "mother" had just provided the milk, the infant monkey would immediately return after feeding to the terry cloth model. This experiment demonstrated that maternal attachment, at least in infant monkeys, is influenced more by the attachment to the softness and comfort of a cloth mother than by the actual gratification of hunger by the wire mother. Recent studies have shown that monkey infants raised in close contiguity with their mothers, separated only by a half-glass, half-wire-mesh partition that allowed free visual, auditory, and olfactory interchange but denied any tactile interaction, still developed a full-blown separation syndrome.

The separation syndrome in monkeys has its more or less exact parallel in humans when children at the age of 2 years or so are separated from their mothers. The syndrome has been identified as a "grief" reaction, generally differentiated from the frustration–aggressivity complex (Robertson, 1958). The syndrome in children separated from their parents has been described as occurring in three phases: the phase of protest, the phase of despair, and the phase of detachment. The first phase usually lasts 1–2 days and is characterized by marked hyperexcitability, mainly of the aggressive type with temper tantrums and continued demands and hostility. Phase 2 lasts for several days during which the child demonstrates profound weeping and withdrawal. In phase 3, the child develops a sense of detachment and unemotionality, with marked indifference to positive or negative occurrences in his surroundings. Clinically, it is certainly more correct to designate the separation syndrome as a "grief reactivity," but it is not wholly implausible to consider it also as the consequence of severe, prolonged, and intractable frustration, leading inevitably to a sense of helplessness and of hopelessness. The psychobiological interpretation of grief and depression suggested here is not too different from the psychodynamic one that postulates depression as being due to aggressive drives directed inwardly against the self in an intrapunitive manner.

The Effects of Childhood Stress

The evidence is not entirely clear whether these developed diatheses in infants are transitory or permanent in the afflicted individuals. For example, the stereotyped behavior of the separation syndrome in monkeys may persist either in an overt form for a given period of time or in a covert form that can be reactivated by a type-related stimulus at some later time. Ordinarily, when monkey infants who have had an acute separation episode from their mothers with concomitant depression are returned to their mothers, they recover fairly rapidly and their subsequent behavioral and social development becomes, so far as investigators have been able to ascertain, quite normal. However, under special circumstances symptoms may persist, or having disappeared, may become reactivated. Young et al. (1973) found that monkeys separated and isolated in infancy (3–4 months of age) from their mothers with subsequent depression, when suffering a second separation and isolation in later life (at 2 years of age), demonstrated far greater huddling and self-clutching than did experimental controls (also separated at 2 years of age but not in infancy). This study, although certainly not conclusive, suggests that adaptational behavioral patterns developed in early life may be reactivated by type-specific or type-related experiences in later life.

Other animal studies similarly support these conclusions. David Levy (1934) compared litter mate puppies who were treated differentially in terms of early feeding patterns. One pair was breast-fed. Another pair, "long feeders," were fed through bottles with a small opening and had access to a nipple-covered finger in between feedings to permit sucking activity gratification. The third pair, "short feeders," were fed through bottles with a large opening that emptied rapidly; these had no access to nipple-covered fingers in the between-feeding intervals. The "short feeders" were most active in sucking activities on each other's bodies, rubber balls, and so forth in the between-feeding intervals; the "long feeders" were intermediate and the breast-fed puppies least active.

Another study in rats using food deprivation during infancy to produce the tendency to hoard food tends to confirm the theoretical formulation that frustration of biological drives in infancy results later in an exaggerated responsivity to that drive. Rats fed irregularly although adequately in infancy, when confronted with a similar episode of irregular feeding in early maturity hoarded twice as much food as control rats fed regularly in infancy and irregularly at early maturity. The fact that the "memory" of the earlier deprivation lasted from infancy to early maturity tends to support the notion of the persistence of emotionally charged childhood memories with consequent effects on behavior.

If one reviews the hierarchical processes through which learning occurs, then it is evident that every new cognitive engram is an elaboration of some old one and retains the basic outlines of the old engram within it. Accordingly, childhood experience is retained throughout life both figuratively, because of the nature of cognitive learning, and literally, because some childhood experiences may remain in a primitive form in the right hemisphere.

Because of continual modifications in cognitive development, however, it does seem improbable that childhood memories should continue to fester and agitate in their original form in the dynamic unconscious. Nevertheless, it seems likely that because of their prominence in shaping future experience, they do play a large role in unconscious activity. It may be that the clinical importance of uncovering unpleasant childhood experience lies not so much in defusing some immense conflictual drama, but rather in familiarizing the patient with some of the significant events in his life that helped form his personality. Furthermore, it seems unlikely that a single childhood event, unless it is overwhelmingly disastrous, determines personality development; a persistent pattern of experience, however, probably does. In this instance, the uncovering of a given childhood experience may be less important for the knowledge of the single event itself than it is for the insight it offers into the patterns of experience one has had in one's formative years.

This point of view has gained increasing credence in recent years as more and more clinicians have found evidence that even severely traumatic experiences in childhood may be absorbed and compensated for if (1) the child is biologically endowed with certain psychological strengths and (2) there are some positive compensatory elements in their life experience (Thomas and Chess, 1984). These findings tend to emphasize biological hereditary factors as very significant in determining adjustment, with traumatic experience in childhood playing a somewhat lesser role than that assigned to it by psychoanalysis.

Psychobiology finds it difficult to conceptualize infantile and early childhood memories as remaining relatively unchanged in their first primitive state in the right hemisphere, despite our previous discussions as to how something like this might occur. It seems to me that the brain is too plastic, with new experiences constantly being registered, for even the most primitive negatively charged engrams to remain untouched, even in the sheltered environs of the psychobiological dynamic unconscious of the right hemisphere. Furthermore, if a strong negative emotional charge on an engram is postulated to be associated with a powerful inhibitory effect on the cognitive component, then that engram would cognitively decay if it were not continually reinforced. Hence, for childhood experience to retain its behavior-influencing effects, it would have to be through constant reinforcement, both of the first negative experience and of its associated decathecting inhibitory treatment. But such repeated experiences in a developing child would inevitably lead to a more sophisticated subjective interpretation of the original traumatic experience, gradually changing the involved engrams from their originally totally primitive context to at least a somewhat more mature one. In these terms, the view of Erik Erikson (1950), that maturation is a lifelong affair, seems very attractive.*

However, even within this context, the Freudian position on the importance of psychosexual development in the historic–experiential sequence is not unreasonable. If sexuality is defined in Freudian terms as the extreme pleasure associated with excitation of limited erogenous zones, then the sequential predominance of the oral, anal, and genital areas in human developmental behavior appears to reflect objective experience. Certainly these erogenous activities become socially conflictual in that order. The only disagreement of psychobiology with this basic psychoanalytic precept is with its overly wide application. We would not even dispute that early psychosexual conflicts might be the most important element in providing the content of the decathected dynamic unconscious; we would only dispute that they were the only contributors to that compartment of mental activity. Furthermore, since we believe that other unconscious activities dominated by positive experiences exercise the greatest influence on normal behavior, the influences of the decathected dynamic unconscious become most significant mainly where there is psychopathology. This is not meant to indicate that the conflicts in the decathected dynamic unconscious do not influence normal behavior; certainly they do. They just do not do so to the same extent as they do in pathological behavior.

The psychoanalytic contributions of René Spitz (1945) and Margaret Mahler (1972), which shift the major areas of psychic conflict from the Oedipal to the pre-Oedipal stages (with particular emphasis on the first six months of life), opens up a *terra incognita* of mental function that is extremely difficult to verify. The general thesis is attractive, but since material presumed to derive from this period is difficult if not impossible to come by even from patients with the most remarkable memories, its formulations are highly theoretical and speculative. Again, psychobiology has nothing definitive to offer. However, even here, these formulations are not necessarily incompatible with the psychobiological model in view of the work of investigators like Young et al. (1973), Denenberg (1981), and Levy (1934), all of whom have demonstrated in animals the lasting effects of infantile experience.

In any event, one must not minimize the influence of early experience on ongoing

---

*D. Milman (personal communication) has suggested that psychoanalysis may be defined as an "imprinting" psychology and learning theory as an "unfolding" psychology. Psychobiology favors the latter position. However, some of the early phenomena of human "bonding" do resemble those of animal imprinting.

mental activities in the psychobiological unconscious. Given the critical role of early experience in cognitive development and given the importance of early emotional experience on the development of positive or negative emotional charge, it would be difficult to exaggerate the influence of these effects even without a conflictual framework. The probably greater channeling of early experiences to the right hemisphere than to the left makes the case for an important role for early experience in ongoing psychobiological unconscious activity even more suggestive.

If these last several paragraphs appear fence-straddling and even somewhat contradictory, such a position may be inevitable where resolution of the issue is not possible. The case for the significance of early childhood experience in later-life psychological adjustment seems clear. The only problem revolves around the Freudian position that such childhood experience is the *only* determinant of adult behavior. Here again, the developmental philosophy of Erikson (1950), which stresses the impact of both maturation and adult experience as well as that of childhood experience on psychological adjustment, seems more compatible with psychobiological principles.

In this connection, it is important to point out in all fairness, that many of the psychoanalytic formulations criticized in these pages have been largely discarded by modern psychoanalysts. The psychoanalytic concepts described here are mainly those formulated early in the development of the science; Freud himself, in later years, changed many of his earlier interpretations. More recent modifications by Hartmann (1958), Spitz (1945), and Erikson (1950) have so changed the theory of psychoanalysis that their particular version is known as "ego psychology." It must be emphasized that ego psychology is by no means a departure from classical psychoanalysis. It is rather a reinterpretation of it, so much within the classical Freudian mold that it itself is now generally accepted as the standard. Nevertheless, because of its emphasis on psychoanalysis as a normal psychology (Hartmann, 1958), on observational studies in childhood (Spitz, 1945), and on the importance of maturation and social influences throughout life (Erikson, 1950), ego psychology fits better with psychobiology than does classical psychoanalysis. For that reason, it will serve as the clinical frame of reference for the study of neurosis in Volume 2 of this series.

19

Psychobiological Mechanisms in Personality Development

Every individual is born with a genetically endowed set of emotional reactivities and of emotional responsivities, where reactivity may be defined as the sensitivity to threats of a specific kind—fear, frustration, or isolation—and responsivity as the reaction to that threat—respectively, anxiety, anger, or depression. Operationally, one can combine the two concepts into a single mechanism where the tendency to demonstrate a given emotional response is considered as a function of the sensitivity to the corresponding threat. Under that paradigm, a low threshold to fear, frustration, or isolation would result in a tendency to respond, respectively, with anxiety, anger, or depression, whereas a high threshold to such threats would be characterized by the absence of correspondingly strong emotional responses. There is some theoretical advantage in separating the parameters of sensitivity and responsivity and in certain cases we shall do so, but from an operational point of view, the concept of threshold is sufficiently specific.

The set of genetically endowed emotional reactivities with which the infant is born is defined as temperament. Through the interaction of the biological organism with life experience, original temperament is modified to mediate between the needs of the individual and the demands of the social environment. The entity emerging from this interaction is personality. This varies obviously with the developmental stage of the individual and with the sum total of his emotional interactions with his particular life experience.

Temperament, like personality, may be characterized along three major parameters. The first of these, emotional style, consists of the pattern of responsivity to the three major types of stress, i.e., anxiety, anger or hostility, and depression. Infants with high thresholds to all of these and with an associated innate propensity for pleasant responsivities—smiling, cooing, resting—are said to have happy dispositions, or more technically, positive temperaments. Conversely, those with low thresholds to any or all threats and an apparent inability to experience pleasure are said to have unhappy dispositions or negative temperaments. Children with positive temperaments tend to be placid and relaxed, whereas those with negative dispositions tend to be tense and irritable.

A second parameter of both temperament and personality is defensive style. This is largely a function of the predominance of either excitatory or inhibitory activity in the normal balance of these two influences in the brain. Behaviorally, this is manifested as a predominance of either approach or avoidance tendencies. Such responsivities may seem to be a function of emotional style, and to an extent they may be, but they are also imposed upon emotional reactivities as still another layer of influences. Thus in an individual with low threshold to frustration and a high level of responsivity of anger and hostility, such emotional responses may be treated extrapunitively, intrapunitively, or impunitively. The first would represent a turning outward of anger, the second a turning inward, and the third a kind of inhibition. These latter effects represent the influence of defensive style.

A third characteristic of both temperament and personality is known as cognitive style. This concept, introduced by Witkin and other psychologists (Witkin and Goodenough, 1981), deals with patterns of cognitive perception that are related to personality characteristics. These are labeled field dependence and field independence. Physiological studies suggest that cognitive style is related to the tendency to respond cognitively with hemispheric specialization (differentiated activity). Cognitive style appears to be related to defensive style, but the physiological mechanisms underlying the two modes of responsivity appear to be different (see pp. 302–304).

The General Characteristics of Temperament

The fundamental biological core of personality is set in the individual's temperament. Temperament is defined as the constitutional element in personality, i.e., the set of inherited behavioral responsivities that are modified and changed by maturation and experience. Experimental evidence indicates that human infants are born with varying proclivities in certain temperamental reactivities. Baughman and Welsh (1962) review the experimental literature and conclude that those reactivities include fear (timidity), aggression, affiliation (the positive movement toward others), self-control (inhibition versus impulsiveness), activity level, perceptual sensitivity, curiosity, persistence, mood, introversion–extraversion, dependence–independence, frustration tolerance, and masculinity–femininity. This list includes most of the significant parameters of personality so that it would seem to imply that personality is almost "fixed" at birth. The point, of course, is quite different. Infants are born with certain tendencies along all personality parameters, and these tendencies are either strengthened or weakened by experience or may actually be reversed.

Baughman and Welsh summarize the evidence for temperament as a biologically defined set of parameters as follows:

> Temperament, like personality, is a construct; its distinguishing characteristic is that it refers to behavior patterns that are determined by constitutional factors whereas personality is not so restricted. Temperamental traits, along with primary-need behaviors,*

provide the foundation materials out of which personality is constructed through interactions with the environment. (p. 143)

An important methodology for evaluating the effects of heredity as opposed to those of the environment is the comparison of concordance of traits between identical and fraternal twins. Assuming that in both cases environmental influence are generally equal, significantly greater concordance between idential twins are attributed to hereditary factors. Such studies are summarized in Table 19-1.

Loehlin (1977) has reviewed the literature for the inheritance of personality traits, as defined by a variety of personality test batteries, in a large number of studies comparing correlations in identical twins versus fraternal twins. As illustrated in Table

Table 19-1 Comparison of Personality Characteristics in Identical (I) and Fraternal (F) Twins.[a]

Study	Number of pairs		Median correlation		No. of scales	Inventory[b]
	I	F	I	F		
Carter (1935)	40	43	.60	.33	4	Bernreuter
Newman, Freeman, & Holzinger (1937)	50	50	.56	.37	1	Woodworth
Vandenberg (1962)	45	35	.55	.00[b]	7	Thurstone
Gottesman (1963)	34	34	.45	.21[b]	31	HSPQ, MMPI
Wilde (1964a)	88	42	.50	.34	4	Amsterdam BV
Gottesman (1966)	79	68	.48	.31	18	CPI
Partanen, Bruun, & Markkanen (1966)	157	189	.26	.18	4	Special
Nichols (1965)						
Males	207	126	.53	.25[b]	24	CPI
Females	291	193	.50	.35	24	CPI
Vandenberg et al. (1967)	111	92	.47	.24	12	Comrey
Shoenfeldt (1968)						
Males	150	53	.40	.36	7	Factors
Females	187	103	.49	.33	7	Factors
Canter	39	44	.37	.15[b]	31	EPI, Foulds, 16PF
Eaves & Eysenck (1975)						
Males	120	59	.42	.21	2	PEN
Females	331	198	.42	.15[b]	2	PEN
Horn, Plomin, & Rosenman (1976)	99	99	.46	.18[b]	18	CPI
Median			.48	.24		

Note. Studies with less than 30 pairs of each kind not included. The Wilde, Partanen, Canter, Horn, and Eaves studies used adult twins, remaining studies used adolescent twins. Partanen and Horn sampled all males; other sexes combined unless indicated. All fraternal pairs like-sexed.
[a]From Loehlin, 1977.
[b]HSPQ = High School Personality Questionnaire; CPI = California Psychological Inventory; MMPI = Minnesota Multiphasic Personality Inventory, BV = Biographical Questionnaire; EPI = Eysenck Personality Inventory; PF = Personality Factor; PEN = Psychoticism, Extraversion, Neuroticism.

*Primary-need behaviors provide the other major variable in personality development. Their implications for such development include such reactivities as oral drives (hunger), need for tactile experience, need for physical comfort and so forth (Murray, 1936).

19-1, the median correlation (see last line in Table 19-1) for identical twins was .48 while that for fraternal twins was .24. The argument could of course be made that these results in themselves do not prove the influence of heredity in determining personality since identical twins might be treated more similarly by their parents than would fraternal twins; thus their higher correlations on personality traits could be due to more similar environments. Loehlin responds to this argument by quoting the findings of Shields (1962), who studied 42 identical twin pairs reared apart and found correlations in personality traits of .61 on the Extraversion scale and .53 on the Neuroticism scale. Similarly, Newman et al. (1937) reported a correlation of .58 on the Woodworth–Matthews Neuroticism scale in 19 identical twin pairs raised apart. The closeness of these correlations to those for identical twins raised together suggest strongly a biological basis for these personality reactivities. These correlations are highly significant for identical twins. However, even at those levels they account for only 30–40% of the variance, thus implying other important influences—maturational, developmental, experiential, and social—in the evolution of personality.

In the consideration of the relative input of heredity and environment in influencing personality development, an important area of study is the natural behavior of newborn infants. Thomas et al. (1968) found that normal newborn infants could be rated on nine different characteristics: activity level, rhythmicity, approach–withdrawal, adaptability, intensity of reaction, threshold of response to stimulation, quality of mood, distractibility, and attention span and persistence. Furthermore, these characteristics persisted proportionately in these children at least until the age of 2 years. Indeed Chess and Thomas (1977) followed these same children to adolescence and found these tempermental traits to persist. Daniel G. Freedman compared differences in Chinese-American, Navaho, and Caucasian-American newborn infants along the parameters of locomotor activity, posture, muscular tone, and emotional reactivity and found the Navaho infants to be most quiescent and passive, and the Chinese-American infants almost equally so, whereas the Caucasian-American newborns showed the most activity. Further, one of his co-workers, Nora Green, found that these patterns of impassivity and emotional hypoactivity persisted in Chinese-American children through the "high arousal age" of 3 to 5 years, when most Caucasian-American children were hyperactive and hyperemotional.

Baughman and Welsh (1962) conclude:

> Human infant behavior is difficult to study if we are looking for temperament, partly because we have not "learned to see" many of the subtleties that exist in infants' behavior patterns. But the likelihood that human infants are born with unique temperaments and that temperament is significantly related to adolescent personality was clearly suggested by Shirley's longitudinal study of babies and Neilson's follow-up (using a matching technique). The accuracy of Escalona's predictions of preschool children's personality characteristics on the basis of infant observations also tends to support the proposition that human infants differ temperamentally, although, it is true, her research did not separate constitutional and environmental determinants. (pp. 143–144)

The list of characteristics described above by Thomas et al. (1968) fall directly into the category of physiological adaptive mechanisms described in Chapter 3, which are essentially elements of the emotional system. It is easy to see how these reactivities can be readily translated into thresholds or tolerances for the three major categories of stress reaction: anxiety, hostility, and depression. The pattern of such reactivities can be seen from these studies to exist already at birth. Although they are unquestionably modified by specific experience, it is the reactivity of a preset organism to a given experience that will both determine how the individual reacts and what permanent effects on personality result.

The Development of Personality

The development of personality is best defined as an ongoing process in which there is a constant interaction of four variables: primary-need behaviors, temperament, maturation, and personal experience. Primary-need behaviors establish the general direction of personality development; temperament provides the biological predispositions in emotional, defensive, and cognitive styles. Maturation constitutes the biological processes of change that are associated with progressive growth from the time of birth until the time of death. Thus maturation or development should be seen not as merely encompassing the physiological changes that occur between birth and the end of adolescence, but truly as the physiological and organic changes that transpire throughout the successive periods of life (Erikson, 1950).

Omitting for the moment the immense influences of experience, there is often the tendency to overemphasize the biological contributions of temperament to the development of personality and to underestimate the biological importance of maturational changes. Again, apart from the effects of experience, maturation is associated with constant and dramatic changes in the biological functions of the individual, comparable to those determined by the genetic influences of temperament. For example, the massive discharge of sex hormones at puberty is frequently associated with dramatic changes in personality. Most remarkable is the frequent occurrence of acute psychological upheavals in adolescence, just as likely to have been ignited by the physiological changes of adolescence as by the behavioral and emotional traumas of that period.

Such dramatic biological metamorphoses are by no means restricted to adolescence. From the time of birth onward to puberty there are rapid progressive physiological changes which are at least as significant as are those of adolescence. These include changes in sleep patterns, in endocrine activities, in rates of growth, in psychological and behavioral activities (Piaget), as well as in a variety of emotional responsivities. In the latter category, Freud's stipulation of the psychological importance of the sequential development of excitation in the three major erogenous zones—the oral, the anal, and the genital—derives from the interaction of social inhibitions with the processes of natural biological maturation.

It is for this reason that the Freudian emphasis on developmental changes in biological sensitivities and responsivities *in a setting of continually pressing societal demands* provides an important context within which the interaction of primary-need behaviors, temperament, maturation, and experience can be considered. This does not necessarily imply that one must totally accept Freud's restriction of that context to the predominantly psychosexual. Neither should one in any way ignore the significant role of maturation and physiological changes in producing psychic conflict during psychosexual development. To develop a comprehensive theory, it is necessary to include Freud's contributions in a larger formulation that encompasses not only psychosexual development but other related and similar areas of motivational–emotional conflict.

The psychobiological position accepts the central role of psychosexual development in personality development, both because psychosexual drives are among the most powerful and because they are among the most socially restricted. However, psychobiology would include as perhaps equally important for normal human development the need in infancy to be touched, the need for cognitive and motor stimulation, the need for emotional security, the need for expression of nonhostile aggressive impulses, the need to control the environment, and the need for intellectual and emotional growth, among others. Certainly, these drives do not lend themselves to the neat formulations of psychoanalysis, but as important elements in the considerations of learning theory and developmental psychologies, they contribute to a more comprehensive theory.

An elaboration of the various types of experience that affect the development of personality is obviously beyond the scope of this book. Given an individual with particular emotional, defensive, and cognitive styles, certain experiences will react positively on his personality development while others will react negatively. For example, an individual with a low threshold for anxiety will respond poorly in an environment that continually excites fear just as an individual with a low threshold for anger and aggression will develop poorly in highly frustrating surroundings. In this way, categorization of experience as constructive or destructive becomes a highly individual matter, determined for each person by his particular pattern of emotional, defensive, and cognitive styles.

The Development of Emotional Style

As delineated in the last chapter, a given sensitivity to certain emotional threats, let us say anxiety or anger, does not in itself signify a specific mode of reactivity to that threat. For example, a low threshold for anxiety may stem from a low threshold for fear, for shame, or alternatively for guilt. Similarly with anger, one may turn one's anger externally (extrapunative), internally (intrapunitive), or tend to repress it (impunitive). The first example is one of sensitivity (threshold) and the second an expression of responsivity (defensive style), but in either case it is clear that single threats may elicit a variety of emotional reactivities.

Accordingly, emotional style must be seen as the consequence of a given temperament, developing in the course of maturation and responding to a variety of experiences in a pattern of reactivity largely determined by the defensive style of the individual. The effects of different defensive styles upon emotional reactivities are best exemplified in the cases of anxiety and anger. Of all emotions, anxiety is the most difficult to defend against, whether it derives from fear, shame, or guilt; so also is the depression deriving from isolation and separation. In each of these cases, the major controlling influence appears to be more on the sensitivity (threshold) and less on the defensive side. With anger, the ultimate emotional characteristic apparently depends less on sensitivity thresholds and more on the defensive style of the individual.

Frenkel-Brunswik (1941) has done an interesting study in which the attempt was made to correlate the strength of underlying drives with specific personality traits. She recorded in her paper that aggression, as rated by several interviewers, correlated positively with exuberance ($r = .30$) and with irritability ($r = .41$). Yet these two latter manifestations correlated negatively with each other ($r = -.52$). With a multiple correlation, aggression showed a highly significant correlation with exuberance or irritability at a level of $r = .73$. Thus aggressive drives can be associated with either exuberance or irritability patterns of behavior. The fact that these behavioral reactivities show such a strong negative correlation with each other but such a strong positive correlation with aggression suggests that a strong association in one direction is associated with a strong inhibitory effect in the other.

Frenkel-Brunswik (1941) goes on to describe other similar intercorrelations with aggressive drives:

> Less drastically, the following patterns point in the same direction. For boys, the intercorrelations of "energy output," "social participation," and "leadership," on the one hand, with "irritability," on the other, are $-.27$, $-.30$, and $-.38$, respectively. The corresponding correlations of these items with ratings on the drive for aggression range from .32 to .46. Multiple correlations, however, are between .66 and .75. Leadership is here the more direct expression of the drive for aggression, whereas tenseness and anxiety are manifestations of aggression of lesser phenotypical similarity to the underlying motive.
>
> In short, adolescents whose ratings on the aggressive drive cluster are high are likely to be either maladjusted, tense, and anxious, or else successful in their overt social activity, say, as leaders; or they may even display both manifestations. (p. 586)

These correlations suggest a selective process in which aggressive drives are stimulated in one direction and inhibited in another, a function highly suggestive of prefrontal and amygdaloid–hippocampal control. The prefrontal amygdaloid–hippocampal paradigm provides us with a mechanism through which basic motivational drives can be channeled into specific personality traits, and suggests a plausible description of the mechanisms by which experience and training may influence personality development (see p. 299).

The question remains whether these defensive reactions are implemented directly on some specific emotional physiological center or whether they are rather effected, as in the case of anxiety, through manipulation of the cognitive component of the internal or external event. In the case of anxiety, inhibitory or distortionary mechanisms exercise cognitive effects to influence the degree to which these emotional ractivities are experienced. In Chapter 16, on psychobiological defense mechanisms, we describe how in the Lazarus et al. experiment (Fig. 16-1) defensive mental sets, both intellectualizing and denying, significantly reduced the anxiety level associated with the viewing of a movie depicting cruel primitive rites. From our analysis there, it appeared that anxiety reduction resulted not from a direct effect of defense mechanisms upon anxiety, but rather from defensive effects, either sensitizing or inhibitory, upon the cognitive vehicles of that anxiety. Although the evidence is less clear in the case of the various defensive treatments of anger, it seems probable that extrapunitive, intrapunitive, and impunitive reactivities are accomplished through direct effects on both the cognitive and the emotional components of the threat. This thesis will be elaborated on shortly.

Psychological defense mechanisms appear to be less effective in dealing with the depression resulting from isolation and separation. Here denial would probably not be an effective defense instrument since it is difficult to deny the absence of gratification of a powerful need. One might more effectively rationalize a separation as not due to one's own fault, e.g., projection, but such rationalizations require a certain maturity. Since the worst effects of separation and isolation occur in early childhood when intellectualizing defenses are less readily available, one can see where separation anxiety and depression would be most difficult to defend against.

The Dynamics of Defensive Style

Emotional style appears to reflect mainly the affective and adaptive elements of emotional reactivity and hence presumably derives from brain stem reactivities. Defensive style, on the other hand, appears to revolve much more about the balance of excitatory and inhibitory responsivities (Nebylitsyn and Gray, 1972). Whether these effects act directly upon emotional expression itself, as may be partially the case in aggression, or alternatively upon the cognitive vehicles that carry the emotion as in the case of anxiety, the final effect is consummated either through some inhibitory action or through some excitatory rechanneling activity.

The most obvious experimental paradigm that encompasses such reactivities is the augmentation–reduction paradigm introduced in Chapter 13. In that model, individuals with a low tolerance to excitation (a form of stress) react by establishing some sort of neural blockade against such excitation so that stimuli of increasing intensity produce evoked potentials with the diminished early components (the P_1-N_1 complex) characteristic of "reducers." On the other hand, individuals with a high tolerance for excitation respond with ever increasing size of P_1-N_1 complex in the evoked potential ("augmenters"). These reactivities are illustrated in Figure 19-1.

As described in Chapter 13, augmenters differ from reducers not only in their reaction to stimuli of increasing intensity, but also in their perception of stimuli of the same intensity. Buchsbaum (1976) has presented evidence that reducers have greater sensitivity to stimuli at low thresholds than do augmenters. He points out, for example, that the P_1-N_1 wave in reducers tends to be greater than that in augmenters at low levels of intensity (see Fig. 13-1). In addition, he found visual thresholds on tachistoscopic presentation to be significantly lower in reducers than in augmenters. He writes:

> Petrie (1960) viewed reduction as operating evenly on all intensities whereas we conceptualized it as operating primarily at high intensities, in individuals who are unusually responsive at low levels. (p. 125)

Buchsbaum suggested that reducing and augmentation might represent different responses at different ends of the inverted U-function curve relating response to stimulus intensity. Responses for perceived and actual intensities of stimuli are illustrated in Figure 19-1. In Figure 19-1A the actual stimuli are of the same physical intensity for

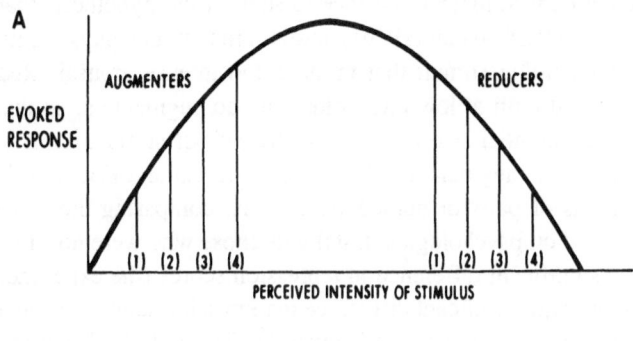

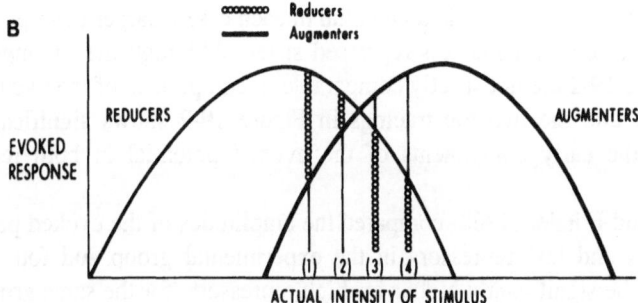

Figure 19-1 Patterns of response of the P_1-N_1 complex of the evoked potential in reducers and augmenters.

both augmenters and reducers, but the *perceived* intensity, particularly in terms of eliciting a defensive response, appears significantly greater at lower real levels of intensity for reducers. When the stimuli are superimposed as in Figure 19-1B, the response curve for augmenters is shifted, as stated by Buchsbaum, toward the end of higher intensity of stimuli. Curve 19-1B suggests that if the stimuli were made weak enough, reducers would become augmenters and if stimuli were made strong enough, augmenters would become reducers. The last prediction was corroborated in a study by Petrie et al. (1963) when a continuous very low noise was used as the stimulus.

There is much evidence to support the existence of these two types of responders both in animals and in humans. Pavlov, working with conditioning in dogs, was probably the first investigator to observe that the strength of the conditioned reflex was proportionate to the strength of the stimulus. However, he also observed that certain dogs showed more or less linear relationship between these two elements (augmenters) while others showed no increase in conditioning with increases in stimulus strength past moderate intensities. Pavlov denoted these animals as having respectively "strong" (augmenting) and "weak" (reducing) nervous systems. However, even the dogs with the strongest nervous systems would level off or even decrease their conditioning responses if the intensity of the stimulus was increased too much. In normal humans, with the standard intensities of visual flashes used, most subjects are augmenters to begin with and then taper off; in other words, they would tend to follow a curve intermediate between those for reducers and augmenters (see Fig. 13-5).

Theoretically, reducers should utilize repression as a major defense mechanism.

There is some electrophysiological evidence to support the hypothesis that repressors may be reducers in the Buchsbaum (1976) paradigm in that they physiologically reduce the magnitude of incoming stimuli that produce too intense arousal. Reducers have greater sensitivity to stimuli at low thresholds than do augmenters, so that the P_1-N_1 wave of the evoked potential at low levels of intensity of stimulation is significantly larger in reducers than in augmenters (Fig. 13-1). Shevrin and Fritzler (1968) studied the evoked potentials of pairs of nonidentical twins, comparing those who were repressors (as measured on psychological tests) with those who were not. In five pairs of twins there was a significant difference in repression scores (the experimental group); in five pairs there was no significant difference in repression scores (the control group). An example of the findings in one case is given in Figure 19-2. The early component (that designated A-B) of the evoked potential in each case is larger in amplitude for the repressed subject than for her less-repressed sister. Although the findings in Figure 13-1 and Figure 19-2 are not strictly comparable, a comparison of the two top tracings in Figure 13-1 and the two top tracings in Figure 19-2 shows significantly higher amplitude of the early components of the evoked potential in both reducers and repressors.

Shevrin and Fritzler (1968) compared the amplitudes of the evoked potentials for high repressors and low repressors in the experimental group and found the early components to be significantly higher for high repressors; for the same group, the late components were significantly lower. There were no significant differences in the control group. The comparisons are shown in Table 19-2.

It is more difficult to account for the lower amplitudes of the late components of the evoked potential in the high repressive group. If the late component does reflect the inhibitory effects of negative emotional valence (Fig. 13-2), it may be that the diminished P_{300} is characteristic of the repressive tendency. If this could be established, this would support the thesis of this book that repression is associated with a lowering of the valence of the cognitive element with a consequent lowered valence for awareness (diminished P_{300}). This finding, together with the presence of larger early components of the evoked potential among repressors, is consistent with the interpretation that repressors tend to be reducers.

Eysenck's Introvert–Extravert Personality Dimensions

Clinical significance is added to these experimental findings by relating them conceptually to the clinical parameters of the introvert–extravert personality dichotomy. Eysenck (1967) found that with a battery of psychological tests, he could describe a spectrum of personality traits that ran from introversion at one extreme to extraversion at the other, with most individuals somewhere in between. Introverts tend to be quiet, unsocial, thoughtful, and serious. Extraverts tend to be active, outgoing, impulsive, and irresponsible. Introverts appear to have an intense inner life with much internal emotional turmoil. Extraverts generally live more superficial lives, gaining most of their excitement from external stimulation.

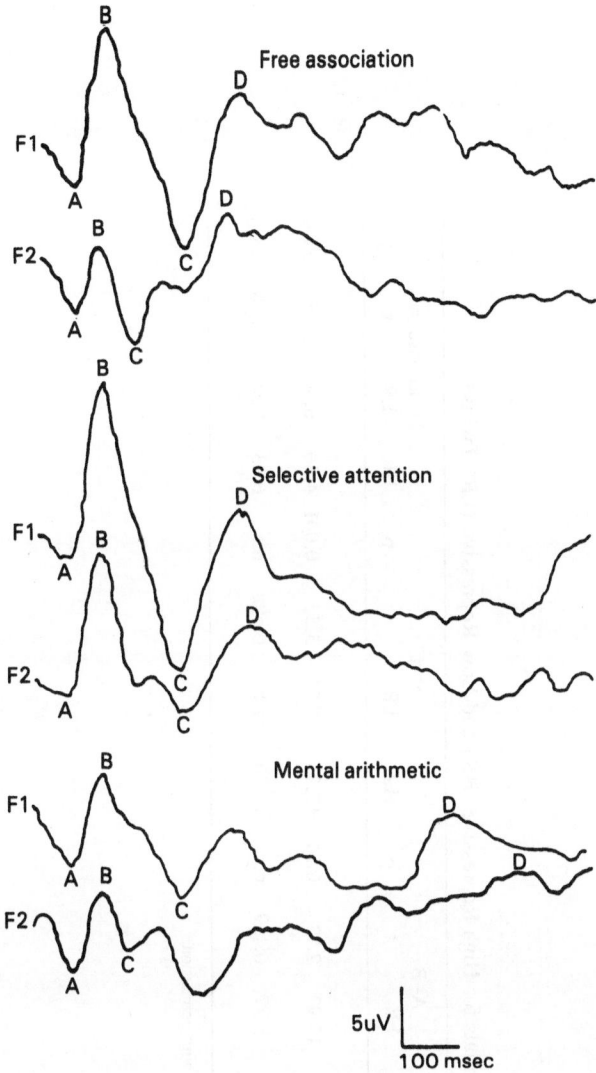

Figure 19-2 Evoked potentials in repressors and nonrepressors. (From Shevrin, 1974. Reprinted with permission.)

The dichotomy of personality described by Eysenck appears to fit the reducer–augmenter paradigm very well. On the basis of this hypothesis, introverts with already high levels of internal arousal would resist increases in arousal by external stimulation and would respond as reducers. Extraverts, on the other hand, with a minimum of internal excitation, would seek as much stimulation from the environment as possible and would be augmenters. Similarly, introverts would tend to act with repression to reduce external involvement while extraverts would tend to respond with sensitizing defenses, i.e., perceptual vigilance.

If in Figure 19-2 the upper curve is considered characteristic of introverts and the

Table 19-2 Evoked Potentials for High Repressive (HR) and Low Repressive (LR) Twins[a]

AER Components	A–B				B–C				D (to baseline)			
	HR	LR	t	p	HR	LR	t	p	HR	LR	t	p
Experimental Group (N=5 pairs)	12.64	10.92	2.73	0.01	17.93	11.74	5.52	0.001	4.50	6.86	2.95	0.01
Control Group (N=5 pairs)	9.87	9.77	0.159	n.s.	11.20	11.87	0.598	n.s.	6.23	5.68	0.688	n.s.

[a]From Shevrin, 1974. Reprinted with permission.

lower curve of extraverts, many of the psychological differences in reactivity between the two groups may be explained. For example, Eysenck found that introverts have lower *auditory* thresholds than do extraverts; Buchsbaum demonstrated lower *visual* thresholds for introverts. Similarly, introverts have been reported, like reducers, to have larger visual evoked potentials to stimuli of low intensity than do extraverts (Boddy, 1978, pp. 242–243). Introverts perceive nociceptive stimuli of moderate intensity to be extremely painful, but react less strongly to stimuli of slowly increasing intensity (Boddy, 1978, pp. 242–243); reducers do the same. Finally, people with established extravert tendencies, alcoholics (von Knorring, 1976), and high scorers on the Sensation-Seeking Scale (Zuckerman et al., 1974) were found to be marked augmenters, whereas highly introverted schizophrenics reacted with marked reduction (Landau et al., 1975).

Behaviorally, introverts should be characterized by the increased use of repression as a defense mechanisms. MacKinnon and Duke (1962) studied the ability of subjects to recollect tasks on which they had cheated (while under surveillance unbeknownst to them) as opposed to tasks on which they had not cheated. Subsequently, subjects were confronted with their cheating. At that time some expressed guilt while others felt no guilt at all. Subjects who felt no guilt remembered the tasks on which they had cheated without any difficulty actually better than they did the tasks on which they had not cheated. On the other hand, subjects who felt guilt had greater difficulty in remembering those tasks on which they had cheated. This study indicates that people who felt guilt for cheating responded by a type of repression (forgetting) while those who felt no guilt actually remembered better (vigilance). Although no specific information on the diagnosis of introversion or extraversion is available in this study, one may operationally assume that those who felt guilt were typically introverted while those who did not were either normal or extraverts. This again suggests that introverts characteristically use repression as the defense mechanism of choice.

Evidence for a somewhat different type of relationship of the augmenting–reducing paradigm to Eysenck's typology has been presented by Inglis (1961) vis-à-vis the kinds of defense mechanisms used by extraverts and introverts in situations of low and high stress. Inglis evolved the mediation–motivational hypothesis which holds that individuals with a lower responsivity to stress (extraverts) react to less stressful stimuli with "vigilance" (augmentation) and to more stressful stimuli with "defense" (reduction). Individuals with a higher responsivity to stress (introverts), according to Inglis, should react to stimuli of moderate stress with repression (reduction). He further postulated that reactions to stimuli of high stress in introverts might lead to increased vigilance through a breakdown of ordinary homeostatic mechanisms (see Chapter 20).

Inglis (1961) reviewed the literature in terms of this formulation and found supportive evidence in several studies with the Zeigarnik (1927) effect. Zeigarnik reported that in a low stress (task-oriented) situation, subjects remembered incompleted tasks significantly more correctly than they did completed tasks. Smock (1956) confirmed this finding, but also reported that when instructions were given that indicated that not completing the task was the fault of the subject (ego-oriented), the task became a high stress one; then completed tasks were remembered significantly more correctly than were incompleted ones, i.e., incompleted tasks were in some way repressed.

Eriksen (1954) compared extraverts and introverts on their performance on the Zeigarnik battery under the same experimental paradigm. Extraverted subjects in the low stress condition remembered incomplete tasks better than completed; in the high stress condition, they tended to suppress the memory of incomplete tasks and did better with completed ones. These results were similar to those of Petrie et al. (1963) on augmenters and were what one expects from inspection of the extravert (augmenter) curve in Figure 19-1B. On the other hand, when Eriksen tested psychasthenic subjects (introverts), he found that in the high stress condition they remembered incompleted tasks better than completed ones. In other words, they responded to high stress not with "memory defense," but rather with "memory vigilance." The results with these introverts at low stress levels were somewhat indeterminate, but tended to fall into the memory defense paradigm, i.e., they remembered the completed tasks better than those left incomplete. Thus they too, like extraverts, showed a reversal in defensive style under high stress.

The Inglis and Eriksen formulations permit us to carry the Eysenck introversion–extraversion paradigm one step further. Using their data and extrapolating back to the augmenter–reducer curves of Figure 19-1, extraverts would follow the augmenter curve of Figure 19-1B at low levels of stress and become reducers at high levels. Introverts, however, who are reducers at moderate levels of stress, apparently suffer a breakdown in the homeostatic mechanism involved and become augmenters at high levels of stress. These relationships will be more clearly illustrated in the next chapter on the neuroses (Chapter 20), in which condition both introverted and extraverted individuals are characteristically exposed to sufficient stress to challenge and reverse their normal homeostatic mechanisms.

Davidson et al. (1980) performed an interesting experiment testing some of these variables although not completely in the context outlined here. They differentiated between two groups of subjects on the basis of psychological testing and interviews— those who had a high need for power and those who apparently had a low need for power. They then tested both groups with power related and neutral visual stimuli at four different intensity levels (in a typical augmentation–reduction paradigm) and obtained their respective batteries of evoked potentials. They found that the high need for power individuals reacted as reducers to both power-related and neutral stimuli whereas the low need for power subjects showed augmentation only to the power-related stimuli.

Davidson et al. (1980) interpret these results to indicate that high need for power individuals feel anxiety with power related stimuli and consequently show a repressive response to power related stimuli of increasing intensity. On the other hand, low need for power subjects feel no such anxiety and show increased interest (augmentation) to power-related stimuli of increasing intensity. This reading seems perfectly plausible as far as it goes. However, that interpretation does not account for the reducing response of the high need for power individuals to neutral stimuli. If we extend the interpretation to assume that the high need for power individuals were probably introverts (reduction with neutral stimuli) with a high degree of guilt about their need for power whereas the low need for power subjects were either normal or extraverts without such guilt, then the findings fall even more neatly into place.

Control of Excitatory–Inhibitory Balance by the Amygdaloid–Hippocampal Complex

There are several speculative hypotheses as to the mechanisms in the brain that may implement augmenting and reducing effects. One possible mechanism is the type of operation encompassed by the Skinner–Yingling prefrontal cortical–thalamic feedback mechanism. Gray (1971) has postulated a similar counterbalancing relationship in the amygdaloid–hippocampal complex where the hippocampus is responsible for most inhibitory (reducing) effects and the amygdaloid for most excitatory (augmenting) effects. Other complexes that show similar antagonistic (excitatory–inhibitory) relationships are the brain stem posterior hypothalamic–anterior hypothalamic complex and the higher level posterior inferior temporal and prefrontal cortical lobe complex. There is evidence to suggest that some or all of these neural centers may be involved in a giant complex feedforward and feedback circuit that ultimately determines the dominant quality (excitatory or inhibitory) in the brain and the direction of such influences.

Throughout this volume, we have referred to the amygdaloid–hippocampal complex as though it were a single entity, involved largely with the executive processes of recognition, memory retrieval, and mental set (Chapter 9). More specifically, this complex was designated as involved in the process of determining the level of consciousness that perceived or retrieved material was destined to achieve (Chapter 12). In terms of its attentional activities, these interpretations of the integrated function of the amygdaloid–hippocampal complex are generally valid. However, that position overlooks the antagonistic interaction between the two components of the complex that leads to such final actions.

As described in Chapter 8, the amygdala is responsible for maintaining the excitatory level of the complex while the hippocampus, in combination with the septum, is responsible for most of its inhibitory activities. The balance between the two elements is best illustrated in the control of anger, rage, and aggressivity. Destruction of the amygdala produces a tame, placid animal, whereas destruction of the septum results in the septal rage syndrome (see Chapter 3). Thus the antagonism between the excitatory effects of amygdaloid activity and the inhibitory effects of the septal–hippocampal circuit is best evidenced in their control of the emotional reactivities of rage and aggression.

The final level of balance between excitatory and inhibitory influences in the brain is determined by the opposition within the amygdaloid–hippocampal complex (where the septum is considered part of the hippocampal circuit). It is at that level that the final pathway of excitatory–inhibitory control of organismic behavior is exercised. That final pathway sets the level not only for behavior, but, through its action upon the anterior and posterior hypothalamic nuclei, upon the level of autonomic nervous sytem activity as well (Isaacson, 1972). Not only does the balance in the amygdaloid–hippocampal complex affect activity levels of the sympathetic and parasympathetic systems, but conversely the activities in those systems affect the balance of excitatory–inhibitory control levels in the amygdaloid–hippocampal complex. A feedback circuit between the two systems, the autonomic nervous system and the amygdaloid–hippocampal complex, represents the lower end of the excitatory–inhibitory control system. The upper end of that system consists of a similar feedback circuit between the prefrontal lobe–temporal lobe complex and the amygdaloid–hippocampal complex, in which the prefrontal lobe and the hippocampus tend to be inhibitory, and the temporal lobe and the amygdala tend to be excitatory.

Thus the excitatory–inhibitory control system consists of three major complexes: the anterior–posterior hypothalamus, the amygdaloid–hippocampal complex, and the prefrontal–temporal cortex. Each complex in turn consists of an excitatory and an inhibitory element. But still another system plays a role here, the previously described thalamic–frontal cortical feedback system with its generally inhibitory effects. This last system should probably be seen, not as separate and distinct, but rather as a component of the prefrontal cortex–hippocampus–anterior hypothalamic inhibitory system with which it is so intimately associated, both anatomically and physiologically (see Chapter 8). In this way, the entire excitatory–inhibitory control system can be viewed as a closely integrated one where the balance of control is established first at each neurological level—brain stem, limbic system, and cortex—and then determined finally through the interaction among the three levels.

Although the balance in excitatory–inhibitory control levels is achieved through the interaction of the complexes at all three neurological levels, the final pathway, at least for behavioral activities, is best reflected in the balance achieved at the amygdaloid–hippocampal level. Here the influences coming both from above and from below are integrated and a suitable level of control activated. Thus, when in future discussions we describe the amygdaloid–hippocampal complex as the control center for excitatory–inhibitory activity, we will be well aware that that level of control is continually affected from both above and below.

An understanding of augmentation–reduction activity follows logically from this anatomical–physiological paradigm. In these terms, augmentation occurs when the excitatory component of the system (the amygdala) is more active, whereas reduction occurs when the inhibitory component (the septal–hippocampal circuit) is more active. Since augmentation is characteristic of the extravert and reduction is more characteristic of the introvert, one would look for evidence of amygdaloid overactivity in the first group and of overactivity of the septal–hippocampal circuit in the second.

Gray (1970, 1971, 1972) has done extensive work relating a variety of physiological and behavioral reactivities in introverts and extraverts to putative levels of dominance of activity in the amygdala as opposed to the septal–hippocampal circuit. At the behavioral level, Gray has equated "active avoidance conditioning" with dominance of amygdaloid influences and "passive avoidance conditioning" with dominance of septal–hippocampal activity. In addition, he postulates that amygdaloid dominance is associated with reward-seeking behavior, whereas septal–hippocampal dominance is characterized more by the desire to escape fear and frustration (see Table 2-1).

Boddy (1978) describes the relationship of these physiological reactivities to behavior with particular reference to active avoidance conditioning and to behavior motivated by the desire for reward as follows:

> Gray (1970, 1971, 1972) has elaborated upon the precise location of the positive and negative reinforcing areas, the processes involved in their activation, the nature of

their influence on different classes of behavior and their relationship to the dimensions of personality. Gray accepts Olds' work locating the reward mechanism in the septal area, lateral hypothalamus and medial forebrain bundle. He claims that this system operates to maximize its own input (which is rewarding, or, in subjective terms, pleasurable) via connections to the motor system which executes approach responses to rewarding stimuli. Gray (1970, 1971, 1972) embodies the novel principle that in addition to active approach to rewards, active escape from punishments is mediated by the same positively reinforcing system. . . . Consistent with this hypothesis Stein (1965) has shown that stimulation of the reward mechanism facilitates avoidance behavior. (p. 250)

Boddy (1978) goes on to explain the mechanisms of passive avoidance conditioning and of behavior motivated by fear and frustration rather than by reward, as follows:

As a complement to the "go" mechanism of the reward system, which energizes approach or avoidance behavior, Gray also postulates a "stop" mechanism which inhibits punished responses, and also responses which were previously rewarded, but are now unrewarded. In other words the "stop" system is the origin of passive avoidance and extinction. In order to sustain this model Gray equates fear, which is the basis of passive avoidance, with frustration, the effect of the nonappearance of an expected reward. Gray not only locates the neural substrate of this mechanism in a system which includes the RAS, medial septal nucleus, hippocampus and basal forebrain, but also identifies a specific pattern of activity, the hippocampal θ-rhythm, with activation of the stop system.* The medial septal nucleus and the hippocampus appear to be the most important structures, the medial septum apparently driving the 7.5–8.5 Hz hippocampal θ-rhythm. This system for behavioral inhibition has been put out of action by lesioning, administration of small doses of sodium amylobarbital (which selectively depresses the septum and hippocampus and blocks hippocampal θ) or blocking the hippocampal θ-rhythm by stimulating the septum at a high frequency. In all of these instances there is a failure of both passive avoidance learning and of extinction of responses to nonrewarded stimuli. In contrast, active avoidance learning is actually improved and rewarded approach learning unimpaired following these treatments. This suggests that normally active avoidance learning is partially antagonized by competition of the stop system commanding that the animal "freeze" in response to fear provoking stimuli. (p. 251)

Extrapolating from these formulations to personality types, Gray argues that introverts show predominance of the septal–hippocampal activity and as a consequence are motivated more by the need to avoid anxiety and frustration tan by the need to seek rewarding experience. As evidence, he cites the neurotic syndromes that develop in introverts, anxiety neuroses, phobias, and obsessive–compulsive syndromes, all of which are characterized by high levels of anxiety. In addition, Eysenck (1967) has observed that introverts are much more readily conditioned to passive avoidance than are extraverts. He reports also that introverts have a greater capacity to attend to faint signals than extraverts, a finding consistent with the greater sensitivity of reducers to faint signals.

The extravert shows the opposite pattern of amygdaloid dominance and of behavior, and is motivated more by the desire for reward than by anxiety. Boddy (1978) writes:

*Gray's research provides further evidence to support our position that θ activity in the hippocampus indicates inhibitory activity. See Chapter 8, p. 119.

The extravert, in contrast to the introvert is not readily conditionable, a lack which Gray attributes to him being "bad on fear." The septo-hippocampal system which inhibits responses that have been punished or have failed to elicit a reward is relatively intensive. Gray goes further and maintains that in the neurotic extravert the reward system is, if anything, over sensitive so that the behavior of the neurotic extravert is almost entirely governed by reward. The consequence of this particular balance can be disastrous for society as these appear to be the ingredients which make up a psychopath. Such an individual fails to become socialized, and lacks the attributes of a conscience, guilt, and remorse, because of his insensitivity to punishment. Consequently the psychopath "lives in the present only. His immediate wishes, affections, disgruntlements rule him completely, and he is indifferent about the future and never considers the past" (Mayer-Gross et al., 1960). (p. 253)

Gray's analysis of the dominance of septal–hippocampal influences in introverts and of amygdaloid influences in extraverts seems compatible with his experimental findings. Obviously these interpretations are not conclusive, but they are consistent with the personality constructs presented in this chapter.

Thus in the introvert–extravert dichotomy, introverts tend (1) to have high initial levels of anxiety, (2) to avoid stress, (3) to be reducers at moderate levels of stress, (4) to use avoidance and desensitizing defense mechanisms as their normal mode of reacting, and (5) to become augmenters under conditions of severe stress. Extraverts, on the other hand, tend (1) to show low initial levels of anxiety, (2) to seek stimulation, (3) to be augmenters at moderate levels of stress, (4) to tend to use vigilance and sensitizing defense mechanisms as their normal mode of reacting, and (5) to become reducers under conditions of severe stress. The physiological mechanism underlying the augmentation–reduction paradigm are unknown, but are considered to reside most likely in the inhibitory–excitatory control mechanisms centered in the prefrontal cortex–thalamic feedback system and in the balance between amygdaloid excitation and hippocampal inhibition in the amygdaloid–hippocampal complex.

The Field Dependence–Field Independence Dimension of Personality: "Cognitive Style"

It appears that still another level of neural activity may be involved in these reactions, namely the hemispheric. In Chapter 16, we described how the left hemisphere appeared to be responsible for sensitizing defense mechanism and the right seemed to activate the more desensitizing defense mechanisms. If that is so, it appears that there is a certain redundancy or alternatively a synergism between the interhemispheric and the hierarchical control systems. Perhaps this is not unexpected since the decathecting of threatening stimuli was said to be accomplished first during upstream processing in the thalamic–basal gangliar complex, secondly by channeling to either the right or left hemispheres, and only subsequently through the actions of the bilateral amygdaloid–hippocampal complexes.

As previously described (Chapter 16), there is substantial evidence that individuals with right-hemispheric dominance favor desensitizing defense mechanisms and those with left-hemispheric dominance, sensitizing defense mechanisms. Gleser and

Ihlevich (1969) found that subjects who favored repressive defenses were significantly more field dependent (i.e., hemispherically undifferentiated) than those who favored intellectualizing defenses. Hemispheric differentiation or undifferentiation indirectly reflects a tendency toward domination of one hemisphere or the other in various behavioral activities. Hemispherically undifferentiated individuals characteristically use both hemispheres for analytic tasks, whereas hemispherically differentiated subjects use the left hemisphere more exclusively for such tasks. Several investigators, using power spectrum measures of lateralization, have shown in a variety of task-specific studies that field-independent (differentiated) subjects show significant left- or right-hemispheric dominance on verbal and spatial tasks, respectively, while field-dependent (undifferentiated) subjects show very little of such EEG differentiation (Oltman et al., 1979). The interrelationship of these behavioral and neurophysiological interactions was illuminated in a study by Buchsbaum and Silverman (1980) who evaluated evoked potential responses to visually presented line stimuli of different angulations (similar to those used in Witkin's Rod and Frame Test). These investigators found that field-independent individuals produced significantly different evoked response patterns for different angulations, whereas field-dependent subjects tended to show similar responses for all angulations. This study indicates that field-independent individuals react more specifically (i.e., more analytically) to external stimuli and field-dependent individuals tend to react more amorphously (i.e., more holistically). These findings are consistent with the interpretation that field-independent individuals have a greater tendency to left-hemispheric dominance than do the field-dependent, who tend to use both hemispheres equally. Similarly, the greater occurrence of intellectualizing defense mechanisms in field-independent individuals seems consistent with the physiological formulation that such behavior is characteristically associated with left-hemispheric dominance.

As described in Chapter 16, the preferential use of sensitizing or desensitizing defense mechanisms depends in part on the functional dominance of one hemisphere or the other. Although the concept of hemispheric dominance is valid when addressing such topics as speech, handedness, and consciousness, the extension of that concept to personality has not proved valid. Essentially all right-handed individuals show left-hemispheric dominance; consequently a dichotomy of personality along the parameter of right- or left-hemispheric dominance would have no meaning.

What does appear to differentiate personality on the basis of hemispheric function is the degree of differentiation between the functions of the two hemispheres. In some individuals, the normal disparity between the cognitive functions of the right and left hemispheres is remarkably active. In verbal activities they use the left hemisphere; in visuospatial activities, they use the right. These individuals are said to show differentiated brain function. Associated with that is a complex behavioral pattern that involves depending more on internal cues than on external, a pattern associated with a variety of other personality characteristics. Such personalities are labeled as field independent because of their general independence from stimuli in the environment. This mode of viewing the outside world as well as the opposite mode of field dependence have been labeled the cognitive style of the individual.

Field-dependent individuals show a less differentiated (i.e., undifferentiated) specialization in the physiological use of their two hemispheres. There appears to be a spilling over of function from each hemisphere to the other. Consequently, on verbal tasks, these individuals show only slight if any dominance of left-hemispheric activity; similarly on visuospatial tasks, they show only slight if any dominance of right-hemispheric activity. This physiological pattern is associated with behavioral responses of greater dependency on external cues for self-orientation and hence a greater need for external stimulation. Clearly there appears to be some clinical correlation between field independence and introversion and between field dependence and extraversion, but the correlation when tested experimentally is only moderate (Evans, 1967; Fine, 1972; Bone and Eysenck, 1972). Apparently, related but different physiological mechanisms are involved: brain stem mechanisms for the introversion–extraversion paradigm and interhemispheric mechanisms for the field dependence–field independence paradigm.

Although degree of hemispheric differentiation is different from hemispheric dominance, the overall effects are similar. Differentiated (field-independent) individuals show greater evidence of left-hemispheric activity in their everyday behavior. They are analytic in intellectual pursuits and more psychologically intellectualistic (Witkin et al., 1962). They also tend to use sensitizing defense mechanisms (Crutchfield, 1955). These effects are similar to those previously described for individuals with increased left-hemispheric activity (Bear, 1979; Gur and Gur, 1975; Fig. 16-2). Undifferentiated (field-dependent) individuals tend to be more holistic in intellectual pursuits and psychologically more emotional (Witkins et al., 1962); they tend to use desensitizing defense mechanisms (Linton, 1962; Gleser and Ihlevich, 1969) similar to those with increased right-hemispheric activity. These findings are consistent with the thesis of hemispheric differentiation of personality and defense mechanisms previously presented in Chapters 14 and 16 (Bear, 1979; Gur and Gur, 1975; Fig. 16-2).

An interesting aspect of cognitive style is the fact that women tend to be more field dependent, i.e., less differentiated than men. There is of course substantial overlap, but as a whole this relationship holds. It is reflected in the fact that when women have strokes affecting their speech centers in the left hemisphere, they are more likely to be able to recover some of their speech faculty than are similarly affected men. This constitutes clinical evidence of the greater equipotentiality of the two hemispheres in women than in men. The physiological basis of that finding has been attributed by DeLacoste-Utamsing and Holloway (1982) to be the result of more effective communication through the corpus callosum in women than in men. They found that the splenium, the major communication tract of the corpus callosum, was significantly larger in females, even at birth, than in males. As a consequence, they reason that the physiological functions of the two hemispheres are more readily shared in females.

The correlation of personality style with cognitive style and the relationship of cognitive style to brain anatomy and physiology provide excellent examples of the ways in which psychobiological studies may contribute to the understanding of human behavior. * Most of the mechanisms described in this chapter have referred mainly to normal behavior. In the next chapter, we shall attempt to demonstrate how the breakdown of these normal homeostatic mechanisms may result, both in animals and in humans, in what has been identified as neurotic behavior.

---

*After this book went to press, I became aware that some of the ideas described in this chapter were previously expressed by Rothbart and Derryberry (1981).

Psychobiological Mechanisms in the Pathogenesis of the Neuroses

This presentation of the psychobiological system has attempted to describe in physiological terms the normal homeostatic mechanisms that insure the physical and psychological survival of the individual. In keeping with the general principles of homeostasis, most physiological and psychological mechanisms are controlled by feedforward–feedback mechanisms that maintain the operation of any particular function at its optimal level. "Optimal" almost always means "moderate" since the human physical and mental organism is usually damaged when the operation of any function goes to one extreme or the other. This basic principle of biological homeostasis was described earlier in this volume in Chapter 3 where the inverted U-shaped curve was cited as prototypical for emotional reactivities (see Fig. 3-1). Since then it has been presented in several situations as governing optimal performance for most biological systems.

This general principle is illustrated diagrammatically in Figure 20-1 where "psychological adjustment" represents a general operational definition of behavioral accommodation to the realities of existence, and "psychobiological homeostatic ac-

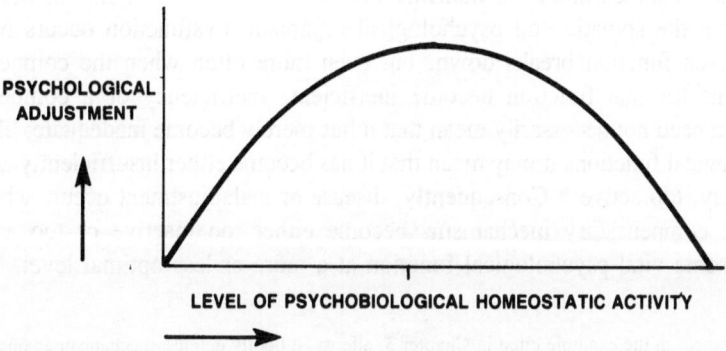

Figure 20-1 Inverted U-shaped curve for psychological adjustment.

tivity" represents almost any modulating function we have described. Optimal adjustment, i.e., optimal psychological performance, occurs when all of the adaptive mechanisms of the organism are operating at their optimal levels, usually somewhere near the middle of their physiological range. Mental health is high when that general level of interaction is achieved and tends to be low when any one major function becomes either underactive or overactive.

On the other hand, the term "normalcy" does not necessarily imply that all conceivable functions are operating at their optimal levels. The behavioral organism, like the physiological organism, must be able to survive even when some one function does go askew; otherwise it would become too vulnerable. For that reason, nature has endowed all biological organisms with compensatory mechanisms that come into play when any given system, for whatever reason, cannot be contained within the normal limits of its operation.

Compensatory mechanisms may be of various sorts. They may involve opposing systems that work toward the same goal of maintaining a particular vital function at a given level. For example, the mechanisms for maintaining normal blood pressure involve the output of the heart and the state of contraction of the arteries. When heart output drops, the arteries constrict to increase resistance and maintain blood pressure at its normal level. When cardiac output is increased above normal, the arteries are relaxed to decrease resistance and still maintain blood pressure at its normal level. In that way, when one function (cardiac output) becomes and remains abnormal, another system, that of arterial constriction, compensates by modulating itself in the opposite direction.

Psychological compensatory mechanisms tend to be less straightforward and more complex. Certainly the most clear-cut example of a psychological compensatory mechanism thus far presented has been that of the defense mechanisms. In those cases where a psychological threat is so great as to produce a level of anxiety that would physiologically and psychologically disrupt performance, the "mind" attempts to reduce that anxiety to manageable levels through the application of sensitizing or desensitizing defense mechanisms. Here, the operations are not simply those of correlated opposition as is the case in physiological compensatory mechanisms. In psychological functions they are certainly more indirect. Nevertheless, they serve the same purpose as do physiological compensatory mechanisms and may be described in similar terms.

In both the somatic and psychological organism, dysfunction occurs not only when a given function breaks down, but even more often when the compensatory mechanisms for that function become inefficient. Inefficiency of a compensatory mechanism need not necessarily mean that it has merely become inadequate; like most other biological functions it may mean that it has become either insufficiently active or alternatively, too active.* Consequently, disease or maladjustment occurs when psychological compensatory mechanisms become either too inactive or too active to maintain some vital psychological function at a more or less optimal level. Thus in

---

*As, for instance, in the example cited in Chapter 3; allergy, a bodily defense mechanism against disease, can itself become fatal when the immune system becomes underactive (AIDS) or overactive (anaphylactic shock).

Figure 20-1, one can correctly substitute "strength of defense mechanisms" for "psychobiological homeostatic activity" as one example.

Since control of defense mechanisms is a function of the combined activity of the subjective and executive self-systems or in psychoanalytic terms, the ego, the ability to maintain compensatory mechanisms at the moderate level of operation has been termed "ego strength." It must again be noted that ego strength does not mean overly strong defense mechanisms; as will be seen, that can lead to psychopathology just as readily as can overly weak defense mechanisms. Ego strength means rather the ability to maintain psychological functions and compensatory mechanisms at a level that permits the individual to function at *his or her* optimal level of psychological and behavioral performance.

Neurosis may be defined then as a state of decompensation stemming from underactivity or overactivity of either a primary psychological function or of a compensatory mechanism, or as is most often the case, both. It is characterized by some deficit in ego strength. This is merely another way of saying that the ego, i.e., the individual's psyche, is not stable or strong enough to maintain psychological homeostasis.

Hereditary Factors in Neurosis

If neurosis is considered to stem from deficits in ego strength, it is legitimate to ask whether such deficits may be genetic, environmental, or both. Our prejudice, of course, leans toward the last explanation, but it is necessary to provide experimental data to support it. Studies by Loehlin (1977) on hereditary influences in personality development were quoted in the last chapter. Although these do bear on the kinds of personality that may evolve (the qualitative aspect), they do not directly address the more pertinent question of ego strength and the tendency to become neurotic (the quantitative factor).

Techniques similar to that of Loehlin have been extended to the study of a variety of neurotic characteristics with somewhat less clear results. Shields and Slater (1960) studied twins with the diagnosis of neurosis or personality disorders. Twenty-nine percent of identical twins were diagnosed as having the same type of neurosis, whereas only 4% of fraternal twins were diagnosed as concordant. Anxiety states showed the highest level of concordance, obsessional states next, and hysterical states least. This is consistent with our psychobiological formulations that anxiety reactions would be the most physiological and hence most determined by heredity. By the same reasoning, one would expect obsessional reactions, which are also characterized by high levels of anxiety, to be more biologically determined than hysterical reactions. These experimental data may necessitate a reconsideration of our thinking as to what extent obsessional reactions are experientially derived and as to what extent hysterical reactions may be hereditary. However, even though the correlation for hysterical reactions was lower than that for the other neuroses, it was still higher than that for normals and consequently still indicative of a significant, albeit somewhat weaker, hereditary effect.

A review of Loehlin's (1977) statistics on genetic factors in personality development as listed in the last chapter (Table 19-1) shows that personality, the variable that determines the kind of neuroses that may develop, certainly shows a strong hereditary influence. Although in only 6 of the 16 comparisons made were there significant differences between identical and fraternal twins, in every case the intragroup correlation was greater for identical twins. It is of particular interest that of the six studies showing significant differences, two, those by Canter (1973) and by Eaves and Eysenck (1975), were on the introvert–extravert scale. As will be shortly described, this is the scale which best differentiates between anxiety related neuroses deriving from introversion (e.g., anxiety states and obsessional states) and hysterical neuroses deriving from extraversion. This lends support to the thesis that both types of neuroses, dysthymic and hysterical, have significant hereditary elements.

Neuroses Secondary to Abnormal Reactivity of Compensatory Mechanisms: Manifestations in Introverts and Extraverts

Utilizing a factor analysis of items relating to the history and symptomatology of a group of neurotics and normals, Eysenck (1961) developed two separate parameters that he considered critical in characterizing normal and neurotic personalities. These were the introversion–extraversion factor and the neuroticism factor. Figure 20-2 illustrates the distribution of normals and of various neurotic categories along this two-dimensional matrix.

Along both continua, the normal population clusters about the mean. There occurs the usual population spread toward the ends of the extraversion–introversion dimension with relatively few at the very extremes. Eysenck characterized extraverts as sociable, active, excitable, lively, and impulsive, whereas introverts tended to be unsociable, thoughtful, and serious. The neurosis parameter represents a breakdown of intrapsychic or intersocial homeostasis, a dimension encompassed under the rubric of ego strength.

Eysenck labeled the neuroses deriving from introversion as dysthymic and those stemming from extraversion as hysterical. Based on a variety of considerations, Eysenck concluded that the major difference between the two groups was the level of arousal at which they were functioning, with the dysthymics operating at a high level and the extraverts at a low. This is an important distinction since the mode of handling excessive arousal is one of the essential elements of adaptation and helps to define extreme opposites of dysfunction.

There is corroborative evidence that dysthymics may be differentiated from hysterics by the general level of arousal in the brain. Of special interest is the well-confirmed finding that obsessive–compulsive characters have a high sedation threshold, an index of high arousal, whereas hysterics show a low threshold. The sedation threshold test involves the administration of sodium pentothal intravenously until speech becomes slurred and/or until there is a diminution in the level of EEG arousal.

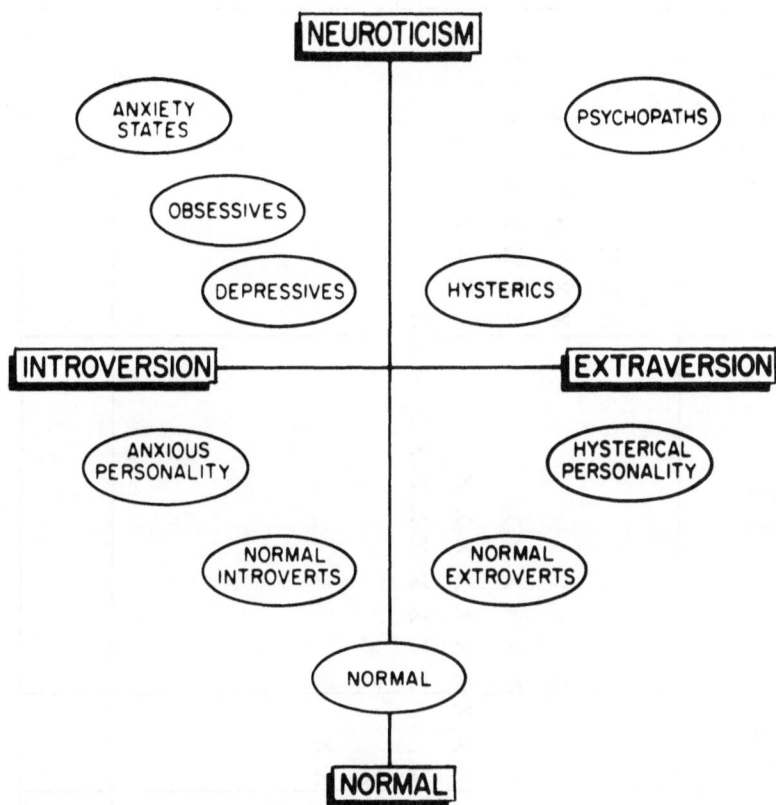

Figure 20-2 Clustering of different neurotic diagnoses on the introversion–extraversion scale. (Modified from Eysenck, 1961.)

The originator of the test, Shagass (1956), first used it to differentiate high-level anxiety patients from low-level patients, a result that it accomplished with great effectiveness; there was a high correlation between the level of anxiety and the sedation threshold. Later, Shagass and co-workers found equally good differentiations on the obsessive–compulsive to hysteria dimension with obsessive patients showing high sedation thresholds and hysterics very low ones. The neurophysiological basis for this is presumably related to the general level of arousal in the brain as a result of which there is a correlation between behavioral anxiety levels and sedation thresholds. These relationships are illustrated in Figure 20-3.

Although Shagass (1956) made his original observations on the distinction between obsessive–compulsives and hysterics, he found that anxiety states and neurotic depressions showed even higher levels of arousal than did obsessive–compulsives (Fig. 20-2). Conversion hysterias and hysterical personalities, on the other hand, showed no higher level of anxiety than did normals. Thus it appears that the dysthymic neuroses, deriving from introverted subjects, were characterized by a breakdown in the compensatory mechanisms existing to prevent the building up of excessive anxiety. On the other hand, in hysterics deriving from the extraverted personalities, such a breakdown does not occur.

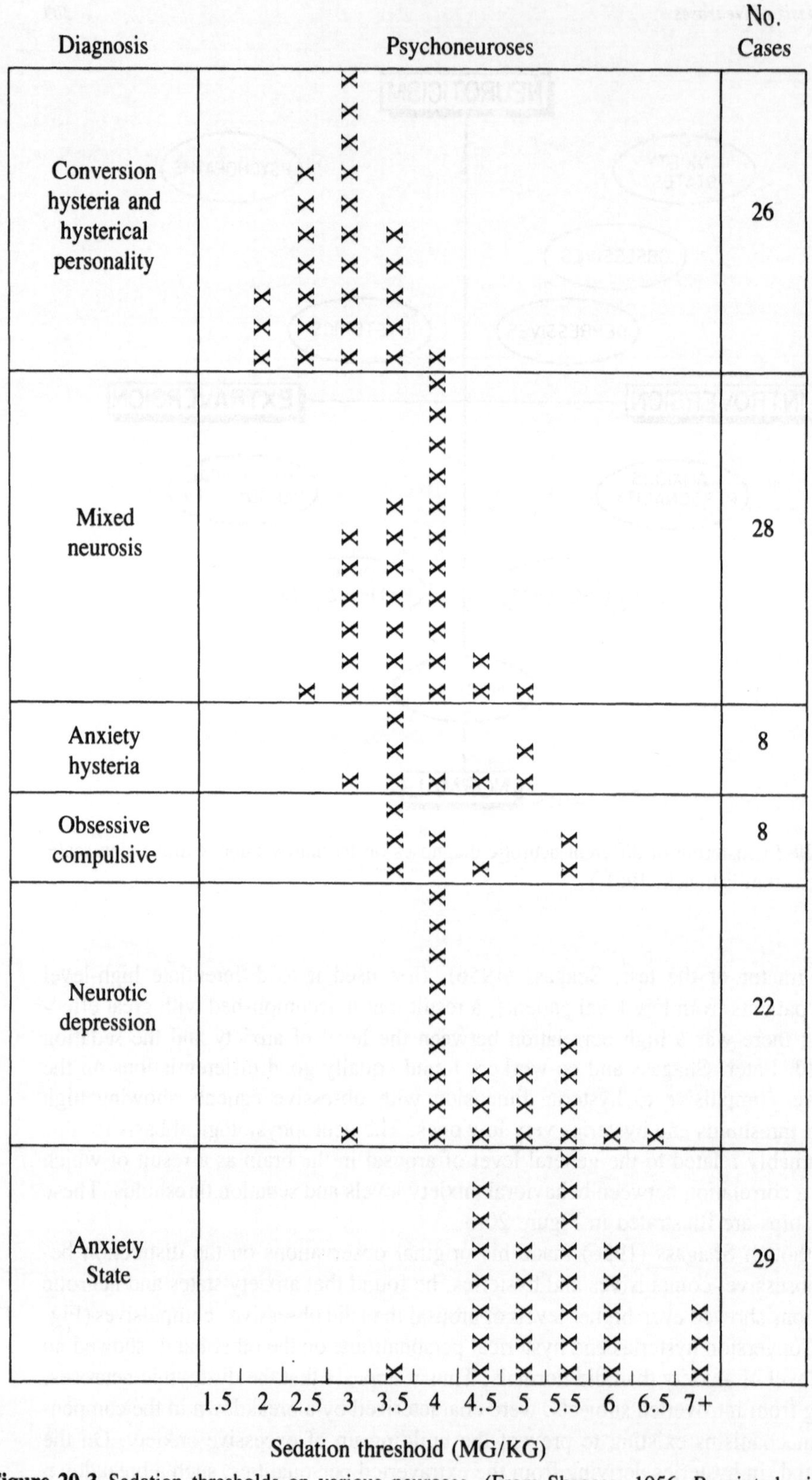

Figure 20-3 Sedation thresholds on various neuroses. (From Shagass, 1956. Reprinted with permission.)

All of these data fit in very well with the physiological reactivities postulated for introverts and extraverts in the last chapter, with particular reference to their relationship to the augmentation–reduction paradigm. Briefly, the key points may be summarized as follows:

1. Under usual conditions, i.e., conditions of low or moderate arousal, introverts tend to be reducers and extraverts augmenters. However, under conditions of extreme stress, introverts tend to become augmenters and extraverts tend to become reducers.
2. Introverts tend to have higher arousal levels under all conditions than do extraverts, but the differential becomes more extreme during stress (neurosis). Under those conditions, the reducing power of extraverts is exercised maximally to depress the level of arousal, while that of introverts decompensates, allowing a marked increase in arousal levels.
3. Introverts are more sensitive to external stimuli (lower sensory thresholds), avoid external stimulation behaviorally, and reduce it physiologically. In neurotic decompensation, their defense mechanisms break down and they are overwhelmed by excessive arousal (dysthymic neurotics). Extraverts are less sensitive to external stimulation, seek external stimulation behaviorally, and enhance it physiologically (augmenters). In neurotic decompensation, as arousal becomes excessive and threatening, they utilize cognitive and adaptational inhibition to maintain physiological (but not psychological) homeostasis.

Homeostatic Decompensation in Dysthymic Neurosis

These interpretations are in keeping with the thesis formulated in the last chapter that introverts are already at the end of their defensive reactivity with even moderate levels of stress (Fig. 19-1B). When additional stress is experienced, the compensatory mechanisms break down completely and severe anxiety results.

The switch over in reduction–augmentation reactivities from reducing tendencies in normal introverts to augmenting in neurotic introverts and from augmenting reactivities in normal extraverts to reducing in neurotic extraverts is consistent with a switch over in amygdaloid–hippocampal control balance at high levels of stress. As postulated in the last chapter, extraversion in normal subjects is associated with the physiological and behavioral reactivities characteristic of amygdaloid dominance while introversion is associated with the reactivities characteristic of septal–hippocampal dominance. Since the development of neuroses is indicative of a breakdown in psychological defenses, it follows that this should be reflected in a comparable breakdown in the normal functional balance between septal–hippocampal and amygdaloid dominance. This is an area of great physiological interest which should be susceptible to testing in neurotic introverts (dysthymics) and extraverts (hysterics).

Some experimental evidence that the reducing mechanisms break down in dysthymic neuroses is provided by a study of repressive activity in dreams. Cohen and Cox (1975) investigated the influence of neurosis and emotionally charged events on

dream production. They used the Neuroticism scale of the Maudsley Personality Inventory and selected those subjects with the highest and lowest scores.* The high-
neuroticism and low-neuroticism subjects were then randomly assigned to a pleasant or
stressful presleep condition. They found a significant correlation between presleep
stress and the occurrence of stressful dreams (as reported the next morning) in high-
neuroticism subjects, but not in low-neuroticism subjects. From this they concluded
that highly neurotic subjects had a deficit in normal repressive function. In these
subjects, not only was there a higher incidence of unpleasant dreams with free recall of
dram material, but there was also the direct incorporation of emotional material into
the dream; this, too, speaks for absence of repression. The correlations between the
emotional content of the presleep experience and the emotional content of the dream
was 0.25 for the high-neuroticism group and 0.14 for the low-neuroticism group, a
highly significant difference.

    These data suggest that nonneurotic subjects were more successful in maintaining
''repression,'' whereas neurotic subjects were less successful. Thus repression must be
seen as a normal reactivity, at least when it is exercised within normal limits; the
breakdown of repressive activity is then viewed as a defect in ego function.

    The extent of the breakdown in defense mechanisms varies among the three
prototypical dysthymic disorders, being greatest in the anxiety states, somewhat less in
the neurotic depressions, and only moderate in obsessive–compulsive neuroses. This
sequence is illustrated in the corresponding level of anxiety existing in each condition
(Fig. 20-3). It appears that the Freudian explanation of neurotic equivalents may be
valid, namely that the ability to express a conflict in some symbolic form, however
pathologically, acts at least partially as a decathecting influence. As will be seen in the
following section, the more extreme symbolic expressions of conflict in conversion
hysterias result in a full decathexis of anxiety with no excessive anxiety resulting
(Fig. 20-3).

The Neurophysiology of Hysterical and Related Clinical Symptomatology

    The situation in extraverts is in many ways the exact opposite of that in introverts.
Extraverts operate on the augmentation side of their curve (Fig. 19-1B) with small to
moderate amounts of stress (excitation), but go onto the reducing side when stress
becomes severe. This represents not a breakdown in compensatory mechanism, but
rather an overreaction. As a consequence, there is no overt evidence of increased
anxiety even in cases of severe hysterical pathology (Fig. 20-3). This of course is
reflected clinically in *la belle indifference* (beautiful indifference) of hysterics, a
condition of apparent total lack of concern despite the presence of severe physical
incapacities.

    In the behavioral aberrations of hysterical neurosis, ordinary psychobiological
explanations appear insufficient. In some of these cases, there may be massive inhib-

---

*Individuals with high scores on this scale tend to be dysthymic neurotics.

itory effects that do not comply with known physiological mechanisms. For example, in hysterical glove anesthesia and paralysis, the area of involvement follows no known anatomical distribution of nerves, but is defined rather by an essentially functional rubric, namely, "the hand." In this case, psychodynamic explanations of an unconscious inability to feel or move the hand appear to make as much or more sense than any presently known psychobiological mechanisms.

Some progress is being made even in this difficult area. Recently, neurophysiological evidence of massive inhibitory actions at the subcortical level has been presented in cases of conversion hysteria. Halliday (1973) has studied visual evoked responses to flashes of light recorded at the occipital cortex in patients with hysterical blindness and has found essentially normal evoked potentials over the primary cortical receiving areas. The presence of an evoked response in the absence of consciousness of light in these patients indicates a block of the stimulus subsequent to the thalamus and not primarily a block of the connection between the optic tracts as they enter the brain stem on their way to the thalamus. Evidence for this interpretation is provided by P. Fenwick (personal communication) who has extended these studies. He writes:

> We had the opportunity of repeating some of the original work on hypnosis. There is no doubt that subjects in a hypnotic trance show minimal change in their EEGs as previously reported. However, visual pattern evoked responses behave quite differently. Deep trance subjects who report that they become blind lose their visual evoked response to pattern reversal whereas they do not lose it with flash stimulation. This would suggest that the visual system handles flash and pattern information differently.

The failure to obtain normal pattern-reversal evoked potentials suggests an inhibitory influence operating below the primary visual receiving areas 17. This finding, together with the normal evoked potential to flash, suggests an inhibitory influence somewhere in the area of the thalamic radiations through which visual impulses are carried from the thalamus to the visual cortex. The putative dynamics for such effects might possibly lie in the interactions underlying inhibitory mechanisms in the prefrontal–thalamic feedback mechanism described in Figure 8-1 or in some aberration of hippocampal function as suggested in the last chapter.

Most important is the fact that hysterical symptoms do not tend to follow lines of physiological disruption, but rather those that would correspond to some more behavioral formulation. This speaks for a complex dysfunctional disruption of normal activity at the unconscious level, the neurophysiology of which appears to be of a different order than that characteristic of episodic unconscious processing.

The unusual patterns of clinical symptomatology in conversion hysterias, in obsessive–compulsive neuroses, and in certain psychosomatic illnesses, e.g., ulcerative colitis and spastic colon, seem at first glance almost beyond psychobiological explanation. In each case, the clinical syndrome has a compelling quality that appears to demand an interpretation delivered in narrative rather than in physiological terms. The glove anesthesia and paralysis of conversion hysteria apparently cannot be explained in physiological terms nor can the obligatory hand-washing of the obsessive–compulsive or the chronic diarrhea of spastic colon. In each instance, the clinical symptomatology is of such a nature as to appear to be explicable only in terms of some complex motivational and emotional scheme. Psychoanalysis, of course, lends itself to such explanations; psychobiology lends a different order of explanations.

Interaction of the Dynamic and the Procedural Unconscious in Hysterical Neurosis

In order to explore the area in which a psychobiological solution to these questions might be sought, one must return to the analysis of the pathogenesis of neuroses touched on in Chapter 17 on the psychobiological model of the unconscious. There it was postulated that highly threatening experiences, particularly in childhood, would be decathected through the inhibition of their cognitive component with a resulting decrease in the associated level of anxiety. Nevertheless, the rekindling of anxiety remains a constant threat and the "psyche" resorts to a mode of behavior that in one way or another will maintain homeostasis. This is what happens in the paralysis of conversion hysteria and in the continuous hand-washing of the obsessive–compulsive syndrome.

But in these cases, the behavioral complex is more than a simple reaction. It is an entire sensory–motor process. Even more, it is the kind of process that falls into the category of a procedural process related to the carrying out of an episodic motivation as much as it is an episodic event in itself. Consequently, it seems that the conflict in these syndromes must lie in the dynamic unconscious with conversion hysteria representing massive desensitizing (inhibitory) effects and obsessive–compulsion representing massive sensitizing (vigilance) effects. It also seems that the mechanisms for the complex sensory–motor deficits or overactivities must lie in the procedural unconscious where such complex activities are organized on an automatic basis rather than in the dynamic unconscious where activities are organized on a cognitive basis. Under these circumstances, the final clinical behavior in both of these syndromes would be the result of an interaction between the episodic conflicts in the decathected dynamic unconscious and the programmatic operations of the procedural unconscious (see Chapters 11 and 17).

Similar explanations might or might not apply to a variety of psychosomatic illnesses where the secondary system involved would be the visceral unconscious rather than the procedural. One can postulate purely autonomic nervous system dysfunctions to account for the symptomatology of psychosomatic disease (see p. 317). On the other hand, a symbolic role for diarrhea in ulcerative colitis and in the irritable colon syndrome cannot entirely be ruled out. The theoretical arena for the organization of such responses would be in the visceral unconscious just as the arena for the symbolic expressions for conversion hysteria and obsessive–compulsive behavior would be in the procedural unconscious.

It may be even more difficult to conceptualize the possible physiological mechanisms through which symbolic acting out could occur in the visceral unconscious than in the procedural unconscious, but it is by no means inconceivable. Apparently, visceral procedural mechanisms involve complex patterns of visceral interactions with those of episodic influences just as do cognitive procedural mechanisms. That this is the case is best illustrated in Lewis Thomas' description of the removal of warts on one side of the body through hypnosis (see Chapter 17 on the visceral unconscious). If suggestion through hypnosis to the dynamic unconscious can bring about such complex visceral operations, it is not inconceivable that conflicts in the dynamic unconscious might bring about similar symbolic reactions in the visceral unconscious.

The massive inhibitory responses of conversion hysteria in which whole systems may be inactivated (hysterical stupors, blindness, paralyses, and anesthesias) may be paralleled by the total inhibition of feelings which is said to be characteristic of extroverted psychopaths. Lykken (1957) studied a group of primary psychopaths, characterized by the inability to express feelings of fear or guilt either clinically or in test situations. He demonstrated that they learned a shock-avoidance task significantly more poorly than did controls; this is consistent with the demonstration by Franks (1960) that hysterics, of whom psychopaths are a subgroup, condition more slowly than normals. Schacter and Latane (1964) replicated this result, but also found that after an injection of epinephrine the group of psychopaths learned the shock-avoidance task more rapidly than did normal controls. Schacter and Latane interpreted this finding to indicate that psychopaths have no efferent system for producing fear (underactivity of the anxiety system), but when such symptoms are produced pharmacologically, they react like normals.

The massive inhibitory effects upon the function of the procedural, emotional, and visceral unconscious predicated in these various examples, i.e., conversion hysterias, psychopathy, and psychosomatic diseases, are, in this paradigm, the products of the breakdown of normal homeostatic mechanisms in the dynamic unconscious. This formulation presumes a variety of prerequisites: (1) an active dynamic unconscious where conflicts are ordinarily resolved; (2) the existence of a variety of conflicts that are insoluble through ordinary normal defensive reactions; (3) the breakdown of ordinary defensive reaction patterns; (4) the adoption of abnormal neurotic defensive modes as a last-stand attempt to reduce anxiety; and (5) the ability of the dynamic unconscious to communicate with the procedural, emotional, and visceral unconscious and thus to transfer the seat of conflict from the dynamic unconscious to still lower levels of awareness. Dysthymic neurosis, particularly anxiety states, would represent a breakdown at level 3. Obsessive–compulsive behavior would fall more in line with the mechanisms at level 4. Conversion hysteria, psychopathy, and possibly psychosomatic illness would come under the rubric of level 5. Under this paradigm, the direction of a neurosis would depend upon the existing personality characteristics of the individual involved as well as upon the nature of the conflict.

The Frustration Dynamic Model and the Pathogenesis of Neurosis

Anxiety neuroses occur among dysthymics when anxiety-reducing mechanisms (the inhibition of the cognitive element of emotional threats) are no longer effective. Hysterical neuroses occur when those same inhibitory mechanisms become so extreme as to be applied not only to the cognitive element of emotional threats, but to entire cognitive–sensory–motor constellations of reactivities in the episodic, procedural, emotional, and the visceral unconscious. In both instances, it is a matter of misapplied compensatory mechanisms, either underactive as in the case of introverted dysthymics or overactive as in the case of extraverted hysterics.

The anxiety resulting from emotional threats cannot always be decathected. As suggested in Chapter 18, the anxiety and depression resulting from separation and isolation in early childhood can hardly be defended against with either sensitizing or desensitizing defense mechanisms. The deprivation is all too real. The resulting anxiety and depression are equivalent to those of neurotic depressions shown in Figure 20-3, and are surpassed only by the level of arousal in acute anxiety states. The underlying dynamic is one of severe frustration of an essential need where the individual is powerless and is reduced to a helpless and hopeless state.

Other forms of frustrating experience may also produce insoluble conflict. One type of neurosis results when an individual continually receives "mixed signals," e.g., has been conditioned to expect that a given action will bring a given treatment (punishment or reward) and that appropriate response will be rewarded by appropriate treatment. Masserman (1950) applied this theoretical formulation to experimental validation by training animals to open a food box in response to a sensory signal. After this response was well learned, Masserman introduced, concurrent with the sensory signal, a strong deterrent stimulus such as an electric shock, an air blast, or with monkeys the sudden appearance of the head of a snake. After many such traumatic experiences, the animals became persistently anxious and developed psychosomatic symptoms, defensive reactions, phobic aversions, sexual deviations, and sensorial disturbances. This experimental paradigm can be viewed equally as conflictual (Masserman) or as frustrating (Rosenzweig).

Liddell (1953, 1954), working within the same theoretical frame of reference, produced similar "neurotic" behavioral syndromes in several animal species through a variety of more cognitive conflictual situations. In one setting, the visual presentation of a circle was associated with a food reward while the stimulus of an ellipse was associated with an electric shock. Animals quickly learned to respond positively to the circle and with avoidance to the ellipse. After these responses were well learned and embedded, the circle was flattened and the ellipse rounded so that the differentiation became extremely difficult. After repeated errors, the animals developed similar neurotic symptomatology to those demonstrated by Masserman's subjects. Other experiments by Anderson and Parmenter (1941) requiring equally difficult experimental distinctions or adherence to rigid time schedules produced similar neurosislike syndromes.

The conflictual type of experimental exposure almost always results in an overtly anxious, hyperactive, unstable, distractable animal comparable to an acute anxiety neurosis in man. Recent studies suggest that these kinds of experiences in human childhood are particularly conducive to the development of psychoses in those individuals who have some predisposition to that type of psychopathology.

One interpretation of the possible dynamic that activates both separation anxiety and depression and conflictual neuroses has been called the "frustration dynamic model." In this model the first reaction is one of extreme frustration from which there is no escape and for which there is no defense. The initial reaction in this phase is one of anger or even rage. When this, too, proves ineffective and futile, the organism goes into a state of chronic anxiety. The continuing anger or rage may be turned outwardly (extrapunitive), inwardly (intrapunitive), or in some way denied (impunitive). With extrapunitive or impunitive reactions, anxiety may be allayed; with an intrapunitive reaction, anxiety and depression result. It is for this reason that on Shagass' chart (Fig. 20-3) neurotic depressions show among the highest levels of anxiety (arousal).

Clinical and experimental evidence provides substantial support for this interpretation. The separation syndrome as described in Chapter 18 is characterized in both children and infant monkeys by a short period of extreme rage followed by a prolonged period of anxiety and depression. The data in experimental conflictual neuroses are less clear, but are not incompatible with those in the separation syndrome. In both cases, frustration occurs at first, but is rapidly converted into a feeling of helplessness which is translated psychologically into anxiety and depression.

The ability to tolerate frustration is a quality of emotional style and presumably derives from the extension of the hereditary influences of temperament. On the other hand, there is no reason to believe that early experience does not markedly influence this largely biological trait. An early childhood where every wish of the child is granted lest he or she go into a temper tantrum is certainly excellent conditioning for low frustration tolerance later in life. Thus tolerance to the many types of frustrating experience of later life is like all other elements of personality, an amalgam of inherited and experienced influences.

The Frustration Dynamic Model and Psychosomatic Disease

The view of neuroses that is most compatible with the frustration dynamic model is that of Masserman who advocated the "biodynamic" approach, a psychology made of about equal parts of psychobiology and psychoanalysis. Masserman's psychology was highly "dynamic" in that it postulated that all behavior, animal and human, was driven by physiological needs which were then translated into psychological motivations. He postulated also that each individual was characterized by his own special armamentarium of motivational, adaptational, and cognitive reactivities that during the course of living experience developed into a unique pattern of needs, desires, attitudes, reactivities, and so forth. These attitudes were frequently idiosyncratic to the demands of reality so that the conflict between them and the prevailing social norms frequently led to neurotic emotional reactions and behavior.

Freedman et al. (1972) describe Masserman's conception of the nature of this conflict as follows:

> Conflict is the clash of two or more motivations accompanied by increasing tension and anxiety and resulting in maladaptive behavior. Neurotic anxieties, depressions, and inhibitions arise in human beings when they are faced with conflicting positive and negative choices. (p. 148)

According to our model, "neurotic anxieties and depressions" would result from the intrapunitive response to frustration while "inhibitions" would result more probably from the impunitive or denial modes of responsivity. On the other hand, extrapunitive reactions would be characterized by a chronic state of anger or hostility or aggression which would be manifest both behaviorally and physiologically. Depending on the mode of defense utilized, three entirely different patterns of behavioral and physiological responsivity might result from essentially similar frustrating experiences.

The behavioral manifestations of intrapunitive and extrapunitive responsivities, as described below, are clinically manifest, but those of impunitive responders are more difficult to detect. Because there is no outward manifestation of anger or hostility, these having been repressed or denied and thus decathected, the pent-up anger, anxiety, or depression that would be regularly expressed by intrapunitive and extrapunitive individuals are released only during periods of extreme frustration. Since repression affects mainly the cognitive elements of an experience and reduces arousal only secondarily during periods of successful repression, smoldering physiological remnants of repressed anger, anxiety, and despair are operative at all times. It is these that are thought to produce in susceptible individuals various psychosomatic illnesses, such as bronchial asthma and ulcerative colitis.

If psychosomatic disease were the product of so specific a mechanism, one might expect all psychosomatic illness to be at least similar in their clinical manifestations, more or less like anxiety states and depressive neuroses. But there are several explanations for the wide spectrum of clinical symptomatology. First would be the multiple influences of the dynamic unconscious on the visceral unconscious. Second, the psychological influences that may lead to a specific psychosomatic reaction can do so only when the physical diathesis for that medical condition already exists. Thus bronchial asthma, which often appears to be a prototypical response for individuals who are characterized by the impunitive response to frustration, occurs only in individuals with a strong family and personal history of allergy. Similarly, individuals who rather than repressing anger and hostility (impunitive) suppress them (a modification of extrapunitive reactivity), tend to develop hypertension, but only if there is a strong family history of hypertension. Thus hereditary physical diathesis is one important element in the diversity of psychosomatic clinical manifestations.

Another reason for such diversity lies apparently in the use of the various modes of defense against frustration. The specific intrapunitive, extrapunitive, and impunitive modes are convenient for description, but do not necessarily describe specific individual reactivities. Each of these may be used to a greater or lesser extent in different situations so that a given individual may be characterized as utilizing one or another modes of responsivity predominantly. As a consequence, there may be a variety of mixed patterns as a result of which anger, anxiety, and depression will be expressed or inhibited to different degrees. Also as evidenced in the work of Frenkel-Brunswik, aggressivity may be expressed behaviorally either as irritability or as qualities of leadership. Similarly, depending on the mode and on the effectiveness of the entire defensive style, differences in the conscious and unconscious manifestations of different emotional reactivities will result.

Still another reason for the clinical variety of psychosomatic symptomatology stems from this last conclusion. If different patterns of conscious and unconscious rage, aggressivity, anxiety, shame, guilt, and depression as well as of positive reactivities such as enthusiasm and happiness exist, then each individual is characterized by a different internal psychologically influenced physiological milieu. As was emphasized in Chapter 3 on the emotions, each emotional reactivity is characterized by a different pattern of discharge in the autonomic nervous system. As a result, individual emotional reactions such as anger, fear, surprise, and happiness are expressed in different patterns of visceral reactivities (Ax, 1953).

Some of these differences in physiological responsivity are illustrated in a study by Ekman et al. (1983). These investigators studied the reactivities of two simple physiological responses, heart rate and finger temperature, under a variety of experimentally induced emotional reactions. The results are illustrated in Figure 20-4. It is evident from using just these two simple parameters that no two emotional reactivities are the same. If one were to add the multitude of other possible physiological indicators of emotional response, the patterns of reactivity of different emotional reactivities would clearly be vastly different from one another.

These psychobiological explanations appear to be sufficient to explain the wide variety of clinical manifestations of psychosomatic disease. If different individuals respond to different kinds of frustration in a variety of defensive modes, then each will

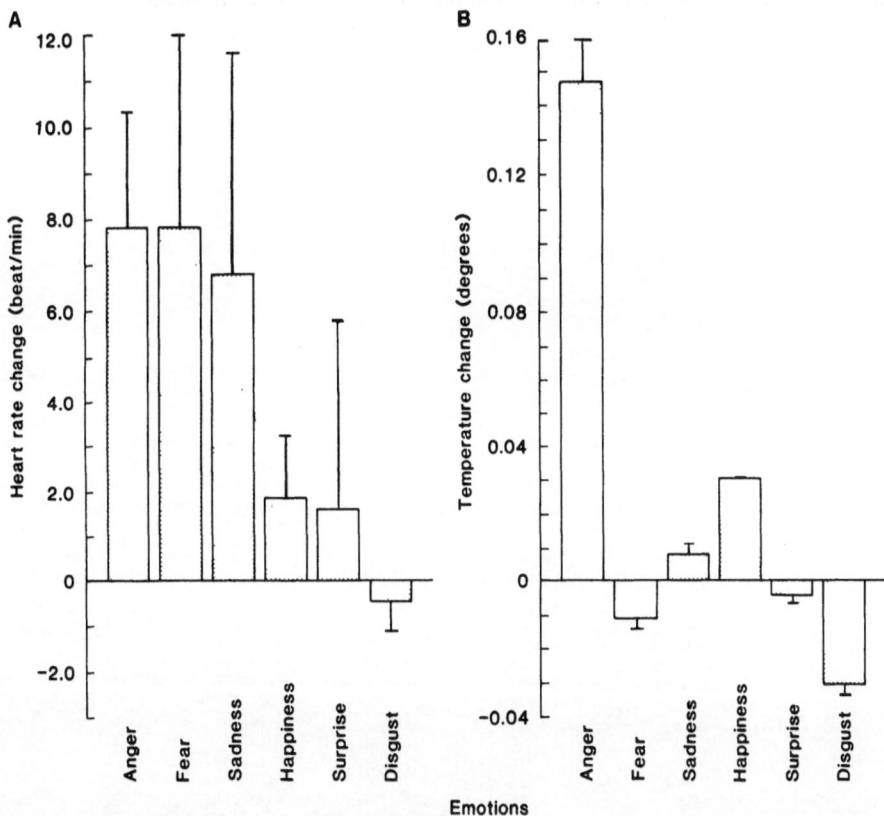

Figure 20-4 Physiological patterns of different emotional responses. (From Ekman et al., 1983. Reproduced with permission.)

have a different internal physiological milieu stemming from psychological influences. Where such influences are congruent with certain hereditary diatheses to psychosomatic illness, they will exacerbate those tendencies and contribute to the development of that disease. Consequently, emotional influences should not be seen as causing psychosomatic illnesses, but rather as contributing to their development.

The mode of interaction between neurotic influences and hereditary diatheses is a complementary one so that the greater either one is, the less of the other is necessary to produce the clinical disorder. It is clear that medically speaking, hereditary diatheses to psychosomatic illness, like neurotic influences, are a variable thing. Depending on the genetic determinants of a given diathesis, i.e., whether they be monogenetic or polygenetic, a syndrome may exist in an all-or-none or in a more-or-less form. Tay-Sachs disease is a monogenetic syndrome; one either has it or does not have it. But the diatheses for psychosomatic diseases, as for the psychoses, are polygenetic so that they may vary from high to slight, depending upon the percentage of critical genes involved.

The principle of interacting genetic and environmental effects, when both contribute toward the development of a specific syndrome, is basic to the understanding of mental and physiological illness. The complementary nature of these two influences, where the sum or the product of the two must reach a certain level before clinical manifestations occurs, is readily understandable. It is of course the basic principle determining the interaction of all environmental and hereditary influences.

21

Hypnagogic States and Transcendent Experience

The foregoing description of the pathogenesis of the neuroses leads along two very interesting lines to a consideration of the subject matter of this chapter "Hypnagogic States and Transcendent Experience." The first line deals with the generation of massive inhibitory effects, mechanisms involved both in the development of hysterical neuroses and in the initiation of transcendent states. The second is concerned more with psychoanalytic methodology for treating neuroses, a technique utilizing altered states of consciousness under which rubric hypnagogic conditions fall. Since the last chapter of this volume deals with psychoanalytic methodology, this chapter provides a convenient bridge between Chapter 20 and Chapter 22.

Still another reason for addressing the subject matter of this chapter is its obvious relationship to unconscious activities of the sort that form the very basis of psychoanalysis. Freud was introduced to the concept of unconscious mental activity through his clinical experience with hypnosis, and the early attempts to probe the dynamic unconscious were mediated through the technique of hypnosis. In view of the important role of hypnosis in the early development of psychoanalysis, it is interesting that the technique not only later fell out of favor but that little effort was made to consider even the theoretical implications of the phenomenon.

Transcendent experience is a by-product of certain hypnagogic states and as such should be considered as still another possible route to the unconscious. Evidence will be presented in this chapter that transcendent experiences, since they are the productions of altered states of consciousness, tap a certain compartment of unconscious experience. As previously stated (p. 184), this may provide psychological benefits of sorts and may account for the great popularity of the use of drugs and other agents in the search for such experience.

The desire and search for transcendent experience has been a universal characteristic of mankind at all times and in all places. Its most common physical manifestations have been in the sexual act and in the taking of various drugs, notably alcohol. Spiritual equivalents exist in the form of religious and esthetic experience in which

321

essentially mental events are somehow translated into physiological reactivities. Other forms of transcendent experience which are neither obviously physical or spiritual involve the achievement of states of altered consciousness as in biofeedback, transcendental meditation, hypnotic fugues, and so on.

Despite the variety of clinical manifestations, all transcendent experiences have certain elements in common. In each case there is a desire to reduce an existing unpleasant state of tension and simultaneously to achieve a highly pleasant state of excitation or relaxation. This paradigm is, of course, the formula for all biological motivation and is in itself insufficient to define transcendent experience as unique. What distinguishes the latter is the intensity of the highly pleasant state of excitation or relaxation achieved, an intensity that borders on or achieves euphoria. What also distinguishes transcendent experience is the fact that associated with it there is an apparent shift in the level of consciousness from β-driven alert consciousness to an $\alpha-\theta$-driven altered state of consciousness (the hypnagogic state). Concomitantly, there are reductions in those mental functions that are critical for reality testing.

As a consequence, the individual escapes from an unpleasant world of reality into a highly pleasant world of unreality. In this way, the search for transcendent experience can become a most powerful defense mechanism for protecting oneself against the exigencies of a hostile world. The tendency to utilize such an extreme defense is partially related to the severity of external stress (e.g., the heavy use of drugs among American soldiers in the Vietnam War), but much more directly to the personality of the individual. Thus factors such as ego strength, extravert–introvert tendencies, and existence of borderline psychotic reactivities will all influence the need of an individual to seek transcendent escapes from reality.

An abortive form of transcendent experience may exist in the absence of a change in level of consciousness. Such maneuvers can be utilized at a lower level of intensity to transform in socially acceptable ways mild-to-moderate tensions into moderate-to-intense pleasures. Thus the moderate tension of sexual desire can be transformed into intense pleasure through the sexual act. The tensions of intellectual uncertainty or esthetic hunger can similarly be transformed, respectively, into spiritual certainty through religion or into esthetic satisfaction through art. Finally, the everyday tensions of life can be reduced and transformed into the highly pleasant states of alcoholic relaxation. Each of these moderate and socially acceptable uses of emotionally transporting experience can be abused and exaggerated into the pathological states of nymphomania and satyriasis, into religious fanaticism and artistic frenzies, and into drug abuse and alcoholism. Only in their extreme form when they are associated with a change in level of consciousness can they be labeled truly transcendent.

The neurophysiological mechanisms underlying transcendent experience involve three major effects: a strong excitation of the pleasure tract (the septum and median forebrain bundle in the brain); a shift of the major energizing focus of the brain from the locus coeruleus to the thalamus with a concomitant shift from predominant β-wave activity to $\alpha-\theta$-wave activity; and a shift from left-hemispheric dominance to right-hemispheric dominance. Of these three effects, the most essential is the shift from a β-driven state of alert consciousness to a $\alpha-\theta$-driven altered state of consciousness. These three effects in moderation are not unique to transcendent experience; in truth, they are characteristic of most intensely pleasurable experience. However, at a certain level of intensity, the effects of pleasurable experience change qualitatively as well as quantitatively with a corresponding change in the state of awareness.

The mechanisms through which purely mental activities can produce transcendent experience as in religious fanaticism, artistic frenzies, hypnotic fugues, and hysterical states can only be speculated on. One must hypothesize that mechanisms in the dynamic unconscious utilize retreat from alert consciousness to an altered state of consciousness as one neurotic method for dealing with insoluble conflict. This is a not infrequent mode for handling threatening external aggression in Western civilization neurotics. It is a standard mode of dealing with overwhelming threats from the outside in certain Eastern societies (e.g., Bali).

The formulation is proposed that physiologically, hypnagogic states are activated through the inhibitory effect of the septal–hippocampal circuit upon amygdaloid control, resulting in a suppression of noradrenergic RAS β-wave activity with a consequent release of α- and θ-wave activity. Evidence for this mechanism derives from consideration of the behavioral consequences of certain psychoactive drugs and from physiological studies in various hypnagogic states.

The Underlying Dynamics of Transcendental Meditation

The prototypical altered states of consciousness, where an α–θ rhythm predominates, occur in transcendental meditation and in the twilight hypnagogic state of normal sleep. As Schuman (1980) writes:

> . . . A composite picture of the progression of EEG changes during a meditation session, derived from studies of Yoga, Zen and TM, appears to be, first, an increase in the abundance of alpha rhythm in the EEG, with well-organized alpha activity appearing in all leads, especially frontal and central; second, an increase in the amplitude of alpha potentials; third, a decrease in the modal frequency of alpha; progressing to, fourth, the appearance of rhythmical trains of theta waves (5–7 Hz). (p. 338)

And later:

> Fenwick and colleagues recently reported that experienced judges could not evaluate any difference on a blind basis between meditation and drowsy EEGs. Raters evaluated EEG records for increased alpha amplitude, decreased alpha frequency, spread of alpha activity to frontal or temporal leads, frontal and temporal bursts, and concurrent alpha and theta activity; if slow, rolling eye movements were present, these changes were considered indicative of drowsiness, and if not, the changes were rated as meditation-related. On the basis of these criteria, judges failed to discriminate meditation-related EEG (Fenwick et al., 1977). (p. 353)

Schuman quotes Banquet (1973) as finding the θ pattern in meditators different from that in drowsiness, in that the former shows runs of θ activity, whereas the latter merely shows an occasional θ wave against a background of mixed frequencies. These differences in patterns of θ waves in meditation and drowsiness are similar to the differences described by Davis et al. (1941) for the θ waves of alcoholism and drowsiness. None of these seem sufficient to establish these states as separate syndromes. It would appear rather that these differences are of lesser significance than the concordance of characteristic physiological and behavioral events, which although somewhat different, are substantially the same.

Meditation appears to be the prototypical transcendent altered state of consciousness in that it is characterized entirely by the subjective qualities of that condition and by an abundant $\alpha-\theta$ rhythm in the EEG. Consequently, a consideration of the conditions necessary for its achievement may provide an understanding of those underlying all transcendent experience.

Schuman (1980) has postulated that two and possibly three conditions are essential for the achievement of a satisfactory meditative state. The first is a low state of arousal that must be maintained before the even lower level of arousal of meditation is achieved. This original low level of arousal is in itself a kind of initiatory relaxation phase in which the major consciousness system is switched from a state of noradrenergic RAS β-wave alert consciousness to a thalamic α-wave altered state of consciousness.

The second necessary condition involves the process by which the initial relaxed state of moderate α rhythm may be further depressed into the meditative state of the slow $\alpha-\theta$ rhythm. According to Schuman (1980), this may be accomplished in one of two ways, both involving attentional mechanisms. The first, so-called mindfulness, involves paradoxically a deep concentration upon mindlessness in an effort to cut off all external stimulation. In a sense it is a conscious attempt to achieve total sensory deprivation. This pattern of behavior requires skill and training, and when applied leads to the most characteristic states of transcendental meditation (TM).

The more common attentional mechanism used is that of "concentration," in which attention is strongly concentrated on an external stimulus, an auditory mantra as in TM or a visual shiny object as in hypnosis. Here there is an initial state of increased excitation secondary to the intense effort of concentration, but again in a paradoxical fashion, the sense of effort is soon converted into a sense of extreme relaxation. These procedures for inducing hypnotic states are extremely revealing about the physiological mechanisms underlying those states and will be re-examined within that context later in this chapter.

The third major factor in determining susceptibility to transcendent experience is that of personality, but the significance of this factor appears to depend as much on the particular type of hypnagogic state to be experienced as upon the personality of the individual involved. In general, individuals who find it easiest to meditate are similar in make-up to those who are most easily hypnotized. Both of these groups tend to be extraverted rather than introverted, to be field dependent rather than field independent, to be augmenters rather than reducers, and to score high on the Zuckerman Sensation Seeking Scale (SSS). Incidentally, subjects in this last category show a preference for activities which produce a marked change in the level of arousal, either toward greater excitement or toward an altered state of consciousness.

The three major categories of hypnagogic types of transcendent experience are (1) the hypnagogic (twilight) state of normal sleep (i.e., stages 1 and 2); (2) the state of TM; and (3) the trancelike state of hypnosis. A fourth state achievable through biofeedback is similar to these hypnagogic conditions, but differs in that there is no shift to the $\alpha-\theta$ state of awareness. Neither are the three hypnagogic states mentioned above entirely the same. However, unlike biofeedback, they do share the essential element of transcendent experience, that of being transported to a different level of consciousness.

Schuman (1980) has comprehensively reviewed the behavioral and physiological characteristics of the three major hypnagogic states. She concludes that despite the fact that they are similar in some of their clinical manifestations, they represent basically different altered states of consciousness. She feels that even though the three states share a common psychophysiological model, that in itself is insufficient to warrant identifying the three conditions as the same. As evidence for her position, she cites the case that in biofeedback an almost identical pattern of psychophysiological reactivity is achieved, but without evidence of any real shift to an altered state of consciousness.

Schuman's thesis is only partially correct. It is true that the major psychophysiological characteristic, namely the nature of the dominant brain wave pattern, is different for the hypnagogic state ($\alpha-\theta$) from that of biofeedback (purely α). This does speak for both qualitative and quantitative difference in the respective altered states of consciousness. However, these may be due to differences in the depth of these conditions and to differences in the mode of induction rather than to any major differences in the nature of each of these states.

The Role of Alcohol and Barbiturates in Transcendent Experience

Still another type of transcendent experience in humans derives from the use of psychoactive drugs, most particularly alcohol and barbiturates. A consideration of the normal and abnormal uses of alcohol and other psychoactive drugs provides a valuable contribution to the subject of transcendent experience because it is in this area that we have the best-controlled data on the nature of the phenomenon and of its underlying biology. The regular use of alcohol and of other psychoactive drugs in almost every primitive culture in which these chemicals were to be found suggests that the effects of such drug use are desirable to all humans and hence responsive to some basic psychological human need. The further putative division of that need into the need in certain individuals for transcendental experience and the need in others to escape pain and tension provides a still larger scope for the drive since it allows fo postulating the operation of different motivations and personalities in different situations (e.g., extraverts versus introverts).

Some evidence for this dual function of the drive for transcendent experiences comes from the study of different kinds of alcoholics and drug abusers. Both social drinkers and alcoholics, when tested on a questionnaire as to the reasons they drink, will offer a wide spectrum of responses. By and large, these may be dichotomized into drinking to relieve anxiety, tension, or depression, or conversely, drinking for its stimulating and transporting effects. In most instances, both elements are present, but usually one or the other predominates.

This differential is better illustrated in individuals who use hallucinogenic and stimulatory drugs as against those who prefer sedative drugs. The former tend to score very high on the Zuckerman Sensation Seeking Scale, whereas the latter tend to show high levels of anxiety and depression. Thus in the former group of sensation-seeking LSD and amphetamine users, one finds mainly thrill-seeking college students and the "hippies" of the 1960s; conversely among alcoholics, one often finds individuals for whom the exigencies of life have proven overwhelming. On the other hand, there is little doubt that in most alcoholics, drinking for the transcendent reality-escaping effects of alcohol was the original incentive and only later did the pain-relieving element become dominant (Kissin, 1972).

Therefore, it appears that generally the key element in drug-induced transcendent experience is not the need to escape pain and tension, although that comes to play a significant role later, but rather the transporting effects of the drugs that raise or lower the individual to a different level of consciousness. "Raise or lower" is an interesting distinction that is best illustrated in the effects of different drugs. Depressant drugs such as alcohol and sedatives, after an initial excitatory phase, produce a state of lowered consciousness similar to the $\alpha-\theta$-driven altered states of consciousness. Conversely, stimulatory drugs such as cocaine and amphetamines produce a hyperexcitatory γ-driven EEG associated with a behavioral state of hyperalert exaltation. The interesting aspect of this dichotomy is that paradoxically both conditions, the hyper-sedative and the hyperstimulant, produce states of euphoria that, although qualitatively different, still share the essential element of transport to a new level of consciousness. Furthermore, there is evidence that the new level of consciousness achieved in both instances may be part of a single phenomenon, even though it is achieved through different mechanisms. This apparently paradoxical statement becomes less so when one considers how closely related the euphorias of extreme excitement and extreme relaxation may be. This relationship returns us again to the paradoxical phenomena of the method of induction of hypnagogic states where both "mindfulness," i.e., total sensory deprivation, and "concentration," i.e., total attention directed onto a single stimulus, are equally effective in achieving a state of relaxation.

Human Sexual Activity as a Transcendent Experience

A similar paradox appears to apply in the area of sexual activity, most particularly in the orgasm. J. Davidson (1980) has reviewed the psychobiology of human sexual experience most comprehensively. In his review, he compares the behavioral and physiological characteristics of animal and human sexual activity and observes that although there are many similarities, there are sufficient differences for the two to be considered as separate and distinct entities. Most importantly, Davidson addresses the question of the subjective elements of human sexuality and concludes that the sexual act, particularly orgasm, is best considered as an altered state of consciousness. He writes:

> Tart (1975) discusses the conditions that are conducive to the "induction" of ASCs in general under the rubric of two sets of forces. The first are those that tend to produce disruption or destabilization of the existing state of consciousness, such as drugs or

any intense physiological procedure—for example, exhaustion, extreme excitation, or other stresses—or removal of normal stabilizing stimuli. The second group comprises patterning forces that tend to substitute an ASC for normal basal states. The latter commonly involve processes of relaxation, as in sleep, meditation, and hypnosis, in which there is reduction of exteroceptive and (presumably) interoceptive sensory input.

"Destabilizing" conditions occur in the case of orgasm. These include intense physical stimulation, exercise, rhythmic motion, and focused attention, all of which tend to disrupt the normal state of consciousness and stop the internal dialogue that is a condition of its maintenance. Major physiological changes that operate here include vasomotor and muscular events and, generally, strong autonomic nervous system activation, which resemble destabilizing events for many other ASCs. The capacity to "let go" of inhibition and of self-consciousness is necessary to some extent for orgasm (Lowry and Lowry, 1976, p. 105), as it seems to be for "mystical" (and other) ASCs (Davidson, 1976). (pp. 252–253)

Davidson goes on to describe the sequence of events that develops during the act of intercourse, which proceed from a series of powerful, almost overwhelming physical sensations to a secondary state of a change in consciousness. Davidson describes as characteristic of the first stage localized physical sensations such as "throbbing in the temples, stomach vibrations, hot or cold feelings in the genitals and elsewhere, expanding feelings in the pelvis leading to release of tension and genital or anal contractions." Associated also were "less localized sensations, such as lightheadedness, dizziness and the desire to sigh; and such sensory phenomena of various modalities as tingling, fluttering, buzzing, tickling, and pulsating and occasionally visual phenomena, for example, spots in front of the eyes."

In a separate category of reactivities, Davidson describes:

> . . . general mood changes, including those clearly recognizable as changes in conscious state. These included, first, such banal experiences as tiredness, release of tension, or sleepiness and some negative manifestations in a few subjects, such as anxiety in the build-up to orgasm. Other mood changes reported were euphoria and peacefulness, as well as experiences clearly belonging in the category of ASCs, such as loss of control (with spontaneous movement in some cases), loss of contact with the environment, apparent lapses of consciousness, and the sensation of being "immersed" in the present or "in limbo," and such hallucinationlike experiences as visualization of lights becoming patterns of color. (pp. 293–294)

This latter condition, Davidson concludes, constitutes an altered state of consciousness, not unlike that found in religious ecstacy. In this connection he quotes from Greeley (1974):

> It is not unreasonable to believe that under some circumstances sexual orgasm can trigger an ecstatic experience. Intercourse does de-automatize somewhat our ordinary reality orientation. It does take us out of ourselves; it is an experience of passionate unity; it is . . . a temporary inertia in fundamental life forces. While it is not the same kind of experience as mystical ecstasy . . . the two experiences are similar enough that it is not surprising that one could lead to the other. (p. 293)

Considerations such as these suggest that transcendent experiences, either of great excitation or of great peacefulness, may derive equally from episodes of overwhelming sensory excitation as in the case of sexual experience, or alternatively from complete relief from sensory excitation as in sensory isolation or with the use of depressant drugs. What seems to apply in each instance is some abrupt and overwhelming disruption in the sensory equilibrium of the organism, either to marked excess or to marked deprivation. Either condition apparently may lead to the development of altered states of consciousness and hypnagogic states. These mechanisms are in keeping with those hypothesized above by Tart (1975).

The Effects of Alcohol and Barbiturates on Brain-Wave Activity

Through the consideration of those hypnagogic states in which both the typical subjective reactions of transcendent experience are present as well as the prototypical $\alpha-\theta$ EEG, it may be possible to postulate the neurophysiological mechanisms through which altered states of consciousness are achieved. With such understanding of the neurophysiology underlying prototypical hypnagogic states, a consideration of those apparently dissociated states where transcendent experience occurs without evidence of the $\alpha-\theta$ rhythms may also be undertaken.

Interestingly enough, some of the most revealing insights into the neurophysiological mechanisms underlying the dynamics of altered states of consciousness and hypnagogic states have come from studies of the pharmacology of alcohol and barbiturate administration. The administration of these drugs to animals and humans is associated with a broad repertory of predictable behavioral activities which may be correlated both in animals and humans with a variety of neurophysiological and biochemical effects. Since alcohol and barbiturates do under certain circumstances produce transcendent effects in humans, the study of their pharmacology is vastly edifying.

The effects of alcohol administration in humans and animals are bimodal in that small doses are excitatory while large doses are markedly sedative. Small doses of alcohol in animals depress the septal–hippocampal inhibitory circuit, as a result of which there is an excitatory effect on the EEG with resultant increased β activity (Story et al., 1961). Large doses in animals enhance the septal–hippocampal inhibitory circuit with consequent depressant effects.

The acute effects of alcohol administration on EEG activity in humans are similarly biphasic. Small doses produce increased β activity. The administration of large doses is followed by a marked increase in α activity, by a slowing in the dominant rate of α activity, and by the appearance of a significant number of θ waves (4–8/sec) particularly during periods of lethargy (Davis et al., 1941). This last EEG pattern is associated with typical altered states of consciousness phenomena such as loss of contact, rambling conversation, and other signs of lethargic intoxication. Davis et al. (1941) describe the θ waves as somewhat different from those in the hypnagogic state of early sleep in that the latter appear to be separate and distinct from α activity, while in alcohol intoxication they appear to exist more as part of a generally slowing continuum.

The effects of barbiturates on septal–hippocampal activity, EEG patterns, and on behavior are similar to those of alcohol, with small doses depressing the septal–

hippocampal inhibitory circuit, while large doses enhance its activity (Gray, 1970). As a consequence, small doses of barbiturates produce a stimulatory effect reflected in increased β-wave activity in the EEG and in behavioral excitability. Larger doses, both by slowing the thalamic α-wave-generating mechanism and by stimulating the septal–hippocampal θ-wave-generating circuit, produce larger quantities of slow α waves and more pronounced θ-wave rhythms (Gray, 1970, 1971, 1972).

The effects of alcohol and barbiturates on the activity of the thalamic α-wave-generating apparatus and on that of the septal–hippocampal θ-wave-generating apparatus perhaps define the basic mechanism underlying the achievement of the full-blown altered states of consciousness characteristic of transcendent experience. The two simultaneous effects associated with high doses of these drugs, i.e., the increase in slow thalamic α-wave rhythm and the enhancement of septal–hippocampal inhibitory power, both contribute to a suppression of noradrenergic β activity with its associated state of alert consciousness. In this way, the combination of increased slow medial–thalamic α-wave-generating activity and of enhanced septal–hippocampal θ activity appear to be responsible for the slow α–θ EEG rhythms of altered states of consciousness and for the subjective transcendent experiences associated with them.

The physiological effects of alcohol and barbiturates on the septal–hippocampal circuit is of particular interest in terms of the effects of these drugs on augmentation–reduction responsivities. Spilker and Calloway (1969) reported that the administration of high doses of alcohol or barbiturates resulted in a marked reduction in the slope of visual evoked responses to stimuli of increasing intensity, a pattern indicative of diminished augmentation. This response was particularly notable among strong augmenters among whom are included alcoholics (von Knorring, 1976) and barbiturate addicts (Zuckerman et al., 1974). The reducing effects of these drugs on known augmenters provides an interesting paradigm for an underlying mechanism in the dynamics of alcohol and barbiturate addiction. Apparently in small doses, these drugs are excitatory, responding to the need of these extraverted individuals for stimulation. However, as in the neuroses, excessive stimulation in extravert addicts may ultimately rise to such a level as to exercise a disruptive influence on the stability of arousal levels. Alcohol and barbiturates apparently represent the "ideal solution" for the extraverted addict since they provide initial stimulation with a built in secondary defense against excessive arousal. There is, in addition, the additional achievement of the transcendent state, the desirable sensation characteristically sought by extraverts.

The bimodal effects of alcohol and barbiturates upon thalamic and septal–hippocampal activities and upon behavior, i.e., initially stimulatory, later sedative and transcendent, is prototypical for a variety of transcendent experiences, to wit, sexual activity, hypnotic trances, and hallucinogenic drug effects. These effects are of special interest in the light that they throw upon the mechanisms involved in the induction of hypnagogic states, namely "mindfulness" and "concentration." The two attentional mechanisms of achieving the transcendent meditative state seem paradoxical since one involves mainly depressive activity while the other involves stimulatory activity followed by depressive activity (not unlike the effects of alcohol and barbiturates). The putative physiological mechanisms involved in these two paradigms are not difficult to postulate. Apparently in the mindfulness condition, the individual is able directly to stimulate the septal–hippocampal inhibiting circuit, thus providing θ-slow-wave activity. This, in conjunction with the α rhythm already existing because of the initiatory low arousal state, leads to further slowing of the α rhythm which in turn leads to θ activity in the septal–hippocampal circuit. The continuous feedback interaction of these two circuits results in the further deepening of the hypnagogic state and of the transcendent experience.

The situation with attentional concentration is initially different, but ultimately the same. Here the initial stage of strong attentional concentration is associated with EEG β-wave activity, indicative of amygdaloid dominance in the amygdaloid–hippocampal complex. But since strong attentional concentration on a single stimulus requires particularly powerful inhibitory action on all other perceptions, major activity in the inhibitory septal–hippocampal circuit is stimulated. Ultimately this activity over-whelms amygdaloid dominance and the feedback circuit between thalamus and septal–hippocampal complex leads to the achievement of a transcendent altered state of consciousness. However, this state, as opposed to that achieved through mindfulness, is characterized by not-infrequent bursts of β-wave EEG activity, suggesting the more tenuous balance of control in the amygdaloid–hippocampal complex.

The third necessary condition for achieving TM, as previously mentioned, is that of appropriate personality. Both the ability to achieve mindfulness and to switch from marked attentional concentration to mindfulness speak for a personal ability to switch from an augmentation to a reduction style of responsivity. This would be consistent with the greater potential of extraverts either to use TM or to be hypnotizable.

The Significance of θ-Wave Activity in Altered States of Consciousness

It appears that increased θ-wave activity in hypnagogic states is indicative of increased activity of the inhibitory septal–hippocampal circuit, with a corresponding depressant effect on the posterior hypothalamus and a reduction in the activity of the noradrenergic locus coeruleus-driven RAS alert consciousness system. We previously described θ activity in the hippocampus as indicative of increased attentional activity (Chapter 8). On the surface, these two conclusions may seem contradictory, but as already suggested in Chapter 8 and 19, they are not necessarily so. Attention is of all activities the most selective, and consequently requires the greatest level of inhibition of irrelevant material. Increased hippocampal activity in attention presumably indicates not so much the stimulatory effects of attending, but rather the active inhibitory effect of screening out all irrelevant matter. The actual level of excitation during attention is set by the amygdala which, as illustrated in Figure 8-2, is as responsible as the hippocampus for the generation of the P_{300} wave in the evoked response.

These reflections on attentional mechanisms help us to reassert the basic formula-tion of the amygdaloid–hippocampal complex as an excitatory–inhibitory balance control center. In attention both elements, the excitatory amygdala and the inhibitory septal–hippocampal circuit, are coactive, both under the driving influence of the locus coeruleus-driven noradrenergic RAS. In altered states of consciousness, the major energy center has shifted from the locus coeruleus to the thalamus and a dopaminergic α-wave pattern now drives the amygdaloid–hippocampal complex. Under the conditions of a dominant thalamic-driven α rhythm, septal–hippocampal circuit activity becomes pre-eminent, θ-wave activity creeps into the EEG, there is further slowing of the α-wave activity, and an altered state of consciousness ensues.

The basic mechanisms through which locus coeruleus-driven β-wave acute consciousness is modified to thalamus-driven α-wave lower-level consciousness vary in different hypnagogic states. For example, in drowsiness the shift is apparently activated through the effects of inhibitory anterior hypothalamic influences on the locus coeruleus (see Fig. 6-4). With drug use it is accomplished mainly through the differential chemical effects of various drugs on different brain centers. With transcendental meditation and hypnosis, it is established by a mental set that deliberately opts to achieve a low arousal resting state. In each case, the thalamus has become the major driving center and the septal–hippocampal circuit the secondarily activated dominant mechanism in the amygdaloid–hippocampal circuit. The role of the amygdala in these activities is more variable. This is clarified in an examination of its activities during atypical episodes of transcendent experience.

The Dynamics of Atypical Forms of Transcendent Experience

The fact that hypnotic states are usually achieved through the use of attentional concentration probably accounts for the absence of a universal α–θ-brain-wave pattern under that condition. From every behavioral point of view, the individual in a hypnotic trance is in a deeper altered state of consciousness than is even the subject in TM. Since the individual under hypnosis is able to perform activities at a moderate level of alertness, it is not surprising that a β-wave pattern of EEG will be superimposed on what must be a basic α–θ-wave energizing system. One must postulate a dissociation of the RAS alerting system from the amygdaloid–hippocampal consciousness alerting system to account for the dual concurrent activities. This may be accomplished through a massive inhibitory action of the septal–hippocampal complex on some functional circuit as postulated for hysterical blindness in Chapter 20, concurrent with continued activity in the amygdala.

What evidence is there that an underlying α–θ state may exist during transcendent experience in the absence of α–θ activity in the EEG? Sexual activity and orgasm appear to offer a paradigm of a transcendent experience during a period of great excitement. The EEG in sexual activity is that of excitement, namely a rapid β- or even γ-brain-wave pattern. Yet Heath (1972), studying brain wave activity with intracranial probes, found spike and slow-wave activity in the septum of one mental and one epileptic patient during the period of sexual excitement and just after orgasm. Thus it appears that even though the dominant EEG pattern during such events is that of marked excitation, intracranial activity at the septal level is consistent with an underlying septal–hippocampal θ state of inhibitory activity.

Evidence for a similar dissociation between hyperexcitability at the cortical level and hypoexcitability at the level of the driving energizing system occurs with stimulant and hallucinogenic drugs.

Mandell (1980) writes:

> The hallucinogens produce high-voltage synchronous activity in hippocampus and septum, but not in amygdala, of cat and man that may last days or weeks after one administration (Adey et al., 1962). Septal and hippocampal synchronous activity in man has been seen on depth recordings in many pleasure states, including the euphoria induced by marijuana smoking (Heath, 1972). Cocaine and the amphetamines, when given chronically, induce hypersynchrony initially in the septal–hippocampal system, with eventual spread to the amygdala and extralimbic structures like the globus pallidus. (p. 399)

Since the use of these drugs is associated with peripheral EEG signs of β–γ-wave activity, but intracranial evidence of increased activity of the septal–hippocampal circuit, it seems reasonable to hypothesize that as in hypnosis and orgasm there is a dissociation in these states between the underlying α–θ energizing system and the more superficial (in these cases) β alerting system. This is not too dissimilar to the dissociation that occurs in REM sleep in which there is also an underlying condition of physical inertness associated with cortical EEG manifestations of extreme reactivity.

The mechanisms through which powerful excitatory drugs such as amphetamines, cocaine, and LSD can produce stimulation of the strong inhibitory septal–hippocampal circuit is not fully understood. Mandell (1980) has postulated that these effects are neurochemical, related to the action of these drugs on serotonin balance in the brain, but this hypothesis is unproven. More directly, one may assume that the powerful stimulating effects of these drugs on brain stem alerting mechanisms raises the general level of arousal so high as to threaten equilibrium. Under such circumstances, a physiological defense mechanism such as activation of the inhibitory septal–hippocampal circuit might be recruited to depress the general level of arousal. Although such a mechanism has not been demonstrated experimentally, it is certainly in keeping with the general principles of organismic homeostasis.

Thus this thesis postulates that the altered state of consciousness associated with transcendent experience is probably a unitary one, initiated by activation of a slowed α-generating system in the median thalamus and concluding in increased activity of the septal–hippocampal θ-generating inhibitory circuit. This feedback circuit can be activated at either end, either through the use of sedative drugs like alcohol or barbiturates that stimulate thalamic α activity or through mindfulness techniques of meditation that directly activate the septal–hippocampal circuit. Other means of achieving such increased activity of the septal–hippocampal circuit are paradoxically processes that increase the excitatory element of the amygdaloid–hippocampal complex to such an extent that the septal–hippocampal inhibitory circuit is compensatorily stimulated to take over. This process apparently applies in attentional (concentration) induction of TM and hypnotic trance and possibly in biofeedback. Finally, a similar defensive activation of the septal–hippocampal circuit appears to occur in sexual activity and in the case of stimulant and hallucinogenic drugs in order to protect the organism from excessive levels of arousal.

The Role of the Internal Reward System in Producing Transcendent States

In the last excerpt, Mandell (1980) quotes Heath (1972) as reporting that the septal–hippocampal inhibitory circuit is strongly activated by highly pleasurable states. Depending on the associated mechanisms involved, highly pleasurable activity can produce a sedated euphoria (e.g., marijuana) or alternatively a highly excitatory euphoria (e.g., orgasm). In each case, the resultant euphorias are qualitatively similar even though one is associated with a high level of relaxation and the other with a high level of excitement.

A similar situation applies with the use of heroin and cocaine, both of which when injected intravenously produce an immediate state of euphoria. However, the feeling associated with heroin is characterized by extreme relaxation whereas that with cocaine is characterized by extreme stimulation. Yet paradoxically, both types of addicts describe the "rush" of either heroin or cocaine injection as being similar to the feeling of an orgasm. Again the inference one draws is that through some common pathway, a great sense of pleasure is produced by stimulation of the median forebrain bundle and septum and a change in awareness is produced by stimulation of the inhibitory septal–hippocampal circuit to provide both the pleasurable and altered state of consciousness aspects of the euphoria.

The known pharmacology of heroin and cocaine bear out this impression. Heroin achieves its pleasurable effects by stimulating of the endorphin receptors and activating the median forebrain bundle and septum, the pleasure–reward system of most vertebrates. Cocaine also produces its pleasurable euphoria through activation of the median forebrain bundle and septum, but through stimulation of its dopamine receptors (see Chapter 2). Consequently, both drugs stimulate the same pleasure system but through different chemical channels. Presumably, it is this maximum stimulation of the median forebrain bundle and septum which in turn excites the septal–hippocampal circuit to produce the transcendent state of euphoria. Probably in sexual activity a similar sequence occurs, but stimulation of the median forebrain bundle and septum would be through neural tracts from the sexual organs rather than through any direct chemical stimulation.

The central role of the septum in activating the sensory experience of euphoria is supported by a substantial body of experimental evidence. Indeed, Olds and Milner (1954) made their original discovery of the brain-reward system through serendipitous stimulation of electrical implants in the rat's septal area. Subsequent testing by electrical stimulation of the septal area in alert humans (Heath, 1963) showed that area to be optimal for eliciting a pleasant sense of euphoria. Heath's (1972) subsequent finding of spontaneous excitation of the septum and hippocampus during highly pleasurable experience is further in keeping with this interpretation. Although there is no evidence that direct stimulation of the hippocampus per se produces euphoria, it appears that stimulation of the septum activates the hippocampus which, through its powerful inhibitory effects, adds the element of transcendence to the underlying sense of pleasure.

The evidence presented in this chapter appears to support the thesis that the brain-reward system has two separate components. First, there is the main tract consisting of areas in: the hypothalamus, thalamus, and basal ganglia (the thalamic–basal gangliar complex); the septal and cingulate nuclei of the limbic system; the medial portions of the prefrontal lobe; and connecting all of these, the medial forebrain bundle. Second, there is a separate offshoot consisting of only the septal area and the hippocampus. The main tract constitutes the true brain-reward system and is responsible for most normal pleasures such as those associated with eating, sleeping, and playing. The septal–hippocampal circuit is apparently activated only when an extreme level of pleasure or pain is being experienced, as in orgasm, sexually or drug induced, or as in physical torture. Excitation of the septal–hippocampal circuit by either extreme pleasure or extreme pain is associated with a sense of euphoria (positive or negative) characterized by a shift in awareness from alertness to an altered state of consciousness. The changes in the nature of experience that occur with sensations of extreme pleasure or extreme pain are very dramatic and play a particularly important role in the pathogenesis of addiction.

Right-Hemispheric Dominance in Transcendent Experience

In addition to the production of an altered state of consciousness and to stimulation of the internal brain reward system, the third characteristic of transcendent experience is a shift in dominant hemispheric activity from the left to the right. This is not unexpected since, as previously described, most states of lowered arousal are associated with such a hemispheric shift. However, the statement of a general principle is not sufficient in itself to prove a thesis that must rather be supported by experimental evidence.

The characteristic switch from left-hemispheric to right-hemispheric type of thinking in twilight states is described by Budzynski (1976) in Chapter 22 of this volume. Similarly, the characteristic dominance of right-hemispheric types of thinking in dreams, both in non-REM and in early and late REM productions, is described by Cohen et al. (1976) and will also be presented in Chapter 22.

Apparently similar effects are found during sexual activity. J. Davidson (1980) writes:

> The idea is gaining support that the right (or nonlanguage) cerebral hemisphere dominates during ASCs. This idea was pursued for the case of meditative–mystical types of experience by drawing analogies with data on dreaming and other states of consciousness characterized by primary-process thinking and/or simultaneous (holistic) instead of the normal sequential form of cognition (Davidson, 1976).
>
> Orgasm would appear to provide an excellent model for testing this hypothesis of left-to-right switching in ASC, but very few observations are yet available on this subject. Recently, however, Cohen, Rosen and Goldstein (1976) recorded left and right parietal EEGs from four male and three female subjects during orgasm produced by self-stimulation. In 8 of 12 experiments, they found a statistically significant change in laterality, as indicated by a large increase in EEG amplitude recorded from scalp electrodes over the right hemisphere during orgasm. The alpha rhythm was

replaced over the right hemisphere by a wave pattern in the 4-Hz range, with minimal effect on left hemisphere alpha. These findings are decidedly preliminary, and it is not clear that the effects noted necessarily indicate right-hemisphere-dominant activity. Nevertheless, the data do indicate a dissociation between right- and left-hemisphere function in orgasm and suggest the likelihood that further investigation would be fruitful. (p. 316)

The EEG changes during orgasm described in the previous excerpt do not in themselves indicate a switch in hemispheric dominance from the left hemisphere to the right, similar to those described by Budzinski (1976) in twilight states and by Cohen (1976) in dreams. On the contrary, the increase in brain wave activity in the right hemisphere during orgasm is of the θ-wave type, indicative if anything of an increase in right-hemispheric electrical power or conversely a decrease in neural activity. Davidson's conclusion that "it is not clear that the effects noted necessarily indicate right-hemisphere-dominant activity" is certainly warranted. On the other hand, the presence of increased θ-wave activity in the right hemisphere under these conditions is certainly noteworthy and as Davidson states "suggest the likelihood that further investigation would be fruitful." The thesis that hypnagogic states and transcendent experience are due specifically to θ-wave activation of the right hemisphere is heuristically attractive, but needs a great deal more substantiation before it can be accepted as more than a hypothesis.

The psychobiological analysis of transcendent experience in this next to last chapter of the volume is valuable, not only because it introduces a subject of human activity at one of the highest levels of complexity, but also because the subject itself in so many ways incorporates the topics and issues thus far described in this volume. The relationship of transcendent experience to psychoanalysis, particularly through the instrument of hypnosis, is also of interest although too complex to analyze in depth at this time. However hypnagogic phenomena appear to represent a kind of bridge between psychobiology and psychoanalytic methodology and as such provide a fitting introduction to our final chapter.

Psychobiology and Psychoanalytic Methodology

As stated in the introduction, the major theoretical thrust of this book has been to structure present psychobiological thinking into a well-ordered system that would explain in physiological terms much of normal and neurotic human behavior. In the course of this effort, it became evident that by far the greatest proportion of mental activity takes place at an unconscious level. This conclusion led to a consideration of the various types of unconscious activity—the episodic, the procedural, and the visceral—and of the interactions between them and consciousness. Inevitably it became necessary to compare this psychobiological model with the Freudian model of the dynamic unconscious in terms of structure, function, and significance.

As a consequence, this book has evolved along two parallel but only somewhat related pathways: the first attempting to describe psychobiological mechanisms that underlie complex modes of human behavior, and the second attempting to relate those mechanisms to psychoanalytic concepts. It may be that the second effort has undercut the first in making it seem like a pseudoscientific attempt to support psychoanalytic theory. I hope this impression is invalid. It seems to me that the psychobiological portions of this book where they do not involve Freudian concepts at all are fairly sound, even though at times somewhat speculative. Those sections can and should be evaluated apart from any consideration of psychoanalytic theory. In these terms, the first two sections of this volume, Section I on the "Fundamentals of Psychobiology" (Chapters 1 through 5) and Section II on "Mechanisms of Conscious and Unconscious Thought Processing" (Chapters 6 through 12) present a purely psychobiological view of the mechanisms underlying conscious and unconscious mental activity.

In Section III on the "Hierarchical and Hemispheric Origins of Repression and Other Defense Mechanisms," where I begin to deal with the overtly Freudian concepts of repression and associated defense mechanisms, it becomes impossible to ignore psychoanalytic theory. But what is one to do. Should one negate the entire area of interaction of emotional and cognitive functions in humans simply because Freud first investigated that area and made it the keystone of his system? That would make no sense either biologically or clinically. Hence one is compelled to examine such effects at the laboratory level and to attempt to extrapolate from there to the clinical.

In my opinion, the evidence that certain types of negative emotional experience result under certain conditions in inhibition of cognitive valence is more convincing than is any evidence to the contrary. This material was covered at some length in Chapter 13. Lieberson (1984) reviews the subject and cites Farrell (1982) as finding that experimental studies support the concept. Lieberson quotes Farrell (1982) as follows:

> Dixon used an apparatus which allowed him to present stereoscopically two spots of light—one brighter than the other—to the left eye of the subject and stimulus words, subliminally presented, to the right eye. The apparatus enabled the subject to control the brightness of the two spots, and he was instructed to work it continuously so that he could "just see the brighter of the two spots but never the dimmer one." It was found that when emotionally disturbing words (whore and penis) were presented subliminally to the right eye, the visual threshold went up and the subject had to increase the brightness of the spot shown to the left eye.
>
> If the experiment is "firmly replicated, it suggests very strongly that some internal control machinery is at work of the sort described by the theory of repression."

Lieberson goes on to state that another experimentalist, Erwen (1985), "claims that this could not test the Freudian theory of repression, which postulates an unconscious mind that is performing the repression." He quotes Erwen (1985) as writing:

> The mere fact that there is discrimination without awareness and that this discrimination affects recognition thresholds does not establish that any subject has defended against threatening material by incorporating it into his unconscious. Repression could be the cause of perceptual defense effects, but there is no firm evidence so far that it is.

What in essence is being objected to here? It seems to me that Erwen accepts the possibility, if not the probability, that the perception of threatening emotional percepts or thoughts might be modified through mechanisms resembling repression or sensitizing defenses. However, what he appears to reject is the idea that such putative repression must be the consequence of active inhibition by a dynamic unconscious. This he considers to be pure conjecture.

But the psychobiological view of the decathected unconscious as described in Chapter 17 is not incompatible with Erwen's position. There the decathected unconscious is not a separate and distinct part of the mind which operates independently from the rest of the mind. It is rather a segment of the entire conscious–unconscious continuum that, because of the nature of the engrams within it, affects behavior differently than does the rest of the continuum. Outside of their negative effect on cognitive valence, the engrams in the decathected unconscious exercise their influence on overt behavior in the same way as do engrams in other parts of the conscious–unconscious continuum, i.e., physiologically. The decathected unconscious, unlike Freud's dynamic unconscious, does not have a life of its own.

If the psychobiological position has any validity at all, then it may contribute somewhat toward demystifying the Freudian unconscious without disrupting its significance. In my opinion, many psychoanalytic concepts of id–ego–superego conflict in the dynamic unconscious may be reformulated in psychobiological terms without detracting from their clinical validity. The last section of this volume, Section IV on "Psychobiology and the Pathogenesis of Neurosis" has attempted to do just this, hopefully with some success.

Concepts such as the dynamic unconscious, the ego, and psychological defense mechanisms are some of the psychoanalytic formulations that are examined psycho-biologically in this volume and reconstituted in psychobiological terms. Other elements of Freudian theory such as the role of psychosexual conflict in neuroses formation, the expunging of neuroses through insight, therapeutic transference, and related themes are obviously beyond the scope of this volume. In that sense this book is limited. Unlike other works in the past, such as Freud's *Project for a Scientific Psychology* (1895), Pribram and Gill's *Freud's "Project" Reassessed* (1976), and Popper and Eccles *The Self and its Brain* (1978), this book is meant to be not a philosophic inquiry into the biological nature of human behavior, but rather an attempt to describe the physiological anlage underlying such behavior.

A Critique of Psychoanalytic Methodology

In the psychobiological approach to psychoanalytic theory, the question as to whether psychoanalytic methodology has scientific validity is of great significance. When addressed in a theoretical vacuum, as has usually been the case, the question has almost always been answered in the negative. Psychoanalytic methodology is different from any other so-called scientific method. It is not experimental in the same sense as controlled laboratory studies; it is not statistical; it has not even been subjected to routine interjudge reliability studies. Perhaps its greatest shortcoming is the claim of its proponents that it can be practiced only by a select few, i.e., by psychoanalysts themselves. This claim is not nearly so outrageous as it may at first seem since physical experiments can be performed only by trained physicists, chemical experiments by trained chemists, and so on. However, the persistently subjective nature of the material and of the doctor–patient relationship, combined with the difficulty in establishing any kind of meaningful controls, have presented even friends of the methodology with problems.

Through the analysis of dreams, parapraxes, and the productions of hypnosis, Freud proved to his own satisfaction that there was indeed a dynamic unconscious; that this unconscious provided the ultimate direction for all individual human behavior; that the unconscious operated in all stages of consciousness—the alert stage (parapraxes), sleep (dreams), and in hypnosis (hypnagogic effects); that the content and machinations of the unconscious ordinarily never came to awareness; that this unconscious was highly irrational; and that unconscious dynamics, beside controlling normal behavior, could produce abnormal symptomatology as well. Having reached these determinations, Freud further concluded that the only way to correct the abnormal activity of the unconscious, which was producing psychopathology, was to bring it to the surface of awareness and to expose it to the cool reason of conscious mental activity.

Since it was in dreams and in hypnosis that Freud had first found evidence of the unconscious, it was natural enough that he should turn to these areas as having the greatest potential for ultimately providing a road to the unconscious. Using these reservoirs of unconscious activity, he derived a methodology for probing into the depths of this material. To put the matter in its most simplistic terms, the psycho-analytic method for probing the unconscious consists essentially in getting clues directly from the unconscious when that level of operation is closest to the surface, i.e., in dreams, hypnosis, and twilight states, and then in allowing the subject to elaborate on those clues through free association. Freud argued that the most direct route, "the royal road to the unconscious," lay in dreams and that the unraveling of the true emotional meaning of dreams could be carried out only by the subject himself, with professional guidance, through free association.

Following this line of argument, one can attempt to analyze the psychobiological mechanisms through which material from the unconscious—particularly negatively charged material from the decathected dynamic unconscious—can be made to rise to the subject's awareness. Although Freud mainly used dreams as this "royal road to the unconscious," we must analyze other transactions in which unconscious material appears to surface and thus to become available to awareness. Such material includes the classical data of REM sleep (dreams) and of altered states of consciousness (twilight sleep, hypnagogic states, sodium pentothal induced states, etc.). However, it also includes the data of free association, parapraxes, and behaviors secondary to various types of psychological defense mechanisms, activities usually associated with alert consciousness. In such a psychobiological analysis, it should become possible to examine the conditions under which material from the deep unconscious can rise to consciousness and awareness.

Repression as a Manifestation of Increased Noradrenergic-Driven RAS Activity

During altered states of consciousness such as early sleep, hypnosis, and twilight states when there appears to be depressed activity of the left hemisphere, right-hemispheric activity becomes relatively greater, with more productions in awareness reflecting the engrams indigenous to that hemisphere. At such times, right-hemispheric material which is more primitive, less logical, more symbolic, and more emotional will filter through impaired consciousness to some level of impaired awareness. Such material might represent right-hemispheric unconscious material deriving from its decathected unconscious, which characteristically is most easily repressed when the alerting system is most active. Thus an active norepinephrine-driven RAS alerting system is the main element in repressive activity since it provides the arousal level necessary to carry negative emotional charge and also stimulates the left hemisphere to be dominant over the right to suppress it.

The argument for the critical role of the alerting system in repression runs as follows. The difficulty that a percept or memory has in entering awareness is in part a function of the intensity of its negative emotional charge; the latter is influenced by the general level of activation in the brain. Thus the more active the norepinephrine-driven

RAS alerting system, the higher the level of arousal and the greater the decathecting repressive effect at the subcortical level. Since the ability of a negative emotional charge to elicit a defensive reaction is related to its ability to produce arousal (the physiological signal of threat), then in states of lower activation (low arousal states) this mechanism will have been relatively deactivated. In such circumstances, all threatening engrams should be less threatening, if only because the organism is not physiologically in a state to register strong emotional responses. Under these latter conditions, the ready passage of decathected engrams from either the right or left hemisphere into impaired awareness seems highly plausible.

Evidence for this interpretation comes from a variety of conditioning and learning studies during states of low arousal, induced either physiologically or pharmacologically. The classic study of this type is that by Masserman and Yum (1946), who investigated the effects of alcohol administration on positive-conditioned-avoidance behavior in cats. In the control situation, Masserman conditioned animals to approach the reward (food) in a positive-conditioning paradigm; he then taught them to restrain from approaching (so as to avoid an electric shock) when a negative cue was flashed. After the administration of sufficient alcohol to make the cats somewhat sluggish, the animals approached the food even with negative cues.

A variety of interpretations of these results are possible. One can postulate that the decrease in avoidance behavior might have been due to the pain-relieving effect of alcohol. This explanation cannot have applied in the conditioned-avoidance experiment where only the conditioned stimulus (the cue) was employed. An alternative explanation is that alcohol depressed the activity of the hippocampus sufficiently to suppress passive-avoidance behavior and thus to produce perseverative responsivities. However, alcohol in large doses enhances hippocampal activity, invalidating that explanation. Consequently, the most plausible explanation appears to be that the decrease in arousal subsequent to alcohol administration reduced the negative emotional charge on the conditioned stimulus sufficiently to permit the animal to approach the reward without anxiety. This reaction would be analogous to a decrease of negative motivational–emotional charge on threatening unconscious stimuli during states of reduced arousal.

According to this formulation, the arousal-reducing effect of sedatives and tranquilizers should result in a general loosening up of both mental and physical behavior. This is, of course, the case. The administration of sodium pentothal as a means of freeing repressed unconscious material is a well-recognized and proven clinical procedure. The ability of tranquilizers to control some of the terrors of agoraphobia so as to improve behavior is almost certainly related to the suppressive effects of such drugs on the emotional charge of the conflictual elements in the environment.*

Increased arousal under stress is presumably achieved through primary activation of the thalamic–basal gangliar complex with subsequent activation of the locus coeruleus and the posterior hypothalamus. The close association of the locus coeruleus-driven RAS with the posterior hypothalamic arousal center and the thalamic–basal gangliar general consciousness center accounts for the equally close association be-

---

*The salutary effects of tricyclic antidepressants in phobias are probably due to their stimulation of the inhibitory actions of the prefrontal lobes, similar to the effects of stimulant drugs in hyperactive children.

tween noradrenergic-driven arousal and alert consciousness (see Chapter 6). It is presumably at this level that inhibition of cognitive valence by negative emotional arousal occurs (see Fig. 13-3). Depression of this system diminishes the suppression of cognitive valence and allows repressed material to surface.

This formulation, which attributes repression to conditions of increased arousal, holds generally for most high arousal situations except for the one in which repression is presumed to be least active, namely during REM dreams. Rapid eye movement dreams are said to probe the deepest levels of the unconscious and thus to be characterized by the lowest levels of repression. Yet REM sleep is a very high arousal state. This paradox may be explained on the basis that REM sleep arousal is cholinergic in origin (see Chapter 6) while the arousal syndrome described above is noradrenergically initiated. These aberrant effects in REM dreams are apparently effectuated through circumvention of the thalamic–basal gangliar complex and through differential activation of the septal–hippocampal circuit in a mechanism now to be elaborated upon.

Noradrenergic and Cholinergic Activation of Hippocampal Function

Winson (1985), who has done much work in this area, has reported that the hippocampus is noradrenergically activated. When that neurotransmitter is depleted as a result of chemical treatment, the "gating" mechanism (the mechanism through which the hippocampus directs incoming information) is incapacitated (Dahl et al., 1983). During REM sleep, norepinephrine activity in the brain is at its lowest ebb. Aston-Jones and Bloom (1981a,b) have reported that the norepinephrine-secreting cells in the locus coeruleus, the cells responsible for activating the amygdala and hippocampus, are almost totally inactive during REM sleep, fire slowly during slow-wave sleep, and fire at their maximum rate (4–5/sec) in the alert condition. Theoretically, during REM sleep there is little or no norepinephrine to activate the hippocampus and hence little or at any rate modified gating activity in that nucleus.

Yet, as previously described, there is during REM sleep marked θ-rhythm electrical activity in the hippocampus, presumably a mark of gating activity. Since there is no specific evidence on this paradox, one can only hypothesize that the gating activity during REM sleep must be cholinergic rather than noradrenergic. If that is indeed the case, then it may also be true that whatever gating activity does exist during REM sleep may be of a different nature than that which occurs with noradrenergic activation in the alert condition.

If we accept the interpretation that the hippocampus is predominantly inhibitory in its effects, then this apparent paradox of hippocampal activity disappears. Within that formulation, the hippocampus under noradrenergic stimulation inhibits the entire inner world ("repression" of the unconscious) and those portions of the external world that are not being attended (Kimble, 1968). With cholinergic activation the hippocampus would still be very active (as manifested by high θ activity), but would be inhibiting the entire outer world and not the inner (release of repression). In both instances the inhibitory activity of the hippocampus would be high (increased θ activity), but the directions of inhibition would be antithetical (see Fig. 22-1).

Since in this paradigm the general level of activation in the brain would be high during REM sleep, unconscious material in both the right and left hemispheres would be stimulated. But because of the almost complete inactivity of the noradrenergic locus coeruleus during REM sleep, the thalamic–basal gangliar complex would lie dormant and repressive activity would not take place. Hence REM dreams should show even less repression than those productions of non-REM slow-wave sleep and twilight states where locus coeruleus activity is at least slight. Consequently, in this formulation, REM dreams should tap deeper unconscious material than non-REM dreams or the productions of twilight states.

These descriptions also help to explain the antirepressive effects of alcohol in small doses. That drug not only reduces the level of activity of the noradrenergic-driven RAS, but also inhibits the normal activities of the hippocampal–amygdaloid complex. Since the latter include activation of the external environment and repression of the internal unconscious, reduction in these activities results in a decreased level of outer awareness (altered states of consciousness) associated with decreased inhibition of repressed material (see Fig. 22-1).

Thus two different modes of antirepressive mechanisms are expressed here: one passive and one active. The passive mode is that which occurs in twilight sleep, non-REM dreams, and in altered states of consciousness. It is characterized by a decrease in conscious awareness and by a decrease of repressive action upon the unconscious. It is associated with the release of only moderate amounts of deep material, since in these states the brain is only moderately active (Figs. 11-2, 11-3, and 11-4). Hence the passive mode of antirepressive activity taps the same reservoir of the unconscious material as do REM dreams, but less completely and less deeply.

The active mode of antirepressive activity, that characterizing REM sleep, may

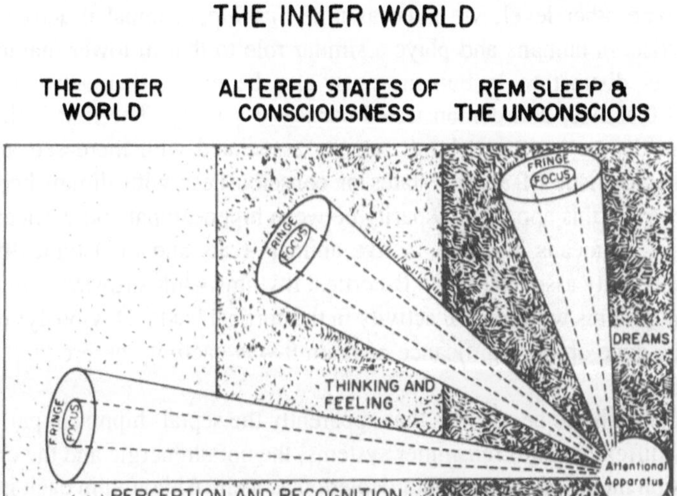

Figure 22-1 Selective functions of the attentional apparatus.

almost be conceptualized as structured specifically to capture the deep repressed material of the unconscious. There is a complete or near complete turning off of the activating effects of the noradrenergic system upon the hippocampus associated with a turning off of the noradrenergic system for attending to the outside world. In its place, there is substituted a cholinergically activated system for attending the inner unconscious. Concomitantly, the entire brain is activated so that all unconscious material is available for entry into the impaired self-awareness system. The results are REM dreams (see Fig. 22-1).

This formulation of the varying roles of the hippocampus in alert consciousness, altered states of consciousness, and REM sleep appears to be compatible with both clinical and experimental evidence. Experimentally, as the animal goes into successively deeper stages of sleep, noradrenergic activity of the locus coeruleus decreases and the animal becomes progressively less conscious. Yet in REM sleep, where noradrenergic activity is essentially nonexistent, there is striking evidence in humans of the vivid mental activity of dreams. During REM sleep, the hippocampus may be activated by the same pontine cholinergic impulses that drive the general REM condition. Mancillas et al. (1986) provided experimental evidence for this by demonstrating that locally applied acetylcholine excites pyramidal cells of the hippocampus much as does norepinephrine. Furthermore, REM mental activity is generated by cholinergic activation and supported by the previously described (p. 88) finding of Karzmar and Dun (1978) that the intrathecal administration of cholinergic substances into the pontine area produces PGO spikes and REM sleep while the administration of atropine sulphate abolishes PGO spikes and REM activity.

One weakness in this formulation is the difficulty in demonstrating θ activity in either the primate or human hippocampus (Winson, 1985, p. 190). Although the absence of such activity has not been fully established, it is possible that in primates and man, θ activity of the hippocampus has been transferred along with certain other activities to other centers in the brain (Isaacson and Pribram, 1975). In the absence of specific evidence either for the absence of hippocampal θ activity in primates or for activity at some other level, we must assume that hippocampal θ activity or some equivalent exists in humans and plays a similar role to that in lower mammals.

One other distinction in humans must also be made, that between presumed hippocampal θ activity and demonstrated cortical θ activity. The first is theoretically considered to denote increased brain activity associated with increased arousal; the second is characteristic of altered states of consciousness with diminished levels of arousal. However, this apparent disparity between hippocampal and cortical electrical rhythms is by no means atypical. Active animals (cats and rats) typically show θ-hippocampal activity associated with β-cortical rhythms while drowsy animals have β-hippocampal rhythms with some θ activity in the cortical leads. Obviously, much more work must be done on the signficance of brain θ-wave activity before these questions can be resolved.

The major point to be made is that apparently the septal–hippocampal circuit can be driven by different neurotransmitter systems, the noradrenergic and the cholinergic, and its function modified by serotonin depletion as well. Although in each instance the overall effect is to stimulate the basically inhibitory actions of this circuit, the mode and direction of inhibitory effect vary greatly with each neurotransmitter. Noradrenergic stimulation is associated with acute attentional activities in the alert stage of consciousness where the inhibitory effects are directed against those elements in the environment which are irrelevant to the event being attended. Cholinergic activation of the septal–hippocampal circuit during REM sleep apparently produces inhibitory effects against the entire external environment. In the use of hallucinogenic drugs, Mandell (1980) has presented evidence that the major pharmacologic action of such drugs is to inhibit serotonin activity in the brain stem, an effect apparently associated with stimulation of the inhibitory actions of the septal–hippocampal circuit. Whether or not this effect is similar to that occurring in REM sleep in which inhibition of pontine serotonergic activity is associated with stimulation of excitatory cholinergic activity is difficult to say, but the changes in awareness with hallucinogen administration are more similar to those in REM sleep than they are to those in normal alert behavior.

Repression and Activity of the Cerebral Hemispheres

A secondary effect of decreased activity of the norepinephrine-driven RAS alerting system is the decreased activation of the left hemisphere. Although low arousal states are associated with a relative shift of power spectral dominance toward the left hemisphere, this apparent paradox is really the result of a greater *decrease* in right-hemispheric activation than in left (see Chapter 15). More important is the fact that left-hemispheric activation is relatively diminished, and with that, its controlling effect on the right hemisphere. In a sense, the Freudian "repressive barrier" may be considered to result in part from the action of the dominant left hemisphere; when that hemisphere is highly active, right-hemispheric activity and consequently right-hemispheric productions in consciousness tend to be suppressed. When both hemispheric activities are depressed, right-hemispheric production, even though less active, are more available to awareness.

Since there is an equally large mass of repressed engrams in the left hemisphere that are released during altered states of consciousness, only part of the total relaxation of repressive effects can be attributed to interhemispheric effects. The release of repressed material from the left-hemispheric unconscious when left-hemispheric activity is reduced must be due to direct hierarchical control effects within that hemisphere secondary to the decrease in the level of arousal. Reduced arousal in left-hemispheric function is even more important for the releasing effects it has on sensitizing defense mechanisms than for those it has on repression, since the former are its chief mode of responsivity. The reduction in arousal levels reduces the effectiveness of the major element in sensitizing defenses, i.e., the detouring of the threatening stimulus through the associational maze in such a way as to avoid reactivating negatively charged memories.

In REM sleep, on the other hand, when the hippocampal mechanisms for scanning the unconscious are at their optimal operational level, the right hemisphere is more electrically active (see Chapter 15) than is the left so that its material is presumably more available. Under such circumstances, repressed material in the right hemisphere should be more receptive to retrieval during REM dreams than during non-REM dreams or in the productions of altered states of consciousness, an interpretation that appears to be supported by clinical and experimental findings.

Experimental Evidence for the Surfacing of Unconscious Data during Dreams

Evidence for such interactions between the hierarchical and hemispheric control systems is forthcoming from the studies of sleep in which customary left-hemispheric dominance is markedly diminished. Goldstein's data on the relative activities of the right and left hemisphere during the different stages of sleep are of interest here (see Fig. 15-2). In the subject followed in that figure, REM periods were predominantly associated with relatively increased right-hemispheric activity (downward deflections) in the early part of the night when sleep was heavy and when the activity of the left hemisphere was at its lowest level. At that time dreams were almost entirely visual and full of imagery (right-hemispheric activity). Later in the night as sleep lightened and the left hemisphere became somewhat more active, the still-predominant downward deflections showed some interspersed upward deflections and dreams became visual–verbal rather than purely visual, i.e., increased left-hemispheric activity.

Thus it would be incorrect to infer that all dreams derive from the right brain; as Hoppe (1977) has pointed out, less "dreamlike" dreams did stem from the left brain in a patient with a total right hemispherectomy. This view is consistent with Cohen's (1976) experimental findings which suggest that REM dreams early in the night (when sleep in general is deeper) tend to stem from the right hemisphere (i.e., are more bizarre and irrational) while those coming late in the sleep cycle (when sleep is generally lighter) stem at least in part from the left hemisphere (i.e., are less bizarre and irrational).

Cohen (1976) writes:

> In addition to REM versus NREM differences in the processing of information, there may be important differences during early and later REM periods. I raise this question in the specific light of preliminary evidence that I recently obtained suggesting a relative increase from early to later REM periods in the prominence or influence of left-hemispheric activity. This evidence is composed of the following: (1) an increase from early to late REM periods in the prominence of left-hemispheric-related dream-content categories (e.g., verbal activity) but not of right-hemisphere-related dream-content (e.g., music); (2) a corresponding increase in the tendency to look to the right; (3) a corresponding tendency for the ratio of left-to-right EEG amplitude (L/R) to diminish; (4) correlations between increase in left- (but not right-) hemisphere-related content, and (a) increase in right looking and (b) decrease in L/R ratio and (5) the failure of subjects with a sinistral bias to fit the observed pattern. These very preliminary results suggest the possibility that information processing shifts in quality during the night, perhaps even favoring different kinds of problems (recent events early versus remote events later?) with somewhat different kinds of treatment emphases (more analogical early versus more analytical later?). (pp. 354–355)

Cohen's (1976) statement indicates that during the progression of sleep, the suppression of the left brain is greatest early in the cycle and becomes less so as the cycle goes on. In close correlation with the evidence of changes in the electrophysiological balance is the nature of the dream productions—right-sided imagery early, but both right- and left-sided late.

The work of Cohen (1976) and others, based on clinical evidence suggesting that dream productions in the early phase of sleep derive mainly from the right hemisphere while those in early morning derive equally from the left hemisphere, is supported by the previously described electrophysiological studies of Goldstein (Fig. 15-2). This finding is of some significance for the interpretation of the content of dreams. If it is valid, it would suggest that most REM dreams that occur in normals and that are remembered are those that occur early in the morning, deriving equally from both hemispheres. In that case, as previously discussed, one would not expect quite the level of bizarreness ascribed to normal dreams by psychoanalysts. On the other hand, in that group of neurotics in whom repressive mechanisms break down (see Chapter 20), one might expect somewhat more bizarre material deriving from the right hemisphere, but still not so bizarre as sometimes appears in the interpretations of psychoanalysts.

These observations lead us to a consideration of the possible biological purposes of REM dreams. They cannot be, as almost seemed to be previously implied, a convenient road to the unconscious for psychoanalysts. Winson (1985) has hypothesized rather that REM sleep is an endogenous mechanism for processing excess cognitive material gathered during the day and for incorporating it into the general unconscious. In support of this position, he quotes the work of Roffwarg et al. (1978) who had subjects wear rose-colored glasses during the day and then tested them to see whether or not their dreams were similarly tinted. These investigators found that after the first day of exposure, only early REM dreams were in color. After 4 or 5 successive exposure days, about 83% of early REM dreams and 44% of late night dreams were in color. A smaller proportion of the productions of stage 1 (twilight) sleep and of non-REM dreams also appeared in color, but less vividly. These findings indicate a carry-over of diurnal conscious activity to nocturnal unconscious activity.

Winson (1985) interprets these results to suggest incorporation and perhaps consolidation of daily experience during REM dreams. This interpretation seems compatible with the data. On the other hand, it also seems compatible with the interpretations in this chapter. These are (1) that early REM sleep is a more physiological state in which daily events are reprocessed in the brain as postulated by Crick and Mitchison (1983) and Winson (1985); (2) that early sleep involves the right hemisphere more (where color perception characteristically occurs); and (3) that the functions of REM sleep are not merely physiological (i.e., to facilitate internal processing), but also psychological (i.e., to allow the individual to have contact with repressed thoughts). As Winson himself writes, "It is also conceivable that REM sleep fulfills two functions. One during early development" (i.e., in infancy) "and a second thereafter" (i.e., in adulthood) (see p. 257). The first would be physiological and the second psychological.

If the biological purpose of REM dreams was only the reorganization and consolidation of daily experience as postulated by Winson (1985), then such dreams would not serve the psychoanalytic formulation of tapping the deep unconscious as postulated by us. Rather, REM dreams would reflect only the specific encounters of the day. The hypothesis presented here that REM sleep represents a turning inward of the "mind" toward the decathected unconscious, particularly that component resident in the right hemisphere, is much more compatible with psychoanalytic thinking. But apart from the logical arguments that both authors have made, what evidence is there for either position?

The just described study by Roffwarg et al. (1978) supports to some extent Winson's position that material learned during the day is incorporated into REM dreams at night. However, the fact that such incorporation occurs mainly in early REM dreams and only partially in later REM dreams is also compatible with our suggestion that the physiological role of such dreams is greatest early in the night and the psychological role of more significance later. Thus, although the Roffwarg et al. (1978) study is generally supportive of Winson's position, it does not necessarily contradict our own.

Rapid eye movement sleep deprivation has been another device used for exploring the function of REM dreams. Subjects who are awakened whenever they show rapid eye movements over several nights begin to show some signs of mental disturbance. Early studies in this area suggested that such disturbance might be severe but later findings have not supported that finding. Fisher and Greenberg (1977), after a comprehensive review of the literature, conclude:

> As one scans the total results that have been laid out, they do suggest that dreaming serves some discharge function. There are inconsistencies and even contradictions in the data, but a major directionality comes through. In various ways it has been shown that if you prevent an individual from dreaming, you upset him psychologically. It is true that the degree of upset was probably exaggerated in earlier reports. One would doubt that disturbance of psychotic proportions is ever really evoked. But in the majority of reported observations at least a small amount of disturbance does appear. One would have to conclude that, at least indirectly, these observations support Freud's hypothesis that the dream helps to maintain psychological equilibrium by providing a partial means for discharging unconscious impulses. (p. 53)

This conclusion obviously favors neither Winson's theory nor my own. If anything, the fact that the consequences of REM deprivation are relatively mild and more psychological than physiological speaks more for our theory. If REM sleep were essential for the consolidation of cognitive engrams experienced during the day, then there should be greater cognitive disturbance than actually occurs with REM deprivation. This does not in any way weaken Winson's conclusion. It merely suggests that the physiological role is only part of the total role REM dreams perform. Perhaps it is as Winson hypothesizes: "It is also conceivable that REM sleep fulfills two functions. One during early development and a second thereafter" (p. 257).

The best evidence for our position, to my mind, lies in the fact that the productions of REM dreams, of non-REM dreams, and of altered states of consciousness are all so similar (see quote from Fisher and Greenberg on p. 184). If indeed they are, then dreams and fantasies must stem from similar mechanisms. Winson's hypothesis postulates that REM dreams are associated with hippocampal θ rhythm, the basis of his physiological mechanism. But the productions of deep sleep (non-REM dreams) and of altered states of consciousness (twilight state fantasies) occur during periods when there is no θ activity in the hippocampus. Therefore, either REM dreams are of a different nature than non-REM dreams and twilight state fantasies, or, if these are similar, (and we shall present evidence for that in the next section) then most likely it is because they tap a common dynamic unconscious, albeit as postulated by us, through different mechanisms. In that case, we would conclude that REM dreams serve a physiological function in infancy and in the early hours of the night but a psychological function in the later dreams of sleep.

To explore in depth the question of just what that psychological function may be is beyond the scope of this book but Fisher and Greenberg (1977) summarize my position admirably. They write:

> A network of scientific results exists compatible with Freud's central concept of dreaming, namely, that it offers an outlet or release for internal (unconscious) tensions. Definitive experiments have yet to be done in which labeled inputs known to arouse unconscious tensions are then traced to focal expressive dream imagery. But within the limitations of our present technology for studying the effects of psychological inputs, the results obtained are approximately what one would expect from the Freudian venting model. (p. 62)

Experimental Evidence for Release of Unconscious Material during Altered States of Consciousness

Recent work by Budzynski (1976) on twilight learning provides further data on these issues. Budzynski performed a series of studies investigating the special properties of the learning process during that period when the subjects were neither fully awake nor deep asleep, a period that he terms the twilight state. He was able to generate a comparable experimental state in subjects through the use of biofeedback mechanisms (monitoring EEG patterns and relating them to a constant state of drowsiness during which the experiments were performed). Budzynski summarizes his findings and his interpretation of them as follows:

> Many of the descriptions of the recall and recognition of material presented during low-arousal states are identical to those attributed to minor-hemisphere learning. In both cases concrete rather than abstract information is processed more effectively. Moreover, when the information is coded in music or rhythm, it is more easily absorbed, as is also said to be the case with minor-hemisphere learning. Finally, there is the observation that following a twilight or low-arousal learning-session, subjects very often cannot verbalize what they have supposedly learned, yet they do well on recognition-comprehension tests. (p. 380)

The similarities in thought process in the phenomenology of some dreams, twilight states, and hypnotic states, and the recurrent evidence of the predominance of right-hemispheric activity in these phenomena, strongly suggests that under conditions of reduced awareness (i.e., left-hemispheric suppression), the right hemisphere is capable of productions that are relatively independent of the other hemisphere. These productions, i.e., some dreams, fantasies, and hypnotic reactions, appear to have different qualities from those characteristic of full awareness. They are driven by α-rather than by β-rhythm activity and they derive mainly from the right hemisphere; consequently, they tap a different reservoir of engrams (motivations and memories) than is ordinarily accessible. It is as though in the neurologically intact individual, the relative suppression of left-brain activity permits right-brain productions to pass through the commissures and surface into impaired awareness. This sequence of events seems compatible with the previously described hypotheses of Doty et al. (1973) and of Kinsbourne (1970), which postulated that increased activity in one hemisphere is associated with a relative inhibition of the other. Since in the alert individual the left hemisphere tends to be more active than the right (Cobb, 1963; Goldstein, 1979; Fig. 15-1, this volume), the normal suppression of right-hemispheric activity would be relieved on occasions of decreased left-hemispheric arousal.

As previously stated, the diminution of activation levels in the two hemispheres would free up not only repressed material in the right hemisphere, but similarly repressed material in the left. However, the latter effects would be secondary only to reduced arousal levels rather than to any specific interhemispheric mechanism. The surfacing of left-hemispheric unconscious material during altered states of consciousness would presumably be of a comparable magnitude to that of right-hemispheric material. Left-hemispheric defense mechanisms such as rationalization, projection, and reaction-formation would be most apparent when the individual is in a state of alert consciousness rather than in a state of suppressed consciousness. Consequently, in altered states of consciousness the absence of sufficient arousal levels to cause circuitous routing of associations, should result in substantial surfacing of suppressed material in the left hemisphere.

The psychobiological hypothesis for the surfacing of material from the dynamic unconscious to impaired awareness during altered states of consciousness returns us to the discussion of the Winson (1985) view of the origin of REM dreams as opposed to our own. In the previous section it was stated that if REM dreams were indeed similar to non-REM dreams and to twilight state fantasies, then because of the absence of hippocampal θ activity in the latter conditions, Winson's thesis of the physiological role of REM dreams was probably only partially correct. The comparison between REM dreams versus non-REM dreams and twilight state fantasies then becomes critical to our discussion. Such a comparison can only be made on the basis of psychological studies—an extensive literature on the subject does exist. The conclusion of Fisher and Greenberg (1977), that these conditions were essentially similar, was reported on p. 184. These authors further quote from Giora (1972) to support their conclusions.

Giora (1972) writes:

> While indulging in daydreams . . . one is momentarily "introverted," and the messages one receives will be assimilated into the ongoing mentation. A fatigued or drowsy man struggles to maintain contact with his surroundings, but he is able to do so only phasically. While sleeping, one will recede from all activity in his relationship with this world. This passivity is the main behavioral characteristic of sleep. But cognition does not cease even in the midst of passivity; we get reports on mental activity from REM as well as from NREM sleep [during which there is an absence of rapid eye movements usually associated with dreaming]; it is only that the level of organization will shift. We may say, therefore, that there are many states of mind, each characterized by a different interaction with the environment and by a specific cognitive organization.
>
> Now what is the function of the cognition typical of the fatigued? Such a question is as legitimate as the question on the function of cognition while being in REM or NREM sleep. Our answer is hinted at in the question; cognition's function is unitary,

but its organization (and effectiveness) is variable. Cognition has many levels, as has wakefulness or consciousness. Actually, the level of cognition is one of the distinctive features of the level of consciousness. They are different aspects of a common essense. (pp. 1071–1072)

Fisher and Greenberg (1977) then continue:

There is little rationale for assuming that continuity does not prevail between processes that occur at different stages of consciousness. It is striking that Fiss et al. (1966) were actually able to show that the characteristic mode of fantasy in the REM state carries over into fantasy obtained directly upon awakening from this state. They report (p. 1069): "Stories produced after interrupted REM sleep were longer, more complex, visual, bizarre, emotional, and vivid than stories produced after interrupted NREM sleep and were more bizarre than stories during control waking periods. . . . The results strongly suggest that the distinguishing properties of a sleep stage are not 'switched off' following awakening but may persist into the waking state."

This constitutes a dramatic affirmation of the continuity between the dream and other types of fantasy. One can see in this instance that the dream and another kind of fantasy mirrored the influence of a specific condition in analogous ways. (p. 65)

The previous conclusions are based on a comprehensive review of both the clinical and experimental literatures and appear to represent the general consensus among researchers in this field. Such being the case, it would seem that the physiological theses of Crick and Mitchison (1983) and of Winson (1985), although probably correct insofar as they go, apply only partially as explanations for the genesis of REM dreams. I believe that the psychological mechanisms described in this volume for REM and NREM dreams and for twilight state fantasies are equally valid and explain a level of phenomenology not explicable by more physiological mechanisms.

Free Association as a Technique for Tapping the Unconscious

If REM dreams, NREM dreams, and twilight state fantasies are reliable techniques for tapping unconscious material, why is it that psychoanalysis relies heavily on free association as its dominant methodology? If our previous speculations have any validity, then there should be some evidence that free association is also a useful instrument for that same purpose. On that subject, Reiser (1984) writes:

The technique of free association serves as the "linchpin" of the psychoanalytic process. One fundamental assumption underlies its use. It is assumed—and clinical experience supports the assumption—that if the patient enters into an agreement with the analyst and does his best to follow the rule of free association, the repressed conflicted motives, and ideas that stem from them, will press for representation in his mind and eventually find expression in his verbalizations. The main features of the contract are (1) to come regularly for sessions of prescribed length; (2) to relax and permit thoughts, ideas, and images to come to mind—without any attempt to control them or in any way judge their possible relevance or therapeutic value; and (3) to verbalize these thoughts as freely as is humanly possible. The use of the couch and positioning of the analyst out of the direct line of vision of the analysand serve to facilitate relaxation and to reduce external sensory input, making it easier for the

patient to attend to ideas coming from within. Optimally, the patient's state of mind
settles into a level of increased inward, and reduced outward attention—very much
like that which obtains in mild drowsiness and states of mind in which reveries and
daydreams flourish. (pp. 36–37)

Within this general construction, it may even be that free association serves a
similar role to that of dreams and twilight fantasies in tapping the brain for psychological material that ordinarily may not be available to left-hemispheric consciousness.
Shevrin and Rennick (1967), in a study of somatosensory evoked potential responses
under a variety of conditions, observed that during free association there were smaller
N_1-P_2 waves and smaller P_{300} waves than those that occurred during selective attention
or mental arithmetic. Reduced N_1-P_2 and P_{300} waves are indicative of reduced arousal
secondary either to generally reduced arousal or more specifically to reduced attention.
Shevrin and Rennick noted as well the presence of regular α waves in the free association tracing; such waves indicate a general state of reduced arousal rather than a shift of
attention. It appears then that free association may involve a lowering of the general
level of arousal which might permit, as in the twilight paradigm, negatively charged
material from both hemispheres to enter impaired left-hemispheric consciousness more
readily (see Fig. 22-1).

The idea that suppressed unconscious material might surface more readily during
free associational interviews if the patient was in a relaxed twilight state is, of course,
hardly new. In the case of Anna O., the primal lode from which all psychoanalytic
techniques were subsequently mined, J. Breuer actually began his "talking cure" with
the patient under hypnosis. As the patient became more accustomed to the therapeutic
milieu, Breuer found this technique no longer necessary since the patient would place
herself in a similar condition through autohypnosis.

In developing the technique of free association, Freud played around with different variations of the "twilight state." Fenichel (1945) writes:

In his early days Freud even asked patients to close their eyes for the purpose of
excluding visual perceptions. Later, however, it turned out that the danger of inducing
the patient to isolate the analytic procedure from "open-eye reality" is usually greater
than the possible gain. (p. 24)

These statements are very interesting. They imply that closing the eyes, by bringing about an altered state of consciousness, did result in some gain (increased access to
hidden material?), but at the cost of suppressing ego activity to the point where it no
longer functioned at a high enough level to translate the primary process symbolism of
the decathected unconscious to the secondary process terminology of consciousness.
Since the major thrust of analytic therapy is just that, namely the translation of primary
process material into secondary process equivalents, the ego must be at least moderately active to accomplish that transition. On the other hand, a partial reduction in the
state of awareness during free association (Fig. 22-1) is probably necessary if deep
material is to be able to surface at all. Thus free association may represent the ideal
level of arousal necessary to free up material from both the left and right hemispheres
yet to keep it under rational control.

Perhaps the most important function of free association is to allow the exploration
of the repertoire of sensitizing defense mechanisms of the left hemisphere that the
individual customarily utilizes in conscious mentation and behavior. We have pre-

viously emphasized that although right hemispheric productions are most severely repressed in the alert conscious state, sensitizing defense mechanisms such as rationalization, projection, and reaction formation are most active under those circumstances. Hence, clinical interviews with the patient acutely alert would be most likely to reveal the operation of sensitizing defense mechanisms. On the other hand, in the alert condition the patient would be least likely to be able to reach beyond his defensive stance to insightful material in his own unconscious since at that time the unconscious is least accessible. Consequently, the conditions of free association, intermediate between those of alert consciousness and the twilight state, would appear to be ideal for probing the unconscious and at the same time, analyzing the customary defensive posture of the patient. This approach is in keeping with the new concepts underlying the *Ego Psychology* school of psychoanalysis.

If these speculations have any validity, then the psychoanalytic methods of dream analysis and free association may be legitimate instruments for tapping the dynamic unconscious, perhaps the only legitimate methodologies available for that purpose. Nevertheless, even if that should prove to be the case, it does not necessarily mean that psychoanalytic interpretations of such material are correct. In fact, psychobiological considerations tend to suggest that some psychoanalytic interpretations are overextended, overly symbolic, and overly bizarre. However, this still does not indicate that Freudian methodology is inadequate to the task it has undertaken. It merely suggests that principles of interpretation rather than the method itself may need re-evaluation.

With these considerations in mind, how should we view the Freudian concept of the dynamic unconscious? In my opinion, it is a tribute to Freud's genius that he was able to abstract from clinical observations on neurotic individuals the physiological and psychological differences between left- and right-hemispheric thought, long before any commissurotomies with their unexpected clinical findings had been performed. It is possible, perhaps even likely, that certain "split personalities" had effected a functional dissociation in their brains through hysterical inhibition of one area or another, in which case Freud's observations and deductions would have been similar to those of Sperry on actually commissurotomized patients. In that event, Freud's deductions leading to his hypothesis of the "dynamic unconscious" could be based on an overinterpretation of legitimate clinical observations.

Having uncovered the existence of an unconscious, more primitive and unstructured than the world of consciousness, Freud developed the theory that most behavior stemmed from or at least was dramatically influenced by mental activity at the unconscious level. Finding further that this primitive unconscious material was more difficult to retrieve (either because it lay in the right hemisphere or because it carried a highly negative motivational–emotional charge), Freud invented the repressive barrier beneath which all repressed highly charged thoughts stewed and simmered. Accordingly, Freud based his entire theory on the concept that the areas of activity below the repressive barrier constituted a special domain, the dynamic unconscious which, characterized by primitive motivations and impulses (the id) doing battle with the ego and superego, ultimately determined all human behavior. Almost as a natural consequence stemming from this basic concept of the dynamic unconscious, the second fundamental principle of psychoanalysis became that of "psychic determinism," the principle that most behavior was the product of the struggle among these various forces in the dynamic unconscious. The development of the concepts of primary and secondary thought processes, characteristic, respectively, of the dynamic unconscious and of the preconscious–conscious domain, completed the basic structure of psychoanalytic theory. Finally, the attribution of the development of the unconscious to early childhood experiences prepared the way for the principles of psychosexual development with all of their inherent complexities.

Despite the seemingly unorthodox manner in which Freud collected his data, the contributions of psychoanalysis have been immense. Because of the development of the psychoanalytic technique, a large body of clinical experience was subjected to a detailed type of analysis never previously practiced. Given the pitfalls of the technique and given the tendencies to extrapolate larger interpretations from smaller data, a comprehensive theoretical system based entirely on clinical observations was developed for the first time. Consequently, it is not surprising that now with the development of new scientific techniques a large segment of that theory is seen to have substantial experimental validity.

My own view of Freud's contributions was expressed by Hilgard in 1952 when he wrote:

> My own position is that Freud and other psychoanalysts have hit upon enough reality so that there is much for us to learn from them, and, with some reworking, there will be a substantial body of scientific generalizations resulting. I say ''resulting'' rather than ''remaining'' for I do not care whether we end up believing that Freud was a scientist or a romanticist. If eventually we are able to make science out of materials that he called strongly to our attention, then we shall owe him that historical debt, whatever the verdict may be about his own formulations. (p. 3)

The material presented in this book, in my opinion, tends more to support most psychoanalytic positions than to negate them. There appear to be physiological mechanisms that are in the main compatible with many psychoanalytic formulations, although by no means with all of them. If for example, one accepts ''primary process'' as characteristic of right-hemispheric-type thinking, then dreams, fantasies, hypnotic states, and the productions of free association tap a similar kind of ''dynamic unconscious'' to that described by Freud. There is throughout the psychoanalytic literature the feeling that much of what is stated has some such validity; there is also the feeling that some is overstated and overextended, a smaller truth expanded into a larger work of creative imagination. In any event, valid or invalid, the attempt to bridge the gap between psychobiology and psychoanalysis should be of some value to both.

Summation

In this first volume, I have attempted to present a psychobiological system that provides a physiological understructure for the better understanding of human thought and behavior. The major thrust here was to develop a working model of a dynamic unconscious, a model that is based on psychobiological principles rather than, as with the Freudian unconscious, on the analysis of clinical productions. However, the very fact that I undertook this enterprise itself indicates that I believed beforehand in the concept of a dynamic unconscious. And indeed I did. But my belief stemmed not so much from readings of Freud as it did from my own conceptions of the biological forces underlying human behavior.

Human behavior, like that of any other organism, must be seen within the context of evolutionary development. Humans belong to the subphylum Vertebrata, to the class Mammalia, to the order Primates, to the family Hominoidea, to the genus *Homo*, and to the species *sapiens*. Each successive advance represents not only biological progress but also a step in the direction of new behavioral characteristics and functions. Although the behavior of a mouse is closer to that of a man than it is to that of a fish, it is still sufficiently removed to make any exact analogy between them invalid. Men are not mice any more than mice are fish. While the primitive reactivities of all may be similar, the complexities developed through evolutionary change produce substantial differences.

Most of these complexities have developed as a consequence of the evolution of the cortex in the brain of man. Chief among the changes has been the vast enlargement of the entire cortex, permitting the enormous increase in the complexity of cognitive function. Of next importance has been the marked development of the prefrontal lobe with not only the addition of new abilities such as improved executive control, but also a shift in homeostatic balance from the predominantly excitatory to the predominantly inhibitory. Third in significance is the increased concentration of self-orienting influences onto the self-awareness center in the posterior inferior parietal lobe. This latter development, together with the increased ability of the entire cortex to elaborate abstract concepts related to the self, creates a more powerful *self-concept* with its implications both for conscious and unconscious mental function. Fourth, is the functional differentiation of the two hemispheres, thus providing, not only the advantages of cognitive specialization, but also increasing the capacity of the right hemisphere as a silent but dynamic unconscious. Fifth, is the development of the speech centers in the left hemisphere, not only permitting better communication among individuals but also introducing the highest level of abstraction, i.e., symbolism, into the mental armamentarium of humans. Finally, the evolution of the cortex has resulted in the development of human society with all of its contingent complexities, the cultural consequence of previous biological evolution.

This brief review is intended not so much as a summary of the contents of this volume as it is a rationale for this present volume and indeed for the entire work. The theme I have tried to develop throughout has been that the dynamic unconscious is, as Lewis Thomas put it "not the kind of Unconscious you read about in books, out at the edge of things making up dreams or getting mixed up on words or having hysterics" (see Chapter 13). Rather it is, with consciousness, the final development in the long history of biological evolution. It is the source of all major art and science and all talent and genius, and the reservoir from which consciousness continually draws its inspirations.

References

Adey WR, Segundo JP, and Livingston RB: Corticofugal influences on intrinsic brainstem conduction in cat and monkey. *J Neurophysiol* 1957;20:1–16.

Adey WR, Bell FR, and Dennis JB: Effects of LSD, psilocybin and psylocin on temporal lobe EEG patterns and learned behavior in the cat. *Neurology* 1962;12:591–602.

Andersen P, and Andersson AA: *Physiological Basis of the Alpha Rhythm*. New York, Appleton, Century, Crofts, 1968.

Anderson JR: Retrieval of information from long-term memory. *Science* 1983;220:25–30.

Anderson OD and Parmenter R: A long-term study of the experimental neurosis in the sheep and the dog. *Psychosom Med Monogr* 1941;2:1.

Aston-Jones G and Bloom FE: Norepinephrine-containing locus coeruleus neurons in behaving rats anticipate fluctuations in sleep-waking cycle. *J Neurosci* 1981a;1:876–886.

Averbach E and Sperling G: Short-term storage of information in vision, in Cherry C (ed): *Information Theory*. Washington D.C., Butterworth, 1961, pp.196–212.

Ax AF: The physiological differentiation between fear and anger in humans. *Psychosom Med* 1953;15:433–442.

Banquet JP: Spectral analysis of the EEG in meditation. *Electroencephalogr Clin Neurophysiol* 1973;35:143–151.

Baughman EE and Welsh GS: *Personality: A Behavioral Science*. Englewood, NJ, Prentice Hall, 1962.

Bear DM: The temporal lobes: An approach to the study of organic behavioral changes, in Gazzaniga MS (ed): *Handbook of Behavioral Neurobiology*, vol 2. *Neuropsychology*. New York, Plenum Press, 1979, pp.75–98.

Begleiter H, Porjesz B, Yerre C, and Kissin B: Evoked potential correlates of expected stimulus intensity. *Science* 1973;179:814–816.

Begleiter H, Porjesz B, and Garozzo R: Visual evoked potentials and affective ratings of semantic stimuli, in Begleiter H (ed): *Evoked Brain Potentials and Behavior*. New York, Plenum Publishing, 1979, pp.127–141.

Begleiter H, Porjesz B, Chou CL, and Aunon JL: P3 and stimulus incentive value. *Psychophysiology* 1983;20:95–101.

Bennett TL: Hippocampal theta activity and processes of attention, in Isaacson RL and Pribram KH (eds): *The Hippocampus. A Comprehensive Treatise*. New York, Plenum Press, 1975, pp.71–100.

Berkson G: Development of abnormal stereotyped behaviors. *Dev Psychobiol* 1968;1:118–132.

Bishop PO: Neurophysiology of binocular single vision and stereopsis, in Jung R (ed): *Handbook of Sensory Physiology*, vol. 7. New York, Springer, 1973, part 3A. pp.255–305.

Blakemore C and Cooper GF: Development of the brain depends on the visual environment. *Nature* 1970;228:477–478.

Blum GS and Barbour JS: Selective inattention to anxiety-linked stimuli. *J Exp Psychol General* 1979;108:182–224.

Blumer D: Changes of sexual behavior related to temporal lobe disorders in man. *J Sex Res* 1970;6:173–180.

Boddy J: *Brain Systems and Psychological Concepts.* New York, John Wiley & Sons, 1978.

Bogen JE: The other side of the brain, II: An appositional mind. *Bulletin of the Los Angeles Neurological Societies.* 1969;34:135–162.

Bone RN and Eysenck HJ: Extraversion, field dependence, and the Stroop test. *Percept Mot Skills* 1972;34:873–874.

Brion S: Korsakoff's syndrome: Clinico-anatomical and physiopathological conditions, in Talland GA and Waugh NC (eds): *The Pathology of Memory.* New York, Academic Press, 1969.

Broadbent DE: *In Defense of Empirical Psychology.* London, Methuen, 1973.

Broadbent DE: The hidden preattentive processes. *Am Psychol* 1977;32:109–118.

Brodmann K: *Verfleichende Lokalizations-lehre der Grosshirnrinde,* 1909, in Clarke E and Dewhurst K: *An Illustrated History of Brain Function.* Sanford Publication, Oxford, 1972.

Bruner JS and Postman L: Emotional selectivity in perception and reaction. *J Pers* 1947;16:69–77.

Buchsbaum M: Self-regulation of stimulus intensity: Augmenting, reducing and the average evoked response, in Schwartz GE and Shapiro D (eds): *Consciousness and Self-Regulation.* New York, Plenum Press, 1976, pp.101–136.

Buchsbaum M and Pfefferbaum A: Individual differences in stimulus intensity response. *Psychophysiology* 1971;8:600–611.

Buchsbaum M and Silverman J: Stimulus intensity control and the cortical evoked response. *Psychosom Med* 1968;30:12–22.

Buchsbaum M and Silverman J: Average evoked response and perception of the vertical. *J Exp Res Pers* 1980;4:79–83.

Budzynski TH: Biofeedback and the twilight states of consciousness, in Schwartz GE and Shapiro D (eds): *Consciousness and Self-Regulation,* vol I. New York, Plenum Press, 1976, pp.361–386.

Burns BD: *The Mammalian Cerebral Cortex.* London, Arnold, 1958.

Butler SR: The effects of commissurotomy on the human encephalogram, in Michel F and Schott B (eds): *Les Syndromes de Disconnexion Calleuse.* Lyon, France, Chez L'Homme Hospital Neurologique 1975, pp. 73–83.

Butler S: Interhemispheric relations in schizophrenia, in Gruzelier J and Flor-Henry P (eds): *Hemispheric Asymmetries of Function in Psychopathology.* Amsterdam, Elsevier/North Holland Biomedical Press, 1979, pp.47–64.

Canter S: Personality traits in twins, in Claridge G, Canter S, and Hume WI (eds): *Biological Differences and Biological Variations: A Study of Twins.* Oxford, Pergamon, 1973.

Chess S and Thomas A: Temperamental individuality from childhood to adolescence. *Pediatrics* 1977;16:218–226.

Chomsky N: *Aspects of the Theory of Syntax.* Cambridge, MA, MIT Press, 1965.

Cobb WA: The normal adult EEG, in Hill JDN and Parr G (eds): *Electroencephalography.* New York, Macmillan, 1963, pp.232–249.

Cohen DB: Dreaming: Experimental investigation of representational and adaptive properties, in Schwartz GE and Shapiro D (eds): *Consciousness and Self-Regulation.* New York, Plenum Press, 1976, pp.313–360.

Cohen DB and Cox D: Neuroticism in the sleep laboratory: Implications for representational and adaptive properties of dreaming. *J Abnorm Psychol* 1975;84:91–108.

Cohen HD, Rosen RC, and Goldstein L: Electroencephalographic laterality changes during human sexual orgasm. *Arch Sex Behav* 1976;5:189–199.

Coyle JT, Price DL, and Delong MR: Alzheimer's disease: A disorder of cortical cholinergic innervation. *Science* 1983;219:1184–1190.

Crick F and Mitchison G: The function of dream sleep. *Nature* 1983;304:111–114.

Crutchfield RS: Conformity and character. *Am Psychol* 1955;10:101–198.

Dahl D, Bailey WH, and Winson J: Effect of norepinephrine depletion of hippocampus on neuronal transmission from perforant pathway through dentate gyrus. *J Neurophysiol* 1983;49:123–135.

Davidson JM: The physiology of meditation and mystical states of consciousness. *Perspect Biol Med* 1976;19:345–380.

Davidson JM: The psychobiology of sexual experience, in Davidson JM and Davidson RJ (eds): *The Psychobiology of Consciousness.* New York, Plenum Press, 1980, pp.271–332.

Davidson RJ: Consciousness and information processing: A biocognitive perspective, in Davidson JM and Davidson RJ (eds): *The Psychobiology of Consciousness*. New York, Plenum Press, 1980, pp.11–46.

Davidson RJ: A newspaper report of current research on repression, by Daniel Goelman in the *New York Times Magazine Section*, May 12, 1985, p.36.

Davidson RJ, Schwartz GE, Saron C, Bennett J, et al: Frontal versus parietal EEG asymmetry during positive and negative affect. *Psychophysiology* 1974;16:212–203.

Davidson RJ, Saron C, and McClelland DC: Effects of personality and semantic content of stimuli on augmenting and reducing in the event-related potential. *Biol Psychiatry* 1980;11:249–255.

Davis PA, Gibbs FA, Davish H, Jetter WW, et al: The effects of alcohol upon the electroencephalogram (brain waves). *Q Stud Alcohol* 1941;1:626.

Deets AC, Harlow HF, Singh SD, and Bloomquist AJ: Effects of bilateral lesions of the frontal granular cortex on the social behavior of rhesus monkeys. *J Comp Physiol Psychol* 1970;72:452–461.

DeLacoste-Utamsing C and Holloway R: Sexual dimorphism in the human corpus callosum. *Science* 1982;216:1431–1432.

Denenberg VH: Hemispheric laterality in animals and the effects of early experience. *Behav Brain Sci* 1981;4:1–49.

Divac I: Magnocellular nuclei of the basal forebrain project to neocortex, brainstem and olfactory bulbs: Review of some functional correlates. *Brain Research* 1975;93:385–398.

Dollard J, Doob L, Miller NE, Mourer OH, et al: *Frustration and Aggression*. New Haven, Yale University Press, 1939.

Donchin E, McCarthy G, Kutas M, and Ritters W: Event-related brain potentials in the study of consciousness, in Davidson RJ, Schwartz GE and Shapiro D (eds): *Consciousness and Self-Regulation*, vol III. New York, Plenum Press, 1981.

Doty RW, Negrao R, and Yamago K: The unilateral engram. *Acta Neurobiol Exp* 1973;33:711–728.

Douglas RJ: Pavlovian conditioning and the brain, in Boakes RA and Halliday MS (eds): *Inhibition and Learning*. New York, Academic Press, 1972, pp.529–554.

Dubos R: *Mirage of Health*. Harper & Row, New York, 1959, p. 110.

Duffy E: *Activation and Behavior*. Wiley, New York, 1962.

Duncan CP: The retroactive effect of electroshock on learning. *J Comp Physiol Psychol* 1949;42:34–44.

Eaves LJ, and Eysenck HJ: The nature of extroversion: A genetical analysis. *J Per Soc Psychol.* 1975;32:102–112.

Eccles JC: *The Understanding of the Brain*. New York, McGraw Hill Book Co., 1963.

Edelman GM and Mountcastle VB: *The Mindful Brain: Cortical Organization and the Group Selective Theory of Higher Brain Function*. Cambridge, MA, MIT Press, 1978.

Ehrlichman H and Weinberger A: Lateral eye movements and hemispheric asymmetry: A critical review. *Psychol Bull* 1978;85:1080–1101.

Ekman P, Levenson RW, and Friesen WV: Autonomic nervous system activity distinguishes between emotions. *Science* 1983;221:1208–1210.

Erdelyi MH: A new look at the new look: Perceptual defense and vigilance. *Psychol Rev* 1974;81:1–25.

Erdelyi MH and Appelbaum GA: Cognitive masking: The disruptive effect of emotional stimulus upon the perception of contiguous neutral items. *Bull Psychon Soc* 1973;1:59–61.

Erickson RP: On the neural basis of behavior. *Am Sci* 1984;72:233–241.

Eriksen CW: Psychological defenses and "ego strength" in the recall of completed and incompleted tasks. *J. Abnorm Psychol* 1954;49:45–50.

Eriksen CW: Perception and personality, in Wipman JM and Heine RW (eds): *Concepts of Personality*. Chicago, Aldine, 1963.

Erikson EH: *Childhood and Society*. New York, Morton, 1950.

Erwen E: Psychotherapy and Freudian psychology, in Modgil S and Midgil C (eds): *Hans Eysenck: A Psychologist Searching for a Scientific Basis for Human Behavior*. London, Falmer Press, 1985.

Evans FJ: Field dependence and the Maudsley Personality Inventory. *Percept Mot Skills* 1967;24:526.

Evarts EV: Unit activity in sleep and wakefulness, in Quarton GC, Melnechuk T, and Schmitt FO (eds): *The Neurosciences. A Study Program*. New York, Rockefeller University Press, 1967, pp.545–556.

Evarts EV: Relation of discharge frequency to conduction velocity in pyramidal tract. *J Neurophysiol* 1965a;28:216–228.

Evarts EV: Neuronal activity in visual and motor cortex during sleep and waking, in Jouvet M (ed):

Neurophysiologic des Etats de Sommeil. Paris, Centre National de Recherche Scientifique, 1965b;pp.189–212.

Eysenck HJ: Classification and the problems of diagnosis, in Eysenck HJ (ed): *Handbook of Abnormal Personality.* New York, Basic Books, 1961, pp.1–32.

Eysenck HJ: *The Biological Basis of Personality.* Springfield, IL, Charles C. Thomas, 1967.

Farrell BA: *The Standing of Psychoanalysis.* New York, Oxford University Press, 1982.

Fenichel O: *The Psychoanalytic Theory of Neurosis.* New York, Norton and Company, 1945.

Fenwick PBC, Donaldson S, Gilles L, Bushman J, et al: Metabolic and EEG changes during transcendental meditation: An explanation. *Biol Psychol* 1977;5:101–118.

Fine BJ: Field-dependent introvert and neuroticism: Eysenck and Witkin united. *Psychol Rep* 1972;31:939–956.

Fisher S and Greenberg RP: *The Scientific Credibility of Freud's Theories and Therapies.* New York, Basic Books, 1977.

Fiss, H, Klein GS, and Bokert ER: Waking fantasies following interruptions of two types of sleep. *Arch Gen Psychiatry* 1966;14:543–551.

Flynn JP: The neural basis of aggression in cats, in Glass DC (ed): *Neurophysiology and Emotion.* New York, Rockefeller Univ. Press and Russell Sage Foundation, 1967.

Flynn JP, Vanegas H, Foote W, and Edwards S: Neural mechanisms involved in a cat's attack on a rat, in Whalen RW, Thompson RF, Verzeano M, and Weinberger NM (eds): *The Neural Control of Behavior.* New York, Academic Press 1970, pp.135–173.

Forster PM and Govier E: Discrimination without awareness. *Q J Exp Psychol* 1978;30:282–295.

Franks CM: Conditioning and abnormal behavior, in Eysenck JH (ed): *Handbook of Abnormal Psychology.* New York, Basic Books, 1960, pp.457–487.

Freedman AM, Kaplan HI, and Sadock BJ: *Modern Synopsis of Psychiatry.* Baltimore, Williams & Wilkens Company, 1972.

Frenkel-Brunswik E: Alternative manifestations of motivational tendencies. *Psychol Bull* 1941;38:585–586.

Freud S: Supplement to the theory of dreams. *Int J Psycho-anal.* 1920;1:354–368.

Freud S: *The Problem of Anxiety.* New York, Norton, 1926.

Freud S (1917): *Mourning and Melancholia,* vol 14, stand ed. London, Hogarth Press, 1957.

Freud S (1895): *Project for a Scientific Psychology,* part 1, stand ed. Hogarth Press, London, 1966;1:295–343.

Gainotti G: The relationship between emotions and cerebral dominance: A review of clinical and experimental evidence, in Gruzelier J and Flor-Henry P (eds): *Hemisphere Asymmetries of Function in Psychopathology.* Amsterdam, Elsevier/North Holland, 1979, pp.21–34.

Galambos L, Sheatz G, and Vernier VG: Electrophysiological correlates of a conditioned response in cats. *Science* 1956;123:376–377.

Galin D: Implications for psychiatry for left and right cerebral specialization: A neurophysiological context for unconscious processes. *Arch Gen Psychiatry* 1974;31:572–583.

Gardiner MF and Walter DO: Evidence of hemispheric specialization from infant EEG, in Harnad S, Doty RW, Jaynes J, Goldstein I, et al (eds): *Lateralization in the Nervous System.* New York, Academic Press, 1977, pp.481–502.

Gazzaniga MS and LeDoux JE: *The Integrated Mind.* New York, Plenum Press, 1978.

Gevins AS, Schaffer RE, Doyle JC, Cutillo BA, et al: Shadows of thought: Shifting lateralization of human brain electrical patterns during brief visuomotor task. *Science* 1983;110:97–99.

Gintzler A: Endorphin mediated increases in pain threshold during pregnancy. *Science* 1980;210:193–195.

Giora L: The function of the dream: A reappraisal. *Am J Psychiatry* 1972;128:1067–1073.

Girvin JP: Clinical correlates of hypothalamic and limbic system function, in Mogenson GJ and Calaresu FR (eds): *Neural Integration of Physiological Mechanisms and Behavior.* Toronto, University of Toronto Press, 1975, pp.412–434.

Gleser CG and Ihilevich D: An objective instrument for measuring defense mechanisms. *J Consult Clin Psychol* 1969;33:51–60.

Glick SD, Jerussi TP, and Zimmerberg B: Behavioral and neuropharmacological correlates of nigrostriatal asymmetry in rats, in Harnad S, Doty RW, Jaynes J, Goldstein L, (eds): *Lateralization in the Nervous System.* New York, Academic Press, 1977, pp.213–250.

Globus A, Rosenzweig MR, Bennett EL, and Diamond MC: Effects of differential experience on dendritic spine counts in rat cerebral cortex. *J Comp Physiol Psychol* 1973;82:175–181.

Goldstein L: Some relationships between quantified hemispheric EEG and behavioral states in man, in Gruzelier J and Flor-Henry P (eds): *Hemispheric Asymmetries of Function in Psychopathology*. Amsterdam, Elsevier North Holland, 1979, pp.237–254.

Grastyán E, Lissák K, Madarasz I, and Donhoffer H: Hippocampal electrical activity during the development of conditioned reflexes. *Electroencephalogr Clin Neurophysiol* 1959;11:409–430.

Gray JA: Sodium amobarbital, the hippocampal theta rhythm and the partial reinforcement extinction effect. *Psychol Rev* 1970;77:465–480.

Gray JA: *The Psychology of Fear and Stress*. London, Weidenfeld and Nicolson (World University Library), 1971.

Gray JA: The psychophysiological nature of introversion–extraversion: A modification of Eysenck's theory, in Nebilitsyn VD and Gray JA (eds): *Behavior*. New York, Academic Press, 1972, pp.182–205.

Greeley AM: *Ecstacy: A Way of Knowing*. Englewood Cliffs, NJ, 1974.

Green JD and Arduini AA: Hippocampal electrical activity in arousal. *J Neurophysiol* 1954;17:533.

Gregory RL: Do we need cognitive concepts?, in Gazzaniga MS and Blakemore C (eds): *Handbook of Psychobiology*. New York, Academic Press, 1975, pp.607–628.

Grillner S: Neurobiological bases of rhythmic motor acts in vertebrates. *Science* 1985;228:143–149.

Gross CG, Rocha-Miranda CE, and Bender DB: Visual properties of neurons in inferotemporal cortex of the macaque. *J Neurophysiol* 1972;35:96–111.

Gur RE and Gur RC: Defense mechanisms, psychosomatic symptomatology and conjugate lateral eye movements. *J Consult Clin Psychol* 1975;43:416–420.

Gur RE and Gur RC: Correlates of conjugate lateral eye movements in man, in Harnad S, Doty RW, Jaynes J, Goldstein L, et al (eds): *Lateralization in the Nervous System*. New York, Academic Press, 1977, pp.261–284.

Halgren E, Squires NK, Wilson CL, Rohrbaugh JW, et al: Endogenous potentials generated in the human hippocampal formation and amygdala by infrequent events. *Science* 1980;210:803–805.

Halliday AM: Evoked responses in organic and functional sensory loss, in Feffard A and Lelord G (eds): Activites evoquels et leur conditionement chez l'honne normal et en pathologie mentale, Paris. *Additions INSERM* 1973, pp.189–212.

Hamilton CR: Investigations of perceptual and anemonic lateralization in monkeys, in Harnad Doty RW, Jaynes J, et al (eds): *Lateralization in the Nervous System*. New York, Academic Press, 1977, pp.45–62.

Harlow HF and Zimmerman RR: Affectional responses in the infant monkey. *Science* 1959;130:421–432.

Harnad S and Doty RW: Introductory overview, in Harnad S, Doty RW, Jaynes J, Goldstein L et al (eds): *Lateralization in the Nervous System*. New York, Academic Press, 1977, pp.xvii–xviii.

Hartmann H: Psychoanalysis and developmental psychology. *Psychoanal Study Child*, 1950;5:7–17.

Hartmann H: *Ego Psychology and the Problem of Adaptation*. New York, International Universities Press, 1958.

Hassler R: Interaction of reticular activating system for vigilance and the truncothalamic and pallidal systems for directing awareness and attention under striatal control, in Buser PA and Rogeul-Buser A (eds): *Cerebral Correlates of Consciousness*. Amsterdam, Elsevier/North Holland, 1978, pp.111–130.

Hayakawa SI: *Language in Action*. New York, Harcourt Brace and Co., 1941.

Heath RG: Electrical self-stimulation of the brain in man. *Amer J Psychiatry* 1963;120:571–577.

Heath RG: Pleasure and brain activity in man. *J Nerv Ment Dis* 1972;152:3–18.

Hebb DO: *The Organization of Behavior*. New York, John Wiley and Sons, 1949.

Hebb DO: *A Textbook of Psychology*, 2nd ed. Philadelphia, W. B. Saunders, 1966.

Heilman KM, and Watson RT: The neglect syndrome: A unilateral defect of the orienting response, in Harnad S, Doty RW, Goldstein L, Jaynes J, and Krauthamer G (eds): *Lateralization in the Nervous System*. New York, Academic Press, 1977, pp.285–302.

Held R and Hein A: Movement produced stimulation in the development of visually guided behavior. *J Comp Physiol Psychol* 1963;56:686–690.

Hilgard ER: Experimental approaches to psychoanalysis, in Pumpian-Mindlin E (ed): *Psychoanalysis, A Science*. Stanford, CA, Stanford University Press, 1952, p.3.

Hillyard SA and Woods DL: Electrophysiological analysis of human brain function, in Gazzaniga MS (ed): *Handbook of Behavioral Neurobiology*, vol 2, *Neuropsychology*. New York, Plenum Press, 1979, pp.345–378.

Hink RF and Hillyard SA: Elctrophysiological measures of attentional processes in man as related to the study of schizophrenia. *J Psychiatr Res* 1978;14:155–165.

Hobson JA, McCarley RW, and Wyzinski PW: Sleep cycle oscillation: Reciprocal discharge by two brainstem neuronal groups. *Science* 1975;189:55–58.

Hohmann GW: Some effects of spinal cord lesions on experienced emotional feelings. *Psychophysiology* 1966;3:143–156.

Holmes DS: Repression or interference? A further investigation. *J Pers Soc Psychol* 1972;22:163–170.

Hoppe KD: Split brains and psychoanalysis. *Psychoanal Q* 1977;46:220–244.

Hoppe KD and Bogen JE: Alexithymia in twelve commissurotomized patients. *Psycho Psychosom* 1977;28:148–155.

Horney K: *The Neurotic Personality of Our Time*. New York, Norton, 1936.

Hubel DH and Wiesel TN: Receptive fields and functional architecture in two nonstriate visual areas (18 and 19) of the cat. *J Neurophysiol* 1965;18:119–189.

Huttenlocher E: Evoked and spontaneous activity in single units of medial brain stem during natural sleep and waking. *J Neurophysiol* 1961;27:152–171.

Inglis J: Abnormalities of motivation and "ego-functions," in Eysenck HJ (ed): *Handbook of Abnormal Personality*. New York, Basic Books, 1961, pp.262–297.

Isaacson RL: Neural systems of the limbic brain and behavioral inhibition, in Boakes RA and Halliday MS (eds): *Inhibition and Learning*. New York, Academic Press, 1972, pp.497–528.

Isaacson RL: *The Limbic System*. New York, Plenum Press, 1974.

Isaacson RL and Pribram KH (eds): *The Hippocampus*, vols 1,2. New York, Plenum Press, 1975.

Iversen SO: Brain lesions and memory in animals, in Deutsch A (ed): *The Physiological Basis of Memory*. New York, Academic Press, 1973, pp.305–364.

Izard CE: The emergence of emotions and the development of consciousness in infancy, in Davidson JM and Davidson RJ (eds): *The Psychobiology of Consciousness*. New York, Plenum Press, 1980, pp.193–216.

Janis IL: Stress and frustration, part I, in Janis IJ, Mahl GF, Kagan J, and Holt RR (eds): *Personality: Dynamics, Development and Assessment*. New York, Harcourt, Brace and World, 1969, pp.3–205.

Janis IL, Mahl GF, Kagan J, and Holt RR: *Personality: Dynamics, Development and Assessment*. New York, Harcourt, Brace and World, 1969.

Janis MG: *A Two-Year-Old Goes to Nursery School: A Case Study of Separation Reactions*. London, Tarstock Publications, 1964.

John ER: *Mechanisms of Memory*. New York, Academic Press, 1967.

John ER, Herrington RN, and Sutton S: Effects of visual form on the evoked response. *Science* 1967;155:1439–1442.

John ER, Bartlett F, Slumokochi M, and Kleinman D: Neural readout from memory. *J Neurophysiol* 1973;36:893–924.

Jones EG, Burton H, Saper CB, and Swanson LW: Midbrain, diencephalic and cortical relationships of the basal nucleus of Meynert and associated structures on primates. *J Comp Neurol* 1976;167:385–419.

Jouvet M: The role of monaminergic neurons in the regulation and function of sleep, in Petre-Inadens O and Schlag JO (eds): *Basic Sleep Mechanisms*. New York, Academic Press, 1974, pp.207–232.

Jung R: Perception, consciousness and visual attention, in Buser PA and Rongeal-Buser A (eds): *Cerebral Correlates of Conscious Experience*. Amsterdam, Elsevier/North Holland 1978, pp.15–36.

Kaada BR: Stimulation and regional ablation of the amygdaloid complex with reference to functional representations, in Eleftheriou BE (ed): *The Neurobiology of the Amygdala*. New York, Plenum Press, 1982, pp.205–283.

Kagan J: Personality development part 3, in Janis IJ (ed): *Personality: Dynamics, Development and Assessment*. New York, Harcourt, Brace and World, 1969, pp.405–574.

Kahneman A: *Attention and Effort*. Englewood Cliffs, NJ, Prentice Hall, 1973.

Kandel ER: Brain and behavior, in Kandel ER and Schwartz JH (eds): *Principles of Neural Science*, New York, Elsevier/North Holland, 1981, pp.1–13.

Kandel ER and Schwartz JH: Molecular biology of an elementary form of learning. Modulation of transmitter release by cyclic AMP. *Science* 1982;218:433–443.

Karczmar AG and Dun MJ: Cholinergic synapses: Physiological, pharmacological and behavioral considerations, in Lipton MA, DiMascio A, and Killman KF (eds): *Pharmacology—A Generation of Progress.* New York, Raven Press, 1978, pp. 293–305.

Kimble DP: Hippocampus and internal inhibition. *Psychol Bull* 1968;70:285–295.

Kinsbourne M: A model for the mechanism of unilateral neglect of space. *Trans Am Neurol Assoc* 1970;95:143.

Kissin B: Alcohol as it compares to other addictive substances, in Keup W (ed): *Drug Abuse: Current Concepts and Research.* Springfield, Charles C. Thomas, 1972, pp.251–262.

Klein D, Moscovitch M, and Vigna C: Attentional mechanisms and perceptual asymmetries in tachistoscopic recognition of words and faces. *Neurophychologia* 1976;14:55–66.

Kling A: Frontal and temporal lobe lesions and aggressive behavior, in Smith WL and Kling A (eds): *Issues in Brain/Behavior Control.* New York, Spectrum Publications, 1976, pp.11–22.

Klüver H and Bucy PC: "Psychic blindness" and other symptoms following bilateral temporal lobectomy in rhesus monkeys. *Am J Physiol* 1937;119:352–353.

von Knorring L: Visual averaged evoked responses in patients suffering from alcoholism. *Neuropsychobiology* 1976;2:233–238.

Kornhuber HH: A reconsideration of the brain–mind problem, in Buser PA and Rougeil-Buser A (eds) *Cerebral Correlates of Conscious Experience.* Amsterdam, North Holland Publishing Co, 1978, pp.319–334.

Kostandov EA and Arzumov YvL: Interhemispheric functional relations in negative emotions in man. *Zh Vyssh Nervn Deyat Pavlova* 1980;30:327–336.

Krettek JE and Price JL: Amygdaloid projections to subcortical structures within the basal forebrain and brainstem in the rat and cat. *J Comp Neurol* 1978;178:225–253.

Kuffler SW: Discharge patterns of functional organization of mammalian retina. *J Neurophysiol* 1953;16:37–68.

Kuhar MJ: *Biology of Cholinergic Function.* New York, Raven Press, 1976.

Kunst-Wilson WR and Zajonc RB: Affective discrimination of stimuli that cannot be recognized. *Science* 1980;207:557–558.

Kupferman I: Hypothalamus and limbic system I, in Kandel ER, and Schwartz JH (eds): *Principles of Neural Science.* New York, Elsevier/North Holland, 1981, pp.431–460.

Landau SG, Buchsbaum MS, Carpenter W, Strauss J, and Sacks M: Schizophrenia and stimulus intensity control. *Arch Gen Psychiatry* 1975;32:1239–1245.

Lasch C: *The Minimal Self: Psychic Survival in Troubled Times.* New York, Norton, 1984.

Lashley KS: In search of the engram, in Society for Experimental Biology Symposium, no. 4: *Physiological Mechanisms in Animal Behavior.* 1950, pp.452–482.

Lazarus RS: A cognitivist's reply to Zajonc on emotion and cognition. *Am Psychol* 1981;36:222–223.

Lazarus RS, Speisman JC, Mordkoff AM, and Davison LA: A laboratory study of psychological stress produced by a motion picture film. *Psychol Monogr* 1962;76:1–35.

Lazarus RS and Alferth E: Short circuiting of threat by experimentally altering cognitive appraisal. *J Abnorm Soc Psychol* 1964;69:195–205.

Lazarus RS, Opton E Jr, Nomikos MS, and Rankin NO: The principle of short circuiting of stress: Further evidence. *J Pers* 1965;33:622–625.

LeDoux JE, Wilson DH, and Gazzaniga MS: Beyond commissurotomy: Clues to consciousness, in Gazzaniga MS (ed): *Handbook of Behavioral Neurobiology.* New York, Plenum Press, vol 2, *Neuropsychology,* 1979, pp.543–554.

Lehman D: Multichannel topography of human alpha EEG fields. *Electroencephalogr Clin Neurophysiol* 1971;31:439–449.

Lenneberg EH: *Biological Foundations of Language.* New York, John Wiley & Sons, 1967.

Lennie P: Parallel visual pathways: A review. *Vision Res* 1980;20:561–594.

Levy DM: Experiments on the sucking reflex and social behavior of dogs. *Am J Orthopsychiatr* 1934;4:203–224.

Libet B, Wright EW Jr, Feinstein B, and Peare DK: Subjective referral of the timing for a conscious sensory experience. *Brain* 1979;102:193–224.

Lieberson J: Putting Freud to the test. *New York Review of Books* 1984;32:24–28.

Liebeskind JC, Guilbaud G, Besson JM, and Aliveras JL: Analgesia from electrical stimulation of the periaqueductal grey matter in the cat. *Brain Res* 1973;50:441–446.

Liddell HS: A comparative approach to the dynamics of experimental neurosis. *Ann NY Acad Sci* 1953;56:164.

Liddell HS: Conditioning and emotions. *Sci Am* 1954;190:48.

Linton HB: *Relations between Mode of Perception and Tendency to Conform*. Unpublished doctoral dissertation. Yale University, New Haven, CT, 1962.

Loehlin JC: Psychological genetics, from the study of human behavior, in Cattell RB and Dreger RM: *Handbook of Modern Personality Theory*. New York, John Wiley & Sons, 1977, pp.329–347.

Lowry TP and Lowry TS: *The Clitoris*. St. Louis, W.H. Green, 1976.

Lukas, JH and Siegel J: Cortical mechanisms that augment or reduce evoked potentials in cats. *Science* 1977;198:73–75.

Lumsden CJ and Wilson EO: *Genes, Mind and Culture*. Cambridge, MA, Harvard University Press, 1981.

Luria AR and Simernitskaya EG: Interhemispheric relations and the functions of the minor hemisphere. *Neuropsychologia* 1977;15:175–178.

Luria AR, Simernitskaya EG, and Tubylevich B: The structure of psychological processes in relation to cerebral organization. *Neuropsychologia* 1970;8:13–18.

Lykken D: A study of anxiety in the sociopathic personality. *J Abnorm Soc Psychol* 1957;55:6–10.

Lynch G: What memories are made of. *Sciences* (New York) Sept/Oct 1985;38–43.

Mack JE: *Nightmares and Human Conflict*. Boston, Little Brown and Company, 1970.

MacKinnon DW and Duke SW: Repression, in Postman L (ed): *Psychology in the Making*. New York, Knopf, 1962.

MacLean PD: The triune brain, emotion and scientific bias, in Schmitt FD (ed): *The Neurosciences Second Study Program*. New York, Rockefeller University Press, 1970, pp.336–349.

Maddi SR: *Personality Theories: A Comparative Analysis*, 3rd ed. Homewood, IL, The Dorsey Press, 1976.

Mahl GF: Conflict and Defense, part 2, in Janis IJ (ed): *Personality: Dynamics, Development and Assessment*. New York, Harcourt, Brace and World, 1969, pp.206–406.

Mahler MS: On the first three subphases of the separation–individuation process. *Int J Psychoanal* 1972;53:333–338.

Mancillas JR, Siggins GR, and Bloom FE: Systemic ethanol: Selective enhancement of responses to acetylcholine and somatostatin in hippocampus. *Science* 1986;231:161–163.

Mandell AJ: Toward a psychobiology of transcendence: God in the brain, in Davidson JM and Davidson RJ (eds): *The Psychobiology of Consciousness*. New York, Plenum Press, 1980, pp.379–464.

Marr D: *Vison: A Computational Investigation into the Human Representation and Processing of Visual Information*. New York, WIT Freeman, 1984.

Marx JL: The two sides of the brain. *Science* 1983;220:488–490.

Massaro DW: *Experimental Psychology and Information Processing*. Chicago, Rand McNally, 1975.

Masserman JH: A biodynamic psychoanalytic approach to the problems of feelings and emotions, in Reynert ML (ed): *Feelings and Emotions*. New York, McGraw Hill, 1950, p.49.

Masserman JH and Yum KS: The influence of alcohol on experimental neuroses in cats. *Psychosom Med* 1946;8:36–42.

Mayer-Gross W, Slater ETC, and Roth M: *Clinical Psychiatry*. Baltimore, Williams and Wilkens, 1960.

Mazziotta JC, Phelps ME, Carson RE, and Kuhl DE: Tomographic mapping of human cerebral metabolism-auditory stimulation. *Neurology* 1982;32:921–937.

McCarley RW and Hobson JA: Clustered discharges of FTG neurons during desynchronized sleep. *Sleep Res* 1974;3:24–32.

McCleary RA and Lazarus RS: Autonomic discrimination without awareness. *J Personal* 1949;18:171–179.

McCormick DA, Clark GA, Lavond DG, and Thompson RF: Initial localization of the memory trace for a basic form of learning. *Proc Natl Acad Sci* 1982;79:2731–2735.

McGaugh JL: A multi-trace view of memory storage processes, in Bovet D, Bovet-Nitti, F, and Oliviero A (eds): *Accordemia Nazionale dai Lincei*, 1968, pp.13–24.

McGinnies E: Emotionality and perceptual defense. *Psychol Rev* 1949;56:244–251.

Meredith MA and Stein BA: Interactions among converging sensory inputs in the superior colliculus. *Science* 1983;221:189-191.

Mesulam MM and Geschwind N: On the possible role of neocortex and its limbic connections in the process of attention in schizophrenia: Clinical cases of inattention in man and experimental anatomy in monkey. *J Psychiatr Res* 1978;14:249-259.

Michel GF: Right-handedness: A consequence of infant supine head orientation. *Science* 1981;212:885-887.

Miller GA: Speech and language, in Steven SS (ed): *Handbook of Experimental Psychology.* New York, John Wiley & Sons, 1951, pp.789-810.

Milner B: Amnesia following operation on the temporal lobes, in Whitty CWM and Zangwill OL (eds): *Amnesia.* London, Butterworth, 1966, pp.112-115.

Milner B, Corkin S, and Tenber HL: Further analysis of the hippocampal amnesic syndrome: 14-year follow-up study of H.M. *Neuropsychologia* 1968;6:215-222.

Mishkin M: A memory system in the monkey. *Philos Trans R Soc London Ser B* 1982;298:85-95.

Mitchell SJ and Ranck JB: Generation of theta rhythm in medial entorhinal cortex of freely moving rats. *Brain Res* 1980;189:49-56.

Monnier M, Hosli L, and Krupp P: Moderating and activating systems on the medio-central thalamus and reticular formation. *Electroencephalogr Clin Neurophysiol* (suppl) 1963;24:97-112.

Morgane PJ: Control of physiological regulations and behavior, in Mogenson GJ and Calaresu FR (eds): *Neural Integration of Physiological Mechanisms and Behavior.* Toronto, University of Toronto Press, 1975, pp.24-67.

Morison RS and Dempsey EW: A study of thalamo-cortical relations. *Amer J Physiol* 1962;135:261-292.

Morrell F: Electrical signs of sensory coding, in Quarton CG, Melneckuk T, and Schmitt FO (eds): *The Neurosciences, A Study Program.* New York, Rockefeller University Press, 1967, pp.452-469.

Moruzzi G and Magoun HW: Brainstem reticular formation and activation of the EEG. *Electroencephalog Clin Neurophysiol* 1949;1:455-473.

Moscovitch M: Information processing and the cerebral hemispheres, in Gazzaniga MS (ed): *Handbook of Behavioral Neurobiology,*vol 2, *Neuropsychology.* New York, Plenum Press, 1979, pp.379-446.

Mountcastle VB: in Edelman GM and Mountcastle VB: *The Mindful Brain: Cortical Organization and Group Selection Theory of Higher Function.* Cambridge, MA, MIT Press, 1978a.

Mountcastle VB: Some neural mechanisms for directed attention, in Buser PA and Rougent-Buser A (eds): *Cerebral Correlates of Conscious Experience.* Amsterdam, Elsevier/North Holland, 1978b, pp.37-52.

Mountcastle VB, Lynch, JC, Georgopoulos, A, et al: Posterior parietal association cortex of the monkey: Command function for operations within interpersonal space. *J Neurophysiol* 1975;38:871-908.

Murray EA and Mishkin M: Amygdalectomy impairs crossmodal association in monkeys. *Science* 1985;228:604-606.

Murray HA: Basic concepts for a psychology of personality. *J Gen Psychol* 1936;15:241-268.

Nauta WJH: Some efferent connections of the prefrontal cortex in the monkey, in Warren JM and Akut K (eds): *The Frontal Granular Cortex and Behavior.* New York, McGraw Hill, 1964, pp.397-409.

Navon D: *Global Precedence in Visual Recognition.* Unpublished doctoral dissertation. University of California, San Diego, 1975.

Nebylitsyn VD and Gray JA: *Biological Bases of Individual Behavior.* New York, Academic Press, 1972.

Neisser U: *Cognitive Psychology.* New York, Appleton, Century Crofts, 1967.

Nemiah JC and Sifneos PE: Affect and fantasy in patients with psychosomatic disorders, in Hill R (ed) *Modern Trends in Psychosmatic Medicine,* 2. New York, Appleton, Century, Crofts, 1970, pp.26-34.

Newman HH, Freeman FN, and Holzinger KJ: *Twins, A Study of Heredity and Environment.* Chicago, University of Chicago Press, 1937.

Nottebohm F: Origins and mechanisms in the establishment of cerebral dominance, in Gazzaniga M (ed): *Handbook of Behavioral Neurobiology,* vol 2. *Neuropsychology.* New York, Plenum Press, 1979.

Oden GC and Massaro DW: Integration of featural information in speech perception. *Psychol Rev* 1978;85:172-191.

Ojemann GA: Asymmetric function of the thalamus in man, in Dimond SJ and Blizard DA (eds): Evolution and lateralization of the brain. *Ann NY Acad Sci* 1977;299:380-396.

O'Keefe J and Black AH: Single unit and lesion experiments on the sensory input to the hippocampal cognitive map, in *Functions of the Septo-Hippocampal System. Ciba Found Symp* 1978;58:179-191.

Olds J: Self-stimulation of the brain. *Science* 1958;127:315-324.

Olds J: Hypothalamic substrates of reward. *Physiol Rev* 1962;42:554–604

Olds J: Multiple unit recordings from behaving rats, in Thompson RF and Patterson MM (eds): *Bioelectric Recording Techniques IA*. New York, Academic Press, 1973, pp.165–198.

Olds J and Milner P: Positive reinforcement produced by electrical stimulation of septal area and other areas of rat brain. *J Comp Physiol Psychol* 1954;47:419–427.

Olds J, Disterhaft JF, Segal M, Kornbluth CL, et al: Learning centers of rat brain mapped by measuring latencies of conditioned unit responses. *J Neurophysiol* 1972;35:202–219.

Oltman PK, Semple C, and Goldstein L: Cognitive style and interhemispheric differentiation in the EEG. *Neuropsychologia* 1979;17:699–702.

Ornstein RE: *The Psychology of Consciousness*. San Francisco, W.H. Freeman & Co., 1972.

Otterson OP: Afferent connections to the amygdaloid complex of the rat and cat: II. Afferents from the hypothalamus and the basal telencephalon. *J Comp Neurol* 1980;194:267–289.

Otto E and Kobryn V: Asymmetry of the quantity and maximum voltage levels of 8/s to 13/s waves in homologous deviations of the EEG in healthy probands. *Psychiatr Neurol Med Psychol* 1969;21:287.

Packer I: Some cognitive and affective characteristics associated with lateral eye movements. Unpublished manuscript. University of Pennsylvania, 1975.

Papez JW: A proposed mechanism of emotion. *Arch Neurol Psychiatr* 1937;38:725–743.

Parasuraman R and Beatty J: Brain events underlying detection and recognition of weak sensory signals. *Science* 1980;210:80–83.

Parent A, Gravel S, and Olivier A: The extrapyramidal and limbic systems relationship at the globus pallidus level. *Adv Neurol* 1979;24:1–11.

Penfield W and Rasmussen S: *The Cerebral Cortex of Man: A Clinical Study of Localization of Function*. New York, MacMillan, 1957.

Perria L, Rosadini G, and Rossi GF: Determination of side of cerebral dominance with amobarbital. *Arch Neurol* 1961;4:173–181.

Petrie A: Some psychological aspects of pain and the relief of suffering. *Ann NY Acad Sci* 1960;86:13–27.

Petrie A, Holland T, and Wolk I: Sensory stimulation causing subdued experience: Audio-analgesia and perceptual augmentation and reduction. *J Nerv Ment Dis* 1963;137:312–321.

Phelps ME and Mazziotta JC: News report on study on hemispheric reaction to music by musicians and non-musicians. *Science* 1982;7.

Phelps ME and Mazziotta JC: Positron emission tomography: Human brain function and biochemistry. *Science* 1985;228:799–809.

Piaget J: *Behavior and Evolution*. Nicholson-Smith D (trans). New York, Random House, 1978.

Picton TW and Hillyard SA: Human auditory evoked potentials II. Effects of attention. *Electroencephalogr Clin Neurophysiol* 1974;36:191–199.

Pomeranz B and Chin O: Naloxone blockage of acupuncture—endorphin implicated. *Life Sci* 1976;19:1757–1762.

Popper KR and Eccles JC: *The Self and its Brain*. New York, Springer Verlag, 1978.

Posner MI: Psychobiology of attention, in Gazzaniga MS and Blakemore C (eds): *Handbook of Psychobiology*. New York, Academic Press, 1975, pp.441–480.

Posner MI: *Chronometric Explorations of the Mind*. Hillsdale, NJ, Laurence Erlbaum Associates, 1978.

Posner MI and Snyder CRR: Attention and cognitive control, in Solso RL (ed): *Information Processing and Cognition*. Hillsdale, NJ, Lawrence Erlbaum Associates, 1975.

Posner MI and Wilkinson RT: On the process of preparation. Paper presented at the meeting of the Psychonomic Society, St. Louis, November, 1969.

Posner MI, Snyder CRR, and Davidson BJ: Attention and the detection of signals. *J Exp Psychol* 1980;109:160–174.

Pradhan SN: Balance between acetylcholine, serotonin, norepinephrine, and dopamine in self-stimulation. *Psychopharmacol Bull* 1974;10:47–48.

Pradhan SN: Aggression and central neurotransmitters. *Int Rev Neurobiol* 1975;18:213–262.

Premack D: On the origins of language, in Gazzaniga MS and Blakemore C (eds): *Handbook of Psychophysiology*. New York, Academic Press, 1975, pp.591–606.

Preston GW: The very large scale integrated circuit. *Am Sci* 1983;71:466–472.

Pribram KH: Mind, brain and consciousness: The organization of competence and conduct, in Davidson JM and Davison RJ (eds): *The Psychobiology of Consciousness*. New York, Plenum Press, 1980, pp.47–61.

Pribram KH and Gill MM: *Freud's "Project" Reassessed.* New York, Basic Books, 1976.

Pritchard RM, Heron W, and Hebb DO: Visual perception approached by the method of stabilized images. *Can J Psychol* 1960;14:67–77.

Raine A, Mitchell DA, and Venables PH: Cortical augmenting–reducing modality specific? *Psychophysiology* 1981;18:700–708.

Rakic P: Local circuit neurons. *Neurosci Res Progr Bull* 1975;13:289–446.

Reiser MF: *Brain, Mind, Body. Toward a Convergence of Psychoanalysis and Neurobiology.* New York, Basic Books, 1984.

Riggs LA, Ratliff F, Cornsweet JC, and Cornsweet TN: The disappearance of steadily fixated visual test objects. *J Opt Soc Am* 1953;43:495–501.

Riklan M and Cooper IS: Thalamic lateralization of psychological functions: Psychometric studies, in Harnad S, Doty RW, Jaynes J, Goldstein L, et al, (eds): *Lateralization in the Nervous System.* New York, Academic Press, 1977, pp.123–136.

Robertson J: *Young Children in Hospital.* London, Tavistock Publications, 1958.

Robinson TE: Hippocampal rhythmic slow-wave activity (RSA, theta). A critical analysis of selected studies and discussion of possible species differences. *Brain Res Rev* 1980;2:69.

Roffwarg HP, Herman JH, Bowe-Anders C, and Tauber GS: The effects of sustained alterations of waking visual input on dream content, in Arkis AM, Antrobus JS and Ellman SJ: *The Mind in Sleep.* Hillsdale, NJ, Lawrence Erlbaum Associates, 1978.

Rolls ET, Sanghera MK, and Roper-Hall A: The latency of activation of neurons in the lateral hypothalamus and substantia innominata during feeding in the monkey. *Brain Res* 1979;164:121.

Rosenblum LA, and Plimpton EH: The infant's effort to cope with separation, in Lewis M and Rosenblum LA (eds): *The Uncommon Child.* New York, Plenum Press, 1981.

Rosenzweig MR: Evidence for anatomical and chemical changes in the brain during primary learning, in Pribram KH and Broadbent DE (eds); *Biology of Memory.* New York, Academic Press, 1970.

Rosenzweig S: The experimental measurements of types of reactions to frustrations, in Murray HA (ed): *Explorations in Personality.* Oxford, Oxford University Press, 1938.

Rosenzweig S: An experimental study of "repression" with special reference to need-perspective and ego-defensive reaction to frustration. *J Exp Psychol* 1943;32:64–74.

Rosenzweig MR, Bennett EL, and Diamond MC: Brain changes in response to experience. *Sci Am* 1972;226:22–29.

Rosvold HE, Mursky AF, and Pribram KH: Influence of amygdalectomy on social behavior in monkeys. *J Comp Physiol Psychol* 1954;47:173–187.

Rothbart MK and Derryberry D: Development of individual differences in temperament, in Lamb ME and Brown AL (eds): *Advances in Developmental Psychology,* Volume 1. Hillsdale, New Jersey, Erlbaum, 1981.

Routtenberg A: The reward system of the brain. *Sci Am* 1978;239:154–164.

Sagi D and Julesz B: "Where" and "What" in vision. *Science* 1985;228:1217–1219.

Sakai K: In Hobson JA and Brazier MA (eds): *The Reticular Formation Revisited.* New York, Raven, 1980, pp.427–447.

Schachter S and Latane B: Crime, cognition and the autonomic nervous system, in Levine D (ed): *Nebraska Symposium on Motivation.* Lincoln, University of Nebraska Press, 1964.

Schneider W and Shiffrin R: Controlled and automatic human information processing I. Detection, search and attention. *Psychol Rev* 1977;84:1–88.

Schuman M: The psychophysiological model of meditation and altered states of consciousness: A critical review, in Davidson JM and Davidson RJ (eds): *The Psychobiology of Consciousness.* New York, Plenum Press, 1980, pp.333–378.

Schwartz GF, Davidson RJ, and Maer F: Right hemisphere lateralization for emotion in the human brain: Interactions with cognition. *Science* 1975;190:286–288.

Segal M and Landis S: Afferents to the hippocampus of the rat studied with the method of retrograde transport of horseradish peroxidase. *Brain Res* 1974;78:1–15.

Shagass C: Sedation threshold: A neurophysiological tool for psychosomatic research. *Psychosom Med* 1956;18:410–419.

Shashoua VE: The role of extracellular proteins in learning and memory. *Am Sci* 1985;73:364–370.

Shepherd GM: Microcircuits in the nervous system. *Sci Am* 1978;238:92–103.

Shevrin H: Brain wave correlates of subliminal stimulation, unconscious attention, primary and secondary process thinking and repressiveness. *Psychol Issues, 8* 1974;monogr 30:56–87.

Shevrin H and Dickman S: The psychological unconscious: A necessary assumption for all psychological theory? *Am Psychol* 1980;35:421–434.

Shevrin H and Fritzler D: Correlates of repressiveness. *Psychol Rep* 1968;23:887–892.

Shevrin H and Rennick P: Cortical response to a tactile stimulus during attention, mental arithmetic and free association. *Psychophysiology* 1967;3:381–388.

Shields J: *Monozygotic Twins*. Oxford, Oxford University Press, 1962.

Shields J and Slater E: Heredity and psychological abnormality, in Eysenck HJ (ed): *Handbook of Abnormal Psychology*. New York, Basic Books, 1960, pp.298–343.

Shiffrin R and Schneider W: Controlled and automatic human information processing, II. Perceptual learning, automatic attending and a general theory. *Psychol Rev* 1977;84:127–190.

Sifneos PE: The prevalence of "alexithymic" characteristics in psychosomatic patients. *Psychother Psychosom* 1973;26:255–263.

Simernitskaya EG: On two forms of writing defect following focal brain lesions, in Dimond SJ and Beaumont JG (eds): *Hemisphere Function in the Human Brain*. New York, Halsted, 1974.

Simon HA: *Models of Thought*. New Haven, Yale University Press, 1979.

Simon HA: Studying human intelligence by creating artificial intelligence. *Am Sci* 1981;69:300–309.

Sitaram N, Wyatt RJ, Dawson S, and Gillin JC: REM sleep induction by physostigmine infusion during sleep. *Science* 1976;191:1281–1282.

Skinner JE and Yingling CD: Central gating mechanisms that regulate event-related potentials and behavior, in Desmedt JE (ed): *Attention, Voluntary Contraction and Event-Related Cerebral Potentials*, vol 1. Basel, Karger, 1977, pp.30–69.

Smith CM and Swash M: Possible biochemical basis of memory disorder in Alzheimer disease. *Ann Neurol* 1978;3:471–473.

Smock CD: Recall of interrupted and non-interrupted tasks as a function of experimentally induced anxiety and motivational relevance of the task stimuli. *J. Pers* 1956;25:589–599.

Snyder F and Scott J: The psychophysiology of sleep, in Greenfield N and Sternbach RA (eds): *Handbook of Psychophysiology*. New York, Holt Rinehart and Winston, Inc., 1972, pp.645–708.

Sokolov EN: Higher nervous functions and the orienting reflex. *Annu Rev Physiol* 1963;25:545–580.

Sperling GA: The information available in brief visual presentations. *Psychol Monogr* 1960;498:74.

Sperry RW: Mental unity following surgical disconnection of the cerebral hemispheres. *Harvey Lect Ser* 1966;62:293–323.

Sperry RW: A modified concept of consciousness. *Psychol Rev* 1969;76:532–536.

Spilker B and Callaway E: "Augmenting" and "reducing" in averaged visual responses to sine wave light. *Psychophysiology* 1969;6:49–57.

Spitz RA: Hospitalism: An inquiry into the genesis of psychiatric conditions in early childhood. *Psychoanal Study Child* 1945;1:53–74.

Squire LR: The neuropsychology of human memory. *Annu Rev Neurosci* 1982;5:241–273.

Squire LR and Cohen NJ: Memory and amnesia: Resistance to disruption develops for years after learning. *Behav Neural Biol* 1979;25:115–123.

Squire LR, Cohen NJ, and Nadel L: The medial temporal region and memory consolidation: A new hypothesis, in Weingartner H and Parker E (eds): *Memory Consolidation*. Hillsdale, NJ, Lawrence Erlbaum Associates, 1982.

Stein L: Facilitation of avoidance behavior by positive brain stimulation. *J Comp Physiol Psychol* 1965;60:9–16.

Stein L, Wise CD, and Belluzzi JD: Neuropharmacology of reward and punishment, in Iversen LL, Iversen SD, and Snyder SH (eds): *Handbook of Psychopharmacology*, vol 8, *Drugs, Neurotransmitters, and Behavior*. New York, Plenum Press, 1977, pp.25–54.

Sternbach RA: Two independent indices of activation. *Electroencephalogr Clin Neurophysiol* 1960;12:609–611.

Story JL, Erdelberg E, and French JD: Electroencephalographic changes induced in cats by ethanol intoxication. *Arch Neurol* 1961;5:565.

Swanson LW and Cowan WM: Autoradiographic studies of the development and connections of the septal area, in DeFrance JR (ed): *The Septal Nuclei*. New York, Plenum Press, 1976, pp.37–64.

Szentagothai J and Arbib MA: Conceptual models of neural organization. *Neurosci Res Prog Bull* 1974;12(3):310–510.

Tart CT: *States of Consciousness.* New York, Dutton, 1975.

Teyler TJ, Roemer RA, Harrison TF, and Thompson RF: Human scalp recorded evoked potential correlates of linguistic stimuli. *Bull Psychonom Soc* 1973;1:333–334.

Thomas, A and Chess S: Genesis and evolution of behavioral disorders from infancy to early adult life. *Am J Psychiatr* 1984;141:1–9.

Thomas A, Chess S, and Birch HG: *Temperament and Behavior Disorders in Children.* New York, New York University Press, 1968.

Thomas L: *The Medusa and the Snail. More Notes of a Biology Watcher.* New York, Viking Press, 1979, pp.76–81.

Thompson RF: *Introduction to Physiological Psychology.* New York, Harper and Row, 1975.

Thompson RF, Mayers KS, Robertson RT, and Patterson CJ: Number coding in association cortex of cat. *Science* 1970;168:271–273.

Turkewitz G: The development of lateral differences in the human infant, in Harnad S, Doty, RW, Jaynes J, Goldstein L, et al (eds): *Lateralization in the Nervous System.* New York, Academic Press, 1977, pp.251–260.

Uttal W: *Psychobiology of Mind.* Hillsdale, Lawrence Erlbaum Associates, 1978.

Van Hoesen GW: The parahippocampal gyrus—New observations regarding its cortical connections in the monkey. *Trends Neurosci* 1982;345.

Victor M, Adams RD, and Collens GH: *The Wernicke-Korsakoff Syndrome.* Philadelphia, F.A. Davis, 1971.

Walker AE: Man and his temporal lobes. *Surg Neurol* 1973;1:69–79.

Warren RE: Association, directionality and stimulus encoding. *J Exp Psychol* 1974;102:151–158.

Weiskrantz L: Hippocampal pathology in man and other animals, in *Functions of the Septo-Hippocampal System.* Ciba Found Symp 1978;58:373–387.

Weiskrantz L and Warrington FK: A study of forgetting in amnesic patients. *Neuropsychologia* 1970;8:281–288.

Whitaker HA and Ojemann GA: Lateralization of higher cortical functions: A critique, in Dimond SJ and Blizard DA (eds): Evaluation and lateralization of the brain. *Ann NY Acad Sci* 1977;299:459–473.

Whitehouse PS, Price DL, Struble RJ, Clark AW et al: Alzheimer's disease and senile demintia: Loss of neurons in the basal forebrain. *Science* 1982;215:1237–1239.

Wickelgren WA: Chunking and consolidation: A theoretical synthesis of semantic networds, configuring in conditioning, S-R versus cognitive learning, normal forgetting, the amnesic syndrome and the hippocampal arousal system. *Psychol Rev* 1979;86:44–60.

Willer JC, Dehen H, and Cambier J: Stress-induced analgesia in humans: Endogenous opioids and naloxone-reversible depression of pain reflexes. *Science* 1981;212:689–691.

Winson J: *Brain and Psyche: The Biology of the Unconscious.* New York, Doubleday, 1985.

Winson J and Abzug C: Gating of neuronal transmission in the hippocampus: Efficacy of transmission varies with behavioral state. *Science* 1977;196:1223–1225.

Witkin HA and Goodenough DR: *Cognitive Styles: Essence and Origins.* New York, International University Press, 1981.

Witkin HA, Dyk, RB, Faterson HF, Goodenough OR, et al: *Psychological Differentiation: Studies of Development.* New York, John Wiley & Sons, 1962.

Wood CC: Auditory and phonetic levels of processing in speech perception: Neurophysiological and information processing analysis. *J Exp Psych Hum Percept Perform* 1975;1:3–20.

Wood CC, Goff WR, and Jay RS: Auditory evoked potentials during speech perception. *Science* 1971;173:1248–1251.

Wood CC, Allison T, Goff WR, Williamson PP, et al: On the neural origin of the P300 in man. Presented at the 5th International Symposium on Electrical Potentials Related to Motivation, Motor and Sensory Processes of the Brain. Ulm-Reisenberg, May 14–18, 1979.

Young LD, Suomi SJ, Harlow HF, and McKinney WT: Early stress and later responses to separation in rhesus monkeys. *Am J Psychiatr* 1973;130:400–405.

Zajonc RB: Feeling and thinking: Preferences need no inferences. *Am Psychol* 1980;35:151–175.

Zeigarnik B: Uber das Behalten von Erledigten und Underledigten Handlungen. *Psychologische Forschungen* 1927;9:1–85.

Zeki SM: The functional organization from striate to prestriate visual cortex in the rhesus monkey. *Cold Spring Harbor Symp Quant Biol* 1976;40:591–600.

Zemach M: *The Effects of Guilt-Arousing Communications on Acceptance of Recommendations.* Unpublished doctoral dissertation. Yale University, 1966.

Zuckerman M, Murtagh T, and Siegel J: Sensation-seeking and cortical augmenting-reducing. *Psychophysiology* 1974;11:535–542.

Author Index

Page numbers in italics indicate reference listings.

Subject Index